AF450149

Bioadhesion
Approaches to Drug Delivery

Bioadhesion
Approaches to Drug Delivery

Amrish Kumar

Senior Research Fellow
Guru Ghasidas Vishwavidyalaya (A Central University)
Bilaspur, Chhattisgarh.

Dinesh K. Mishra

IPS Academy, College of Pharmacy, Indore (M.P.)

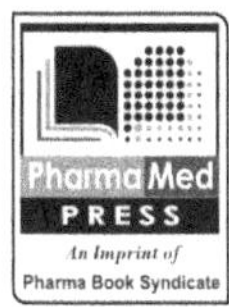

PharmaMed Press
An imprint of Pharma Book Syndicate

A Unit of BSP Books Pvt. Ltd.

4-4-309/316, Giriraj Lane,
Sultan Bazar, Hyderabad - 500 095.

Bioadhesion: *Approaches to Drug Delivery by Amrish Kumar and Dinesh K. Mishra*

© 2016, *by Publisher*

Third Reprint 2019

Published by

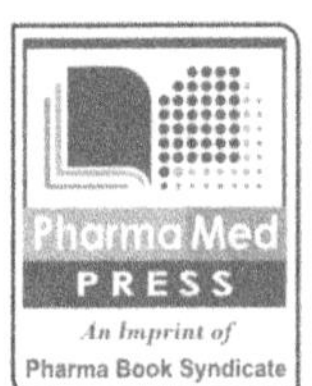

PharmaMed Press

An imprint of Pharma Book Syndicate

A Unit of BSP Books Pvt. Ltd.

4-4-309/316, Giriraj Lane, Sultan Bazar, Hyderabad - 500 095.

Phone: 040-23445600, 23445688; Fax: 91+40-23445611

E-mail: info@pharmamedpress.com

www.pharmamedpress.com/pharmamedpress.net

ISBN: 978-93-5230-128-7 (Hardback)

FOREWORD

Safe and effective drug delivery is the most desirable attribute of any drug delivery system. This premise is most acceptable when the approach employed is based on natural principle. Bioadhesion is a natural process for prolonged retention of desired material in the body and similar approach is employed in current dosage form design of novel drug delivery systems. Because of inherent advantages of bioadhesion approach to drug delivery a number of research reports are already available in the literature testifying the overwhelming superiority of approach and hence critical review of burgeoning literature has become a difficult task. The book entitled "Bioadhesion: Approaches to Drug Delivery" is a timely critique to help understand the phenomenon of bioadhesion and its pharmaceutical ramifications to the researchers in the field in particular and to the scientific community, students and teachers in general. All the chapters have been intelligently designed and adequately elaborated. Figures and Tables further enhance the utility of the book.

The author in his debut book publication has devoted lot of efforts in bringing out this very useful research book and deserves appreciation.

Bhopal, 14 December 2015

Prof. N. K. Jain
Emeritus Fellow (UGC)
Rajiv Gandhi Technical University
BHOPAL

PREFACE

Bioadhesive formulations have emerged as valuable contender for the treatment of various complicated modalities in modern health care. This textbook is intended to provide a basic grounding in the field of bioadhesive drug delivery to undergraduates and post graduates who are interested in a future career in formulation and development. It attempts to convey the fascinating concepts of bioadhesion which can be utilized for drug delivery through different routes of administration. The first two chapters explain the basic principles of bioadhesion. Both of the chapters are designed to provide students with a clear and concise introduction to bioadhesion process aided with suitable diagrams for better understanding. Chapter 3 is focused on the bioadhesive materials utilized for the preparation of drug delivery systems. The role of physicochemical properties of these polymeric materials is described in order to tailor a bioadhesive system to achieve desired properties for effective drug release at the site of application/absorption. Chapter 4 gives an introduction to different routes of administration which offers suitable characteristic mucosal or biological surfaces utilized for the application of bioadhesive formulation. A brief account of different types of bioadhesive formulations is also incorporated in this chapter. Chapter 5 covers the methods practiced for the evaluation of bioadhesive systems to predict their bioadhesive properties. Simple and clear diagrams are used to illustrate the principles involved and working of different experimental models and devices. Chapters 6, 7, 8 & 9 provide a detail account of commonly studied bioadhesive formulations. Attempt has been made to cover all the aspects i.e. basic principle, materials, methods of preparation, evaluation of bioadhesive properties and their applications with particular emphasis on therapeutic delivery.

The book can be helpful to students, teachers as well as research scientists who intend to learn and practice bioadhesive dosage forms.

We wish to express our sincere gratitude to Mr. Bhushan Hatwar for initiation of proposed edition and constant motivation. We are thankful to Dr. Sunil Jain, Dr. Anuja Mishra for their sincere support and help during proof reading and editing of book. We thankfully acknowledge publication of this book by PharmaMed Press, Hyderabad.

Dinesh K. Mishra
Amrish Kumar

Contents

Chapter 1

Introduction to Bioadhesive Drug Delivery

Chapter 2

Basic Concepts of Bioadhesion

CHAPTER 3

BIOADHESIVE POLYMERS

Chapter 4

Bioadhesive Drug Delivery System

Chapter 5

Evaluation of Bioadhesive Formulations

CHAPTER 6

BIOADHESIVE NANOPARTICLES

CHAPTER 7

BIOADHESIVE MICROSPHERES

CHAPTER 8

BIOADHESIVE NANOGELS

CHAPTER 9

BIOADHESIVE PATCHES/FILMS

Introduction to Bioadhesive Drug Delivery

Patho-physiology of diseases that are currently among the leading causes of death now require much more than just a stethoscope for diagnosis and a pill for treatment. The developing generation of therapeutics needs to combine with a degree of intelligence; the ability to sense and respond to their environment at the desired site of action. Dosage forms, when combined with intelligent polymers (i.e. bioadhesive, pH responsive) have the ability to sense and respond to external stimulus and with the advent of nanotechnology; these polymers can be fabricated on microsize, nanosize and on the same size scale as cellular and sub-cellular processes.

Recently, the formulation scientists applied the bioadhesion phenomenon for the development of novel and smarter systems for the delivery of therapeutics in order to maximize the effectiveness with minimal or no adverse effects. When a bioadhesive drug delivery system come in contact of application/absorption site, an intimate interaction between the biological surface and bioadhesive delivery system has been established. This course of action prolongs the residence of therapeutic agent for better absorption and superior performance. This prolonged residence time can result in enhanced absorption and in combination with a controlled release of drug also improved patient compliance by reducing the frequency of drug administration. In carrier technology microspheres, nanospheres, liposomes, nanoparticles, etc., offers an intelligent approach for drug delivery by coupling the drug to a carrier particle which modulates the release and absorption of the drug from the carrier system. In recent years, types of such mucoadhesive drug delivery systems have been developed for both systemic as well as local effects by different routes i.e. oral, buccal, nasal, rectal and vaginal routes **(Table 1.1)**.

Bioadhesion is relatively new and emerging opinion in drug delivery. It keeps the delivery system adhering to the underline absorption surface. This phenomenon is facilitated with the aid of bioadhesive polymers and these polymers lead to the possible development of novel drug delivery systems with modified drug release patterns. Bioadhesive drug delivery systems show various merits over conventional drug delivery systems. In the recent years the interest is growing to develop a drug delivery system with the use of a bioadhesive polymer. Such systems that are developed using bioadhesive polymers that will attach to related tissue or to the surface coating of the tissue for targeting various absorptive mucosal surfaces such as ocular, nasal, pulmonary, buccal, gastric, vaginal etc., are known as bioadhesive/mucoadhesive delivery systems.

Table 1.1 Some commercially available bioadhesive drug formulations

Brand	Company	Bioadhesive polymer	Dosage form
Buccastem[®]	Reckitt Benckiser	PVP, Xanthum gum and locust been gum	Buccal tablet
Corlan pellets[®]	Cell Tech	Acacia gum	Oromucosal pellets
Suscard[®]	Forest	HPMC	Buccal tablet
Gaviscon liquid[®]	Reckitt Benckiser	Sodium Alginate	Oral liquid
Orabase[®]	Conva Tech	Pectin, gelatin	Oral paste
Nyogel[®]	Novartis	Carbomer and PVA	Ocular gel
Zidoval[®]	3-M	Carbomer	Vaginal gel
Corsodyl gel[®]	GalaxoSmithKline	HPMC	Oromucosal gel

Mucosal surfaces are highly permeable membranes allowing rapid absorption of drug into the systemic circulation with avoidance of first pass metabolism. The well-organized uptake offers several paybacks over other methods of drug delivery and allows active agents to avoid some of the body's natural defense mechanism. The focal idea of bioadhesion was derived from the need to localize drugs at a definite site in the body. Habitually the extent of drug absorption is restricted by the residence time of the drug at the absorption spot. For e.g. in ocular drug delivery system, less than 2 min are available for drug absorption after instillation of a drug solution into the eye, since it is removed rapidly by the solution drainage and hence the ability to extend the contact time of an ocular delivery system in front of the eye would undoubtedly improve the bioavailability. In oral drug delivery, the drug absorption is restricted by the gastrointestinal transit time of the dosage form. In view of the fact that many drugs are absorbed only from the upper small intestine, localizing oral drug delivery system in the stomach or in the duodenum would extensively improve the drug absorption. To overcome the relatively short GI retention time and improve localization for oral controlled drug delivery system, bioadhesive polymers which adhere to the mucin or the epithelial surface are valuable and lead to significant improvement in oral drug delivery. By involving the bioadhesive polymers in novel drug delivery systems improvement is also expected for other mucus covered sites of drug administration.

In biological systems, four types of bioadhesion **(Figure 1.1)** could be speculated:

1. Normal cell-normal cell adhesion i.e. cell fusion or cell aggregation.
2. Cell (normal/pathological)-foreign substance adhesion i.e. cell adhesion onto culture dishes or adhesion to a variety of substances including metals, woods and other synthetic materials.
3. Normal cell-pathological cell adhesion i.e. adhesion of pus cell to normal cell.
4. Biological surface-adhesive material adhesion i.e. adhesion of artificial substances to biological substrates such as adhesion of polymers to skin or other soft tissues.

Bioadhesive drug delivery system implies attachment of a drug carrier system to a specific biological site or the surface and this biological surface may be epithelial tissue. If this attachment or adhesion is with a mucus layer, it is referred as mucoadhesion.

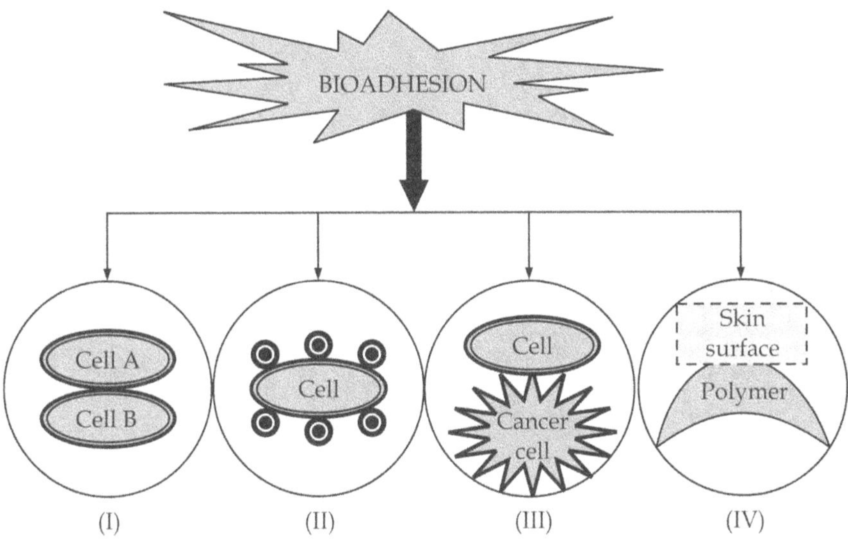

Figure 1.1 Types of bioadhesion: (I) Normal cell – normal cell, (II) Normal cell – foreign substance, (III) Normal cell – pathological cell, (IV) Biological surface – adhesive substance

1.1   BIOADHESION AND MUCOADHESION

Bioadhesion/Mucoadhesion can be defined as an experience of interfacial molecular attractive forces amongst the two surfaces i.e. biological substrate and adhesive polymers of natural or synthetic origin. This interfacial interaction results into adherence of polymeric material to the biological surface and keep it at the site of adhesion for a longer duration. Practice of bioadhesive polymeric systems for biomedical purposes are not new; the utilization of adhesive bandages, surgical glues etc., witnessed the presence of bioadhesive products from a long time. The human gut housed several bacterial species, this bacterial adhesion results due the interaction between mucin (present in mucus lining of gut mucosa) and lectin resembling structures (present on bacterial cell surface). In common, a variety of biopolymers shows the bioadhesive property and has been utilized for a choice of therapeutic purposes in medicine. Broadly, bioadhesive polymers can be categorized under two groups i.e. specific and non-specific. The polymers with the capability to adhere to specific chemical structure of biological molecules comes under specific bioadhesive polymers e.g. Lectins, fimbrin. On the other side, non-specific bioadhesive polymers bind to both i.e. cellular and mucosal surfaces e.g. Poly-acrylic acid and Cyano-acrylates.

Bioadhesion is the course of action which explains the interaction between an adhesive polymer (natural/synthetic) with a biological substrate.

The interaction of adhesive polymers with mucosal layers instead of other cellular layers is acknowledged as *mucoadhesion* **(Figure 1.2)**.

The substrate possessing bioadhesive assets can help in devising a delivery system proficient of delivering a bioactive agent for a prolonged period of time at a specific delivery location. The literature provided in this book gives a good insight on bioadhesive polymers, the phenomenon of bioadhesion and the factors which have the ability to affect the bioadhesive properties of a polymer.

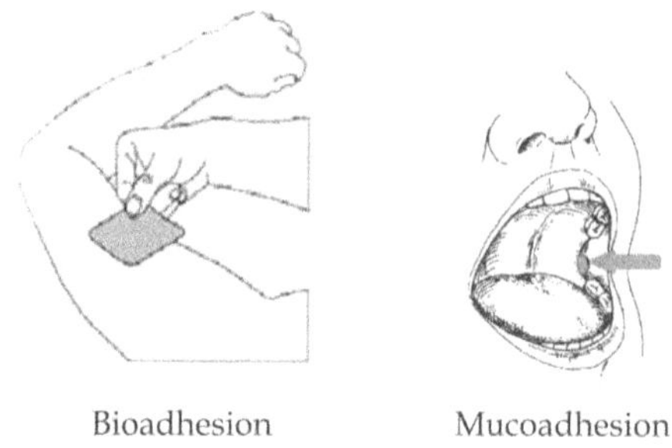

Figure 1.2 Bioadhesion and Mucoaadhesion

1.2 HISTORY OF BIOADHESION

The utilization of bioadhesive polymers for the development of pharmaceutical formulations has been tried in 1947 to deliver penicillin to the oral mucosa. In that attempt, gum tragacanth and dental adhesive powders were incorporated in formulation to deliver bioactive agent to mucosal surface of oral cavity. Later on, carboxy methyl cellulose and petrolatum were reported for the development of bioadhesive preparations. With the advancement in bioadhesive drug delivery systems a mucoadhesive formulation Orahesive® was marketed which consists of sodium carboxy methyl cellulose (SCMC; finely ground), gelatin and pectin as bioadhesive component. Subsequently, another bioadhesive formulation Orabase® based on blend of poly methylene/mineral oil entered into the clinical trials. A newer bioadhesive system was also developed in which SCMC and poly-isobutylene were blended to coat a polyethylene leaf, this coating supplements the shielding of bioadhesive layer by polyethylene backing film and minimizes the physical interference due to surrounding environment.

In the development wave of bioadhesive polymers, a range of other bioadhesive polymers from natural or synthetic resources were reported with their applications in pharmaceutical delivery systems. Sodium alginate, guar gum, hydroxy ethyl cellulose (HEC), karya gum, methyl cellulose (MC), retene, tragacanth and polyethylene glycol (PEG) etc., demonstrated their potential for bioadhesive application for drug delivery purpose. The period of 1980s witnessed the exhaustive use of hydroxy propyl cellulose (HPC) and SCMC as a bioadhesive component in pharmaceutical formulations. From that time, the use of acrylated polymers in the formulations intended for bioadhesive delivery, increases many-fold. The effect of molecular level structure modification of these polymers on bioadhesive properties has also been investigated by several researchers in order to develop more effective bioadhesive polymers for therapeutic delivery.

1.3 MERITS OF BIOADHESION/MUCOADHESION

Bioadhesion promotes the residence time of dosage form in addition to improved intimacy of contact between the delivery system and biological surfaces. These attributes of bioadhesive systems attracted the scientific community to utilize them for enhanced effects with localization of therapeutic agents at the site of absorption/application. These delivery systems are also capable to control the rate and extent of drug release, that's why there is a possibility to be utilized as a platform for the development of sustained release systems.

1. Prolongs the residence time of the dosage form at the site of absorption. Due to an amplified residence time it enhances absorption and hence the therapeutic efficiency of the drug.

2. Surface characteristics can be easily manipulated to accomplish both passive and active drug targeting after parenteral administration. Drug is protected from degradation due to acidic surroundings in the GIT and drug bioavailability is increased due to the avoidance of first pass metabolism.

3. The controlled and sustained release pattern of the drug during the transportation and at the site of localization altering organ allocation of the drug and succeeding clearance of the drug so as to attain enhanced drug therapeutic efficacy and diminution in side effects.

4. Controlled release pattern and particle degradation characteristics can readily modulated by the choice of matrix constituents. Drug loading is comparatively high and drug can be integrated into the system without any chemical reaction; this is a vital factor for preserving the drug activity.

5. Site specific targeting can be achieved by attaching targeting ligands to exterior of particles or make use of magnetic guidance.

6. The system can be used for various routes of administration including oral, nasal, parenteral and intraocular etc.

7. Tremendous accessibility and reduced dosing due to lengthen residence time of the dosage form at the intended site and absorption to allow once or twice a day dosing.

8. Superior patient compliance due to ease of drug administration.

9. Quicker onset of action is achieved as the mucosal surface offers rapid absorption due to enormous blood supply and good blood flow rates.

10. These dosage forms smooth the progress of intimate contact of the formulation with the underlying absorption surface. This allows adaptation of tissue permeability for absorption of macromolecules, such as peptides and proteins. Addition of penetration enhancers such as Sodium glyco-cholate, Sodium taurocholate and L-lysophosphotidyl choline and protease inhibitors in the mucoadhesive dosage forms resulted in healthier absorption of peptides and proteins.

1.4 DEMERITS OF BIOADHESION/MUCOADHESION

Based upon the therapeutic requirement i.e. local or systemic action, several demerits are associated with the drug delivery through bioadhesive systems.

1. In case of local delivery, the bioadhesive system may possibly flush-off by biological fluids (saliva/lacrimal fluid) or ingested food stuffs resulting into rapid elimination or termination of local effect. In that condition frequent dosing is required, this nullifies the advantage of prolonged residence associated with bioadhesive systems.

2. As the majority of bioadhesive systems for local delivery are available in solid or semisolid form, they lack the uniform distribution over the intended biological surface. There may be possibility that some area of intended biological surface may remain deficient in terms of effective therapeutic levels.

3. Patient compliance is compromised in some cases e.g. application of bioadhesive system for buccal delivery may be irritable due to the 'mouth feel' effect as it resembles a foreign stuff over buccal mucosa.

4. For systemic delivery the relative impermeability of biological surface with regard to drug absorption, especially for large hydrophilic biopharmaceuticals, is a major concern.

1.5   RECENT DEVELOPMENTS IN
BIOADHESIVE DRUG DELIVERY SYSTEMS

The scope of bioadhesive polymers in pharmaceutical arena covers a wide range of applications **(Table 1.2)**. The expansion of bioadhesive drug delivery systems for oral, topical, nasal, ocular, vaginal and rectal delivery, itself witnessed the potential of these systems. The basic principles involved in bioadhesion process can be applied for the development of drug delivery systems with controlled release of medicaments. Advantages associated with oral mucoadhesive drug delivery systems e.g. prolonged residence time for enhanced absorption of incorporated drug, lower dosing frequency etc., markedly influences the oral bioavailability. The successful implementation of bioadhesive systems for therapeutic purpose depends on the physicochemical properties of the polymers which contribute towards the bioadhesion phenomenon. The physiological factors such as mucin flow, mucin turnover rate and the pathological condition of biological surface at the site of application/absorption are also considered for the development of bioadhesive drug delivery systems. In the current scenario, several *in-vitro* and *in-vivo* techniques are available to evaluate the bioadhesive properties of such delivery systems. Hydrophilic, anionic molecules with high molecular weight e.g. carbomers are choice of bioadhesive polymers which are commonly studied for the development of bioadhesive systems. In recent years, the rise of second generation bioadhesive polymers grabs the attention for the development of bioadhesive system with better control over the bioadhesive properties for effective therapeutic delivery.

Table 1.2 Scope of bioadhesive drug delivery systems

- Novel formulation approaches to oral mucoadhesive drug delivery systems
- Bioadhesive formulations for nasal delivery
- Development of bioadhesive buccal patches
- Bioadhesive formulations for vaginal delivery
- Ocular bioadhesive drug delivery systems
- Bioadhesive preparations as topical dosage forms

1.5.1 Developments in Bioadhesive Nanoparticulate Drug Delivery Systems

In the previous 35 years, the expansion of nanotechnology has opened a number of innovative vistas in medical sciences, particularly in the field of drug delivery. New multifunctional moieties are approaching for treating diseases. The biotechnology has also produced several powerful drugs, but numerous of these drugs encounter problems delivering them in biological systems. Their therapeutic effectiveness is significantly spoiled owing to their incompatibilities and specific chemical structure. The input of today's nanotechnology is that it allows genuine advancement to accomplish sequential and spatial site-specific delivery. The market of nanotechnology and drug delivery systems based on this technology will be extensively felt by the pharmaceutical industry. In recent years, the figure of patents and products in this field is escalating appreciably. The most straight advance application is in cancer treatment with quite a few products in market such as Caelyx®, Doxil®, Transdrug® and Abraxane®.

Paul Ehrlich (1854–1915), working on immunologist, summarized the lectures delivered by Herter at Johns Hopkins University and published few articles in 1904 in Boston Medical and Surgical Journal, the immediate predecessor of New England Journal of Medicine. These publications brighten the view of immunochemistry and explain the side-chain theory of antibody development. He also explains the *in-vitro* mechanism of immune hemolysis. However, later findings of other researches challenged those publications and remained controversial in the view of a clinical journal. Beside of all, Ehrlich's contributions and findings related to infectious diseases and his concept of 'magic bullet' revolutionized the delivery of chemotherapeutic agents. The theory of Paul's magic bullet has turned out to be veracity with the authorization of several forms of drug-targeting systems for the treatment of certain cancer and infectious diseases. Nanoparticulate drug delivery systems with the concept of bioadhesion may produce fruitful outcome in this direction.

Even though the mammoth amount of work has been done on this drug delivery platform, the center of attention has been primarily on the formulation of gastro-retentive dosage forms; hence, work must be done to take advantage of this drug delivery system for various other approaches like drug targeting and site specific drug delivery systems. Bioadhesive drug delivery systems is one of the most significant novel drug delivery systems with its collection of advantages and it has a lot of prospective in formulating dosage forms for a choice of chronic diseases.

2 Basic Concepts of Bioadhesion

Adhesion can be defined as the bonds created by making contact between a pressure responsive adhesive and a surface. The American Society of testing and materials has define it as the status in which two surfaces are seized together by interfacial forces, which may consist of valence forces, interlocking action or both. Bioadhesion is defined as capability of a material to adhere with a biological tissue for an extended phase of time. In the case of polymer attached to the mucin film of a mucosal tissue, the expression "mucoadhesion" is used.

Bioadhesion may be classified into three types based on phenomenological scrutiny, rather than on the mechanisms of bioadhesion.

Type I: Bioadhesion is characterized by adhesion taking place between biological objects without association of artificial materials. Cell fusion and cell aggregation are first-class examples.

Type II: Bioadhesion can be represented by cell adhesion onto culture dishes or adhesion to a diversity of substances including metals, woods and other synthetic resources.

Type III: Bioadhesion can be described as adhesion of artificial substances to biological substrates such as adhesion of polymers to skin or other soft tissues.

2.1 THE BIOADHESIVE/MUCOSA INTERACTIONS

For adhesion, molecules are required to attach with the interface. These attachments can come to pass in the following ways:

2.1.1 Ionic Bonds

Where two oppositely charged ions catch the attention of each other by means of electrostatic interactions to figure a well-built bond (e.g. in a salt crystal).

2.1.2 Covalent Bonds

Where electrons are communal, in pairs, connecting the bonded atoms in order to fill up the orbital in both and create strong bonds.

2.1.3 Hydrogen Bonds

In this interaction a hydrogen atom, when covalently bonded to electronegative atoms such as oxygen, fluorine or nitrogen carries a minor positive charge and is consequently attracted to other electronegative atoms. The hydrogen can therefore be thought of as being communal and the bond created is usually weaker than ionic or covalent bonds.

2.1.4 Van-der-Waals Bonds

It is the weakest forms of interaction that come up from dipole–dipole and dipole-induced dipole attractions in polar molecules and dispersion forces with non-polar substances.

2.1.5 Hydrophobic Bonds

More specifically described as the hydrophobic effect, these are indirect bonds (such groups only come into sight to be attracted to each other) that come about when non-polar groups are present in an aqueous solution. Water molecules neighboring to non-polar groups form hydrogen bonded structures, which lowers the system entropy. There is consequently amplification in the tendency of non-polar groups to associate with each other to minimize this effect.

2.2 MUCUS STRUCTURE, FUNCTION AND COMPOSITION

Mucus, covering almost all the mucosal surfaces is viscous in nature with slight adhesive property owing to its composition. This viscous secretion is synthesized by specialized goblet cells composed of glandular columnar epithelial cells, lining cavities/surfaces of organs in direct contact or open to foreign matters e.g. buccal, gastrointestinal tract, oral, nasal, ocular, vaginal and rectal cavities/surfaces. Mucus perform several functions including protection of underlying hydrated epithelial layer, lubrication of cavity surfaces for easy movement of substances and exchange of gases and nutrients between epithelial cells and permeable gel layer. Due to its viscosity and adhesiveness it also entraps the pathogens and other deleterious stuffs. The inherent properties of mucus prove it is a marvelous biological lubricant, available for various processes of human body.

Maximum proportion of mucus is consists of water with more than 95% fraction. Another major and biologically important constituent for bioadhesive interactions is mucin, composed of high molecular weight glycoproteins which are responsible for the high viscosity of mucus. Some other minor constituents i.e. lipids, mucopolysaccharides and proteins are also present with a fraction of less than 1%. The glycoproteins of mucin form a densely entangled polymeric network which involves non-covalent interactions. These non-covalent entanglements markedly influence the rheological properties of mucus. At neutral pH, anionic nature of mucin is owed to the presence of sialic acid and sulphate groups on glycoproteins. The non-mucin portion of the mucosal secretion contains IgA, lactoferrin, lysozyme etc., not confirmed but some of them contribute towards bacteriostatic property of mucus.

2.3 THEORIES OF BIOADHESION

A number of theories have been projected to enlighten the fundamental mechanisms of adhesion. In a particular system, one or more hypothesis can equally well elucidate or contribute to the configuration of bioadhesive bonds.

2.3.1 Wetting Hypothesis

Wetting theory is predominantly appropriate for liquid bioadhesive systems. It analyzes adhesive and contact behavior in expressions of the aptitude of a liquid or paste to spread over a biological system. According to this theory, the lower contact angle between the liquid bioadhesives and biological/mucosal surface give rise to a superior affinity for bioadhesive interaction. If a liquid material is sandwiched between two substrate surfaces, it may act as an adhesive and hold the both substrates together. The capability of the adhesive to spread spontaneously on mucin influences development of intimate contact among the mucoadhesive and mucin and consequently influences the mucoadhesive potency. The thermodynamic exertion of adhesion is a function of the surface tension of the surface in contact as well as the interfacial tension. A small value of interfacial tension would represent a more intimate contact between the two surfaces.

This theory can more easily explained by the example of spreading of a liquid bioadhesive polymer over a biological surface **(Figure 2.1)**. According to the Young's equation, for adequate spreading contact angle (θ) should ideally be zero, which can be represented in terms of interfacial tension ($\yen$)

$$\yen_{bs} = \yen_{pb} + \yen_{ps} \cos \theta$$

where subscripts b, s and p represent biological surface, surrounding biological contents and bioadhesive polymer respectively, for spontaneous wetting to occur,

$$\yen_{bp} \geq \yen_{pb} + \yen_{ps}$$

Further, spreading coefficient ($S_{p/b}$) can be calculated by

$$S_{p/b} = \yen_{bs} - \yen_{pb} - \yen_{ps}$$

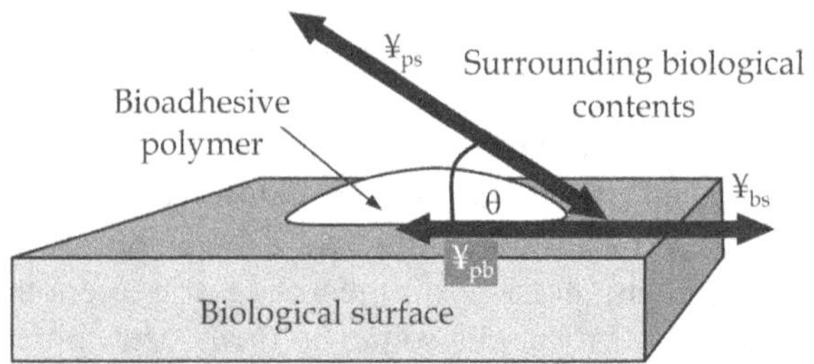

Figure 2.1 Schematic representation of interfacial tensions at biological surface and bioadhesive polymer interface

For effective bioadhesive bonding, maximization of interfacial tension at biological surface-surrounding biological contents interface and minimization of interfacial tension at other two interfaces is required. This condition is maintained by keeping positive value for spreading co-efficient. Several methods i.e. Wilhelmy plate method can be used for the calculation of interfacial tension at bioadhesive polymer-biological surface interface and given by the equation

$$\yen_{pb} = \yen_p + \yen_b - 2F\,(\yen_p\,\yen_b)^{1/2}$$

where, F represents the parameter for interaction

With the help of these mathematical relationships one can predict the intensity of bioadhesive bonding and calculation of spreading co-efficients for various bioadhesive polymers over different biological surfaces. This information is useful for the selection of bioadhesive polymers for different routes of administration.

Spreading coefficient is also expressed in terms of adhesive and cohesive forces involved at the interface. The exertion of adhesion expressed in terms of surface and interfacial tension ($\yen$), is defined as the energy per square centimeter released when an interface is created. The work done for adhesion (W_a) is given by the equation:

$$W_a = \yen_B + \yen_P - \yen_{BP}$$

where, B and P represent the biological membrane and bioadhesive formulation respectively.

The work done for cohesion (W_c) is given by the equation:

$$W_c = 2\yen_B \text{ or } \yen_P$$

The spreading coefficient ($S_{P/B}$) for spreading a bioadhesive polymer P over a biological substrate B is given by the equation:

$$S_{P/B} = \yen_B - (\yen_P + \yen_{BP})$$

As stated earlier $S_{P/B}$ should be positive for effective bioadhesive bonding between a bioadhesive polymer and biological surface. Both spreading coefficient and bioadhesive work directly influence the nature of the bioadhesive bond and thus provide essential information for the development of bioadhesive drug delivery systems.

2.3.2 Diffusion Hypothesis

The diffusion hypothesis assumes the diffusion of the polymer chains, present on the substrate surfaces, across the adhesive interface; in this manner forming a networked structure **(Figure 2.2)**. According to this hypothesis, the bioadhesive polymeric chains and the mucus glycoprotein chains interact to an adequate profundity which results into semi-permanent bioadhesive bonding. The polymer initially brought into intimate contact among mucus and in excess of time, the concentration gradient across the interface causes the diffusion of the chains of the bioadhesive into the mucus layer and also the diffusion of the glycoprotein chains of the mucus into the bioadhesive polymer. The contact period and diffusion coefficient markedly influence the depth of bioadhesive polymer chains infiltration through the mucus. At such interface, diffusion coefficient is affected by molecular weight of cross-linked network and decline sharply with the increase in the density of cross-linking.

The rate of the diffusion is reliant on the chemical potential gradient and the diffusion coefficient of a macromolecule through a cross-linked network. The chains that have diffused transversely serve as anchors to give support in securing semi-permanently the bioadhesive appliance in place. An appropriate interpenetration distance is required for high-quality bioadhesion that in the region of end to end distance of the macromolecular chains.

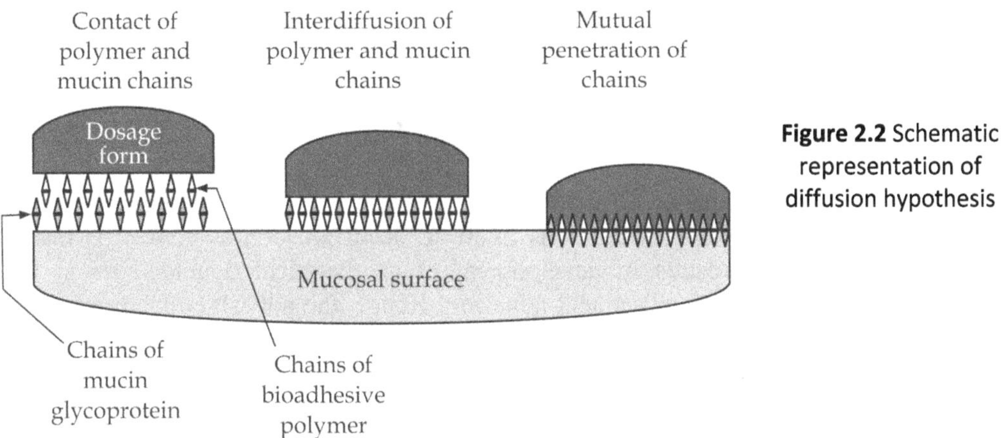

Figure 2.2 Schematic representation of diffusion hypothesis

Although the inter-diffusion in compatible polymers has been verified by radiometric studies, the exact depth of penetration requisite to accomplish adequate mucoadhesion is not acknowledged but it is believed to be in the range of 0.2-0.5 μm. However, the depth of penetration (P_D), can be given by the relationship

$$P_D = (tD_p)^{1/2}$$

where, t represent time of contact and D_p stands for diffusion coefficient of bioadhesive polymer in mucosal secretion.

As stated in earlier hypothesis, diffusion coefficient relies on molecular weight of the polymeric chains and decrease markedly with increase in cross-linking density. It concludes that the flexibility and mobility of bioadhesive polymeric chain fragments and mucosal glycoproteins controls the inter-diffusion process to a great extent.

2.3.3 Electronic Hypothesis

The electronic assumption proposes transfer of electrons along with the surfaces resulting in the development of an electrical double layer in this manner giving rise to attractive forces. As per the concept of this hypothesis, the different electronic structures of bioadhesive polymer and mucosal glycoproteins set up the basis for mutual electron relocation which results into the contact between them. This process of electron relocation give rise to the formation of an electrical double layer at the interface **(Figure 2.3)** bioadhesion is observed as a result of attractive forces across the electrical double layer.

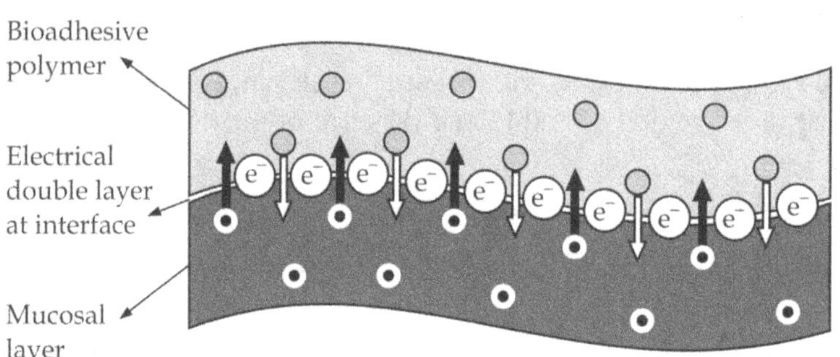

Figure 2.3 Schematic representation of electronic hypothesis

The mucin glycoprotein and bioadhesive polymers acquire different electronic structure; therefore electronic relocation is likely to occur as soon as contact is made. This electron relocation results in development of an electrical double layer at the adhesive interface by way of subsequent adhesion. Hence, the adhesive-mucin interface can be treated as a capacitor, which tends to be stimulate as soon as the two surfaces are in close contact and discharged when they are separated.

2.3.4 Adsorption Hypothesis

The adsorption hypothesis proposes the occurrence of intermolecular forces, viz. hydrogen bonding and Van-der-Waals forces, for the adhesive interaction surrounded by the substrate surfaces **(Figure 2.4)**. This hypothesis explains the bioadhesion process on the basis of surface forces generated at atomic level when two surfaces i.e. bioadhesive polymer and biological surface, comes in contact of each other. These surface forces give rise to two types of chemical bonds.

(a) Primary chemical bonds are undesirable in case of bioadhesion for drug delivery purpose due to their higher strength owed to formation of permanent covalent bonding.

(b) Secondary chemical bonds includes the non-covalent forces e.g. hydrogen bonding, hydrophobic bonding, van der Waals forces and electrostatic forces.

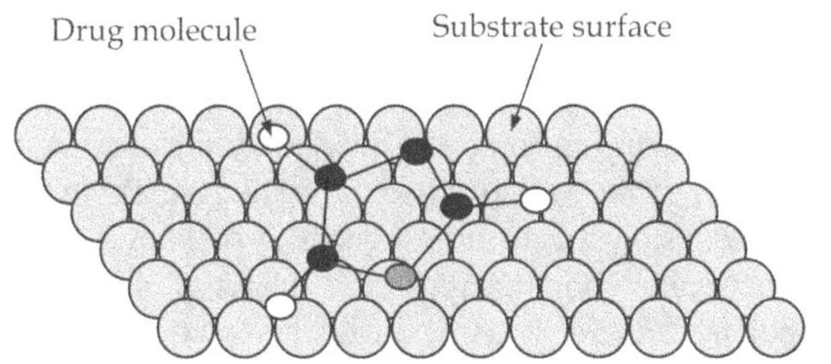

Figure 2.4 Schematic representation of adsorption hypothesis

The affection of adhesive to biological tissues on the source of a group of interactions recognized as 'secondary forces'. The Van-der-Waals forces of attraction are the summation of all attractions among uncharged molecules. These attractive forces arise from

- Polar or keesom forces developed owing to orientation of permanent dipoles in two molecules.

- Induction Debye forces developed due to induced dipole and permanent dipole.

- Dispersion or London forces developed due to the changes in the charge distribution in the region of non polar molecules.

2.3.5 Fracture Hypothesis

This is the most practical assumption for studying bioadhesion in the course of tensile experiments, based on analysis of forces required for the separation of two surfaces involved in bioadhesion phenomenon. The maximum tensile strength (T_M) generated during detachment can be given by the ratio of maximum force (F_M) required for the detachment to the total surface area (A_T) covered by the bioadhesive polymer.

$$T_M = F_M/A_T$$

For a harmonized mono-component bioadhesive system, fracture strength (S_F) which equally corresponds to maximum tensile strength (T_M), can be calculated by the equation:

$$S_F = T_M = (G_F\, E/C_l)^{1/2}$$

Where, (G_F) represent fracture energy, E stands for Young's modulus of elasticity and C_l represents the critical length of crack. G_F can be obtained by following mathematical expression:

$$G_F = W_R + W_I$$

where, W_R is reversible work of adhesion corresponds to energy required to rise a new fracture and W_I is irreversible work of adhesion and corresponds to work of plastic deformation at tip of rising fracture. W_R and W_I can be expressed in terms of per unit area of fracture surface. The elastic modulus of the system (E) is correlated to stress (s) and strain (e) through Hooke's law,

$$E = [F/A_0/\Delta_I/I_o]_{\Delta t \to 0}$$

In this equation, stress is equal to the charging force (F) divided by the area (A_0) and strain is equal to the chain thickness (Δ_I) of the system divided by the original thickness (I_0). Above equation suggests that the system being investigated is of known physical dimensions and composed of a particular homogenous-bulk material. Taking into consideration these equations cannot be functional to evaluate the fraction site of the multi constituent bioadhesive bond between a polymer microsphere and either mucus or mucosal tissue. For such evaluation, the equation requires extension to accommodate proportions and elastic module of each constituent.

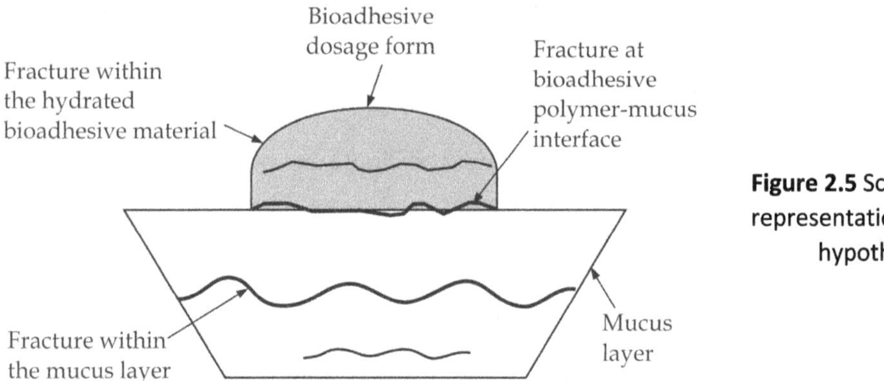

Figure 2.5 Schematic of representation fracture hypothesis

On the other hand, it has been demonstrated that fracture occurs at the interface hardly ever, but as an alternative occurs close to it **(Figure 2.5)**. Regardless of these restrictions, for the reason that the fracture theory deals only with analyzing the adhesive force necessitate for separation, it does not assume or involve entanglement, diffusion or interpenetration of polymer chains. Following equation is used to compute the fracture strength of adhesive bonds involving rigid bioadhesive materials in which the polymer chain may not penetrate the mucus layer.

$$D = D_0 \exp^{(-E/RT)}$$

where, D_0 is a constant which is not affected by the temperature and E represent experimental activation energy for diffusion/mobility of segmental polymeric chain.

Fracture hypothesis is based on the difficulty observed to separate two surfaces involved in bioadhesion process. According to this hypothesis, the corresponding adhesive strength is given by:

$$G_F = (E/C_l)\, l\, h$$

where E represents Young's modulus of elasticity, G_F is the fracture energy and C_l corresponds to post separation critical crack length.

2.3.6 Mechanical Hypothesis

The mechanical hypothesis explains the diffusion of the liquid adhesives into the micro-cracks and irregularities present on the rough substrate surface in this manner forming an interlocked structure which gives rise to adhesion **(Figure 2.6)**. In addition to this mechanical effect, enhanced plastic and viscoelastic immoderation of energy due to higher surface area at interaction site is also consumed to significantly strengthen the bioadhesive bonding.

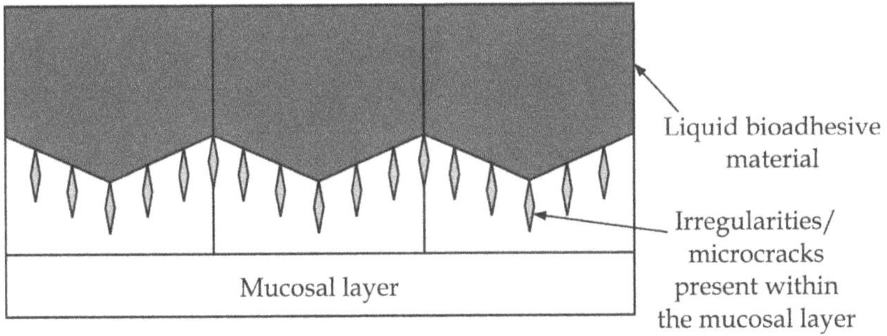

Figure 2.6 Schematic representation of mechanical hypothesis

2.3.7 Cohesion Hypothesis

The cohesive hypothesis proposes to facilitate the observable fact of bioadhesion are primarily due to the intermolecular interactions between like-molecules. The attraction force between the similar molecules of a material is termed as cohesive force and the phenomenon is called as cohesion. These intermolecular attraction forces hold the bioadhesive material as a single mass **(Figure 2.7)**. The final bioadhesive strength of a polymer is represented by the combination of adhesive and cohesive forces working at the site of interaction. The failure of bioadhesive bonding is also observed which is caused by:

(a) ***Separation of bioadhesive material from substrate***: Adverse biological conditions e.g. higher turnover rate, damaged mucosal/biological surface, pathological state etc., may cause this type of bioadhesive bonding failure **(Figure 2.8 a)**.

(b) *Split up of bioadhesive material*: Some bioadhesive materials have greater adhesive and cohesive forces in comparison to cohesive force of substrate which may lead to such type of partial failure of bioadhesive bonding **(Figure 2.8 b)**.

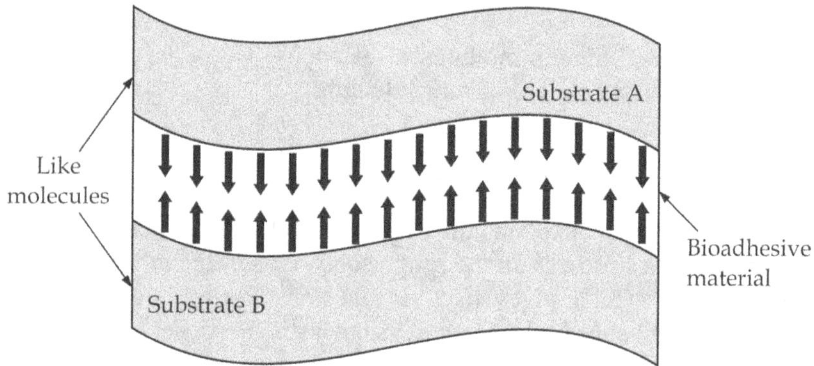

Figure 2.7 Schematic representation of cohesion hypothesis

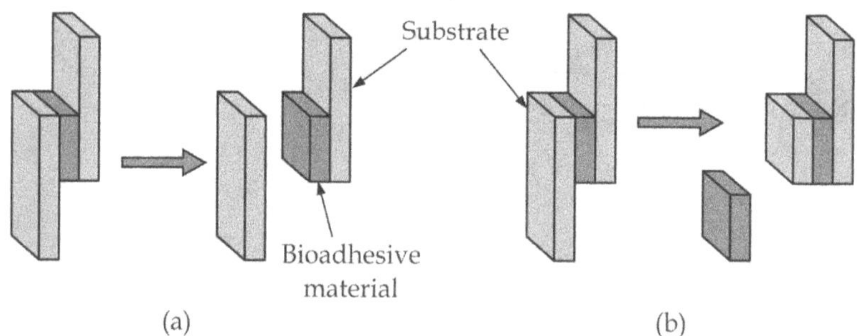

Figure 2.8 (a), (b) Schematic representations of adhesion failure modes

All the above discussed hypotheses categorized the bioadhesion process into two groups i.e. Chemical which include adsorption and electronic hypothesis and Physical which include diffusion, wetting and cohesion hypothesis. In conclusion, all hypotheses suggest two main progressions for bioadhesive bonding; first wetting or contact with biological fluids and second development of physico-chemical interactions.

As acknowledged above, bioadhesion may take place either by physical or by chemical interactions. These interactions can be further classified as hydrogen bonds, Van-der-Waals force and hydrophobic bonds which are considered as physical interactions while the formation of ionic and covalent bonds are classified as chemical interactions.

2.4 MECHANISM OF BIOADHESION

As acknowledged, bioadhesion is the affection of the drug along with appropriate carrier to the mucus membrane. Bioadhesion is a complex phenomenon which involves wetting, adsorption and interpenetration of polymer chains. The mechanisms accountable in the formation of bioadhesive bonds are not completely recognized, however on the basis of research in the proposed area of the mechanistic processes involved in bioadhesion between hydrogels and mucosa can be illustrated in three steps **(Figure 2.9)**:

Step 1: Wetting and swelling of bioadhesive polymeric chains

Step 2: Interpenetration and entanglement of bioadhesive polymer chains with mucosal glycoprotein and

Step 3: Formation of weak chemical bonds

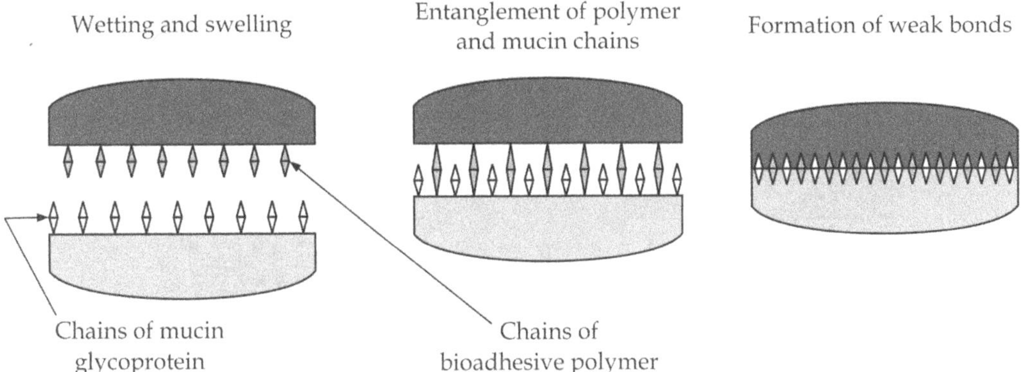

Figure 2.9 Stages of interaction between a bioadhesive polymer and mucin glycoprotein

Step 1: Wetting and swelling

The process of wetting and swelling initiates instantly after the application/spreading of bioadhesive dosage form over biological substrate or mucosal surface leading to an intimate acquaintance between them **(Figure 2.10)**. This process can be easily demonstrated by application of bioadhesive formulation i.e. tablet or gel over the buccal or vaginal mucosal surfaces. Bioadhesives are capable to adhere to or bond with biological tissues facilitated by the surface tension and forces that present at the site of adsorption or contact. The affinity towards the surrounding aqueous biological media makes the bioadhesive polymeric component to swell.

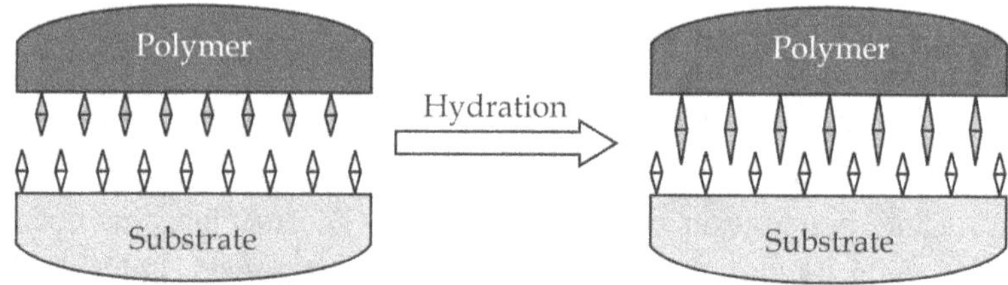

Figure 2.10 Swelling of a polymer

Step 2: Interpenetration and entanglement

The superficial surface of human mucosal linings contains high molecular weight polymeric chains of glycoproteins. These chains of biological surface intermingled and entangled with the polymeric chains of bioadhesive polymer leading to formation of semi permeable bonding between the duos **(Figure 2.11)**. The degree of penetration of these polymeric chains into each other decides the strength of bioadhesive bonding. For effective and strong bioadhesive bonding with biological surfaces, polymers must have analogous to the chemical structure of mucosal glycoproteins. The solubility of bioadhesive polymer in mucosal secretions is also a determinant for the strong bioadhesive bonding.

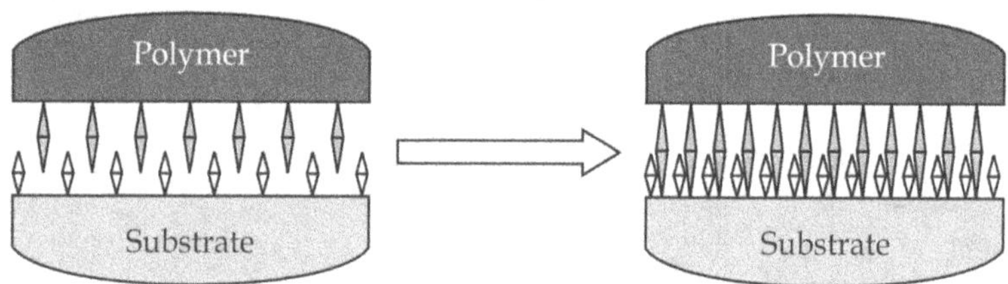

Figure 2.11 Interpenetration of polymer chains

Step 3: Formation of weak chemical bonds

At this stage, entangled polymeric and mucin glycoprotein chains form weak chemical bonds by compromising primary bonds e.g. covalent bonds and other secondary interactions e.g. hydrogen bonding and Van-der-Waals forces **(Figure 2.12)**. Both type of interactions i.e. primary and secondary, actively contribute towards the bioadhesiveness of such delivery systems in biological environment.

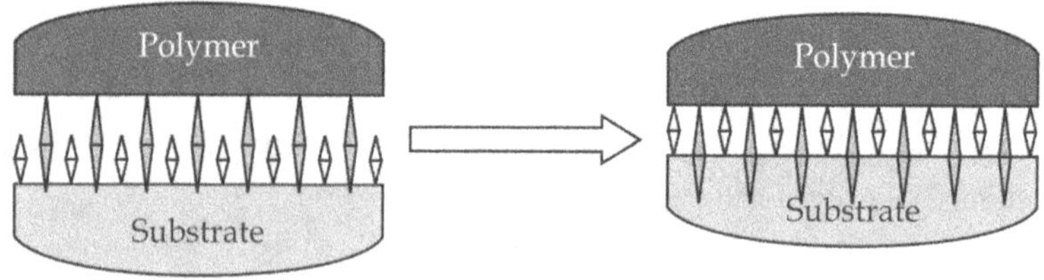

Figure 2.12 Formation of weak chemical bonds between the entangled polymer chains

The shorter residence time of dosage forms over the mucosal surfaces is owed to its rapid turnover rate and natural lubrication property. The residence time for different mucosal routes utilized for therapeutic delivery is generally less than an hour and even averaged in minutes for several mucosal sites. To amplify the residence time, one can incorporate a bioadhesive component in formulation to practically localize the dosage form and increase the time of contact for more effective absorption. On molecular level, bioadhesion can be elucidated based on molecular interactions. The interaction involving two molecules is composed of attraction and repulsion. Attractive interactions arise from Vander Waals forces, electrostatic attractions, hydrogen bonding and hydrophobic interactions. Repulsive interactions occur due to electrostatic and steric repulsion. For bioadhesion to occur, the attractive interaction should be superior to non-specific repulsion.

2.5 FACTORS AFFECTING BIOADHESION

Contingent on the various assumptions of bioadhesion it can be concluded that the bioadhesive polymers can be tailored by varying the constraints which controls the interaction between the polymers and the biological/mucosal layer. Several parameters which can modify the bioadhesive property of a particular polymer are analysed and their effects are recorded with factual evidences **(Table 2.1)**.

Table 2.1 Factors affecting bioadhesion

Polymer related factors	Environmental factors	Physiological factors
• Molecular weight of polymer • Chain length of polymer • Spatial arrangement • Polymer chain flexibility • Hydration of polymer • Hydrogen bonding • Functional group contribution • Polymer surface charge and degree of ionization • Active polymer concentration	• pH • Applied strength • Interaction time • Swelling • Selection of model substrate surface	• Mucin turnover • Diseased state

2.5.1   Polymer Related Factors

The interaction between mucin layer and a bioadhesive polymer can be expressed as the contribution of following factors:

2.5.1.1   Molecular weight of polymer

Bioadhesive polymers normally hooked on the mucosal layer and consequently adhere to the mucin coat by crafting intermolecular entanglements. In the course of interaction between bioadhesive polymer and mucosal layer, the molecular interpenetration of polymeric chains varies with an inversely proportional relationship to their molecular weight i.e. the penetration power of low molecular weight polymers is superior to the high molecular weight polymers. On the other hand, intermolecular entanglements are directly proportional to the molecular weight of bioadhesive polymers, owing to the high density of polymeric chains available for entanglement with mucin glycoproteins surface chains. Therefore, bioadhesiveness of a polymer might be enhanced by increasing the molecular weight of polymer chain.

For biomedical purposes, generally high molecular weight polymers ($\geq$1,00,000 D) exhibit enduring bioadhesive property. This fact can be well demonstrated by the example of polyethylene glycol (PEG). Low molecular weight PEG (20,000 D) fails to exhibit sufficient bioadhesive strength for biological surfaces. When the molecular weight of PEG is increased to 2,00,000 D, it shows better bioadhesive strength in similar conditions and at the level of 4,00,000 D its bioadhesiveness amplified exceptionally. Another polymer, polyoxyethylene shows stupendous bioadhesive property at molecular weight of 70,00,000 D in comparison to low molecular weight grades, for the development of buccal bioadhesive systems. This trend further extends to dextrans (1,95,00,000 D and 2,00,000 D), poly (acrylic) acid (~7,50,000 D) and polyoxyethylene oxide (40,00,000 D) which shows superior bioadhesiveness over their low molecular weight grades.

2.5.1.2 Chain length of polymer

Polymer chain length has a significant function in bioadhesiveness. The bioadhesive property of a polymer is increased with the increase in the chain length of the polymers. A flexible polymer chain facilitates the improved penetration and entanglement of the polymer chain with that of mucosal layer in this manner improving the bioadhesive property of a particular polymer.

2.5.1.3 Spatial arrangement

Spatial conformation of polymer molecules is also a noteworthy factor. Accompanied by MW and length of the polymer chains, spatial arrangement of polymer chains may also impart a vital accountability. As mentioned earlier, dextrans of 1,95,00,000 D and 2,00,000 D MW exhibit good bioadhesive properties. The proficiency of both dextrans and PEG (MW 200,000 D:) have been ascertained comparable bioadhesive effectiveness. The helical or linear conformation of polymers is also accountable to bioadhesive potency. Several active groups, predominantly responsible for the bioadhesive interactions may possibly shielded in helical conformation which results into decreased bioadhesive potency of the polymer.

2.5.1.4 Polymer chains flexibility

Interpenetration and entanglement are significantly governed by the polymer chain flexibility. As hydrophilic polymers evolve as more and more cross linked mass, the mobility of the individual polymer chain diminishes; furthermore with the increase in cross linking density, the effective length of the chain which can infiltrate into mucus, shrinks even further and bioadhesive strength is declined. A flexible polymer chain facilitates penetration and entanglement of the polymer chain with their counterpart on mucosal/biological surface consequences into enhanced bioadhesive property. Flexibility of the polymer chains is usually affected by the degree of hydration and crosslinking density of polymer network. Increase in crosslinking density results into the reduction in flexibility of the polymer chains. On the basis of this fact the bioadhesiveness of a polymer can be improved by tethering of long flexible chains in combination with high crosslinking density. In contemporary times this recognizable piece of information was exploited to develop tethered poly (ethylene glycol) poly (acrylic acid) hydrogels with superior bioadhesive properties.

2.5.1.5 Hydration of polymer

Another factor that significantly affects the bioadhesive potency of polymeric complex is the degree of hydration. At the same time as hydration is vital for relaxation and interpenetration of polymer chains, excess hydration may possibly lead to diminished bioadhesion and/or retention owing to the development of slippery mucilage. Keeping these facts in mind, to achieve prolonged bioadhesive effect the cross linked polymers that only permit a definite degree of hydration may be beneficial.

Besides the reduced flexibility of the polymer chains, crosslinking consequences in the reduced diffusion of water into the cross linked polymer matrix. However adequate hydration of the polymer complex is requisite for the absolute opening of the inter-polymeric apertures available in polymer matrix in addition to the mobilization of the polymer chains. For this reason exceedingly cross linked polymeric matrix restricts the interpenetration of polymer and mucin chains amongst themselves which in turn results in decline in bioadhesive strength of polymer.

However several polymers demonstrate bioadhesive property in hydration limited environment. In such environment, bioadhesive property is owed to be an outcome of a combination of capillary action and osmotic forces between the dehydrated polymer and the wet mucosal surface which function to dehydrate and reinforce the mucus layer. Even though this type of "sticking" also comes under the bioadhesion process but they must be clearly differentiated and not be compared with 'wet-on-wet' bioadhesive process which require attachment of swollen polymers to biological/mucosal surfaces.

2.5.1.6 Hydrogen bonding

Extent of hydrogen bonding among the functional groups of the polymers and mucosal layer also plays a prominent role to exert bioadhesiveness. Generally, bioadhesion property of a polymer is directly proportional to hydrogen bonding i.e. stronger bioadhesion forces can be achieved with higher extent of hydrogen bonding. Hydroxyl, carboxyl and amino groups are involved in the formation of these interactions. Examples of the polymers which have the capability to form strong hydrogen bonds include poly vinyl alcohol, acrylic derivatives, celluloses and starch. Usually, physical entanglements and hydrogen bonding contribute to create strengthened network; for that reason polymers with elevated density of existing hydrogen bonding groups accomplished more powerful interactions with glycoproteins present in mucus.

2.5.1.7 Functional group contribution

The functional groups of polymer may render the polymer chains as polyelectrolytes. The phenomenon for the attachment and bonding of bioadhesive polymers to biological substrates generally started as interpenetration followed by secondary non-covalent bonding between substrates. As the secondary non-covalent bonds are predominantly hydrogen bonds, the potential of bioadhesive polymers having hydrophilic functional groups such as, carboxyl (COOH), hydroxyl (OH), amide (NH_2) and sulphate groups (SO_4H) is comprehensively acknowledged for targeted drug delivery.

2.5.1.8 Polymer surface charge and degree of ionization

The charged conferred on functional groups of polymer chain has a noticeable effect on the bioadhesive potency which can be confirmed by cell-culture-fluorescent probe system. Anionic polyelectrolytes have been found to form stronger bioadhesive interactions in comparison to neutral polymers.

2.5.1.9 Active polymer concentration

The concentration of the polymer plays a significant part in the event of bioadhesion. Low concentration of polymers results in poor bioadhesion due to insufficient and unstable interaction between the polymer and mucosal layer. However for several polymers like poly vinyl pyrrolidone and poly vinyl alcohol, at very high polymer concentration the extent of solvent diffusion into the polymer network decreases due to the formation of the highly coiled structure in that way limiting interpenetration of the polymer and mucin chains with the subsequent reduction in the bioadhesive property. For solid dosage forms such as tablets higher concentration of polymer is required for stronger bioadhesion force. In general, for drug delivery purpose a polymer concentration in the range of 1-2.5% may produce sufficient bioadhesiveness.

2.5.2 Environmental Factors

The factor related to surrounding environment markedly influences all the events during the progression of bioadhesion. These factors include

2.5.2.1 pH

pH is always a factor of concern as the biological pH varies to a great extent within the body and influences the surface charge of both mucus and polymers. The charge density of mucus fluctuates depending on pH due to the difference in dissociation of functional groups on polymer chains resulting into a change in bioadhesive property. As admitted previously that bioadhesive property depends on functional groups which can ionize to provide a charge distribution on the polymer chains. The ionization of functional groups depends on the pH of the surrounding environment. Hence bioadhesive property can be tailored by changing the pH of the external environment. For example, chitosan a cationic polyelectrolyte exhibit astonishing bioadhesive property at neutral or alkaline pH. The result of some investigations reveals that the pH of the medium significantly affects the degree of hydration.

2.5.2.2 Applied strength

The initial stress functioned at the interface of bioadhesive polymer and biological membrane can influence the intensity of interpenetration. If excessive stress is employed for an adequate extended period polymers turn out to be bioadhesive even though they do not have attractive interaction with mucin. To set down a solid bioadhesive system, application of a definite strength is necessary. The effectiveness of bioadhesive polymers is directly proportional to the applied strength.

2.5.2.3 Interaction time

The interaction time between the polymer matrix and the mucosal layer can also influence the bioadhesive property. Initial increase in interaction time favors the hydration of the polymer matrix and subsequent interpenetration of the polymer chains. The initial interaction time between bioadhesive polymer and the mucus layer governs the extent of swelling and interpenetration of polymer chains. The bioadhesive strength of a polymer increases with the increase in initial interaction time.

2.5.2.4 Swelling

The swelling property is associated with the nature of polymer itself and also depends on the environment at the site of action. Swelling provide the space for disentanglement of polymer chains which results into higher extent of interpenetration as disentangled and interaction free chains easily interpenetrate into the mucus layer. Polymer concentration and availability of aqueous medium both affects the extent of swelling. Higher the extent of swelling of polymeric matrix greater the period of adhesion. However excessive swelling causes a decline in bioadhesive property.

2.5.2.5 Selection of the model substrate surface

The handling and treatment of biological substrates at the time of evaluation of bioadhesiveness is an important factor, since physical and biological variations may possibly arises in the mucus gels or tissues under the experimental conditions.

2.5.3 Physiological Factors

The physiology of the mucosal layer may vary according to the patho-physiological state of the human body. The physiological factors which exert their effect prominently on the bioadhesive property of a polymer matrix include

2.5.3.1 Mucin turnover

The mucin turnover is supposed to restrict the residence time of the bioadhesive polymer on the mucus layer irrespective to the bioadhesive strength of polymer.

2.5.3.2 Diseased state

The pathological conditions also have effect on bioadhesiveness of a polymer because in diseased state such as common cold, gastric ulcers, ulcerative colitis, etc., there is significant change in the physicochemical properties of mucus.

2.6 BIOADHESION AND DRUG ABSORPTION

Absorption of drug from the dosage form is the series of action by which a drug moves from site of administration and progressed into the general circulation. To exert its effect on the target tissue a drug has to circumvent several biological membranes which act as the limiting barriers for the movement of drug and other molecules among the cells. The biological membranes generally consist of matrix of proteins surrounded by a phospholipid bilayer. Drug absorption varies according to the physicochemical properties of drugs, type of formulation (e.g. tablet, capsule, solution) and routes of administration such as oral, parenteral or rectal. Various hypotheses are given for the absorption of drug through biological membranes which includes passive diffusion, facilitated passive diffusion, active transport and pinocytosis.

2.6.1 Passive Diffusion

In the process of passive diffusion the transport of molecules through the biological membranes governs by the concentration gradient i.e. concentration of the drug molecule.

Diffusion is the affinity of molecules to blowout into an available gap. The majority of drug molecules are transported across the membranes by diffusion from a high concentration region such as gastrointestinal fluids to one of an inferior concentration such as blood **(Figure 2.13)**. Due to the lipophilic nature of the biological membranes lipophilic drugs competently diffuses across the membrane in comparison to hydrophilic drugs. Smaller molecules are also capable to infiltrate the membrane more rapidly than outsized ones.

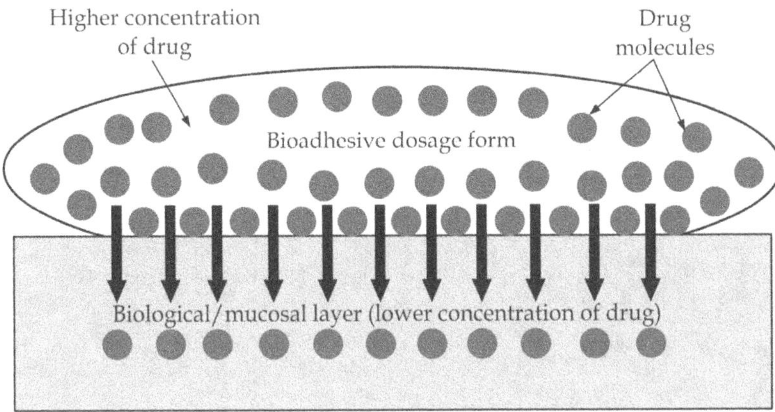

Figure 2.13 Passive diffusion

2.6.2 Facilitated Passive Diffusion

The transport of drug molecules with the assistance of carrier proteins through the biological barriers is termed as facilitated passive diffusion **(Figure 2.14)**. But all molecules do not interact with the proteins of biological membranes rather they exhibit specificity and only interact with certain molecules. This carrier-mediated transportation of molecules depends on the availability of carrier proteins; this signifies that after a particular time when the entire carriers will be involved in interaction then the process convert into saturated system. The transport of glucose from blood is a classic example of this type of diffusion.

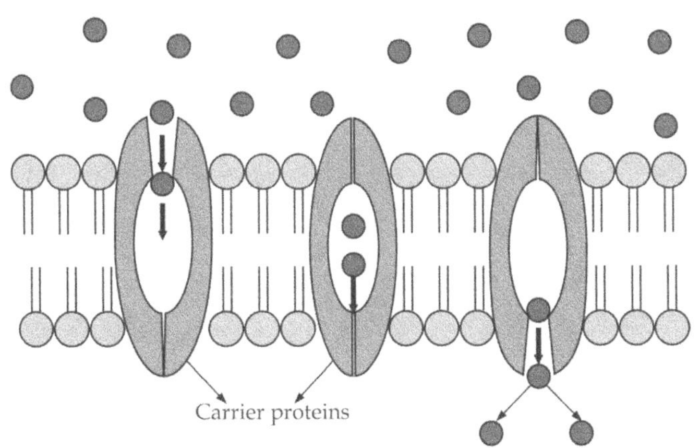

Figure 2.14 Facilitated passive diffusion

2.6.3 Active Transport

The transportation of molecules against the concentration gradient i.e. from inferior to greater concentrations is known as active transport **(Figure 2.15)**. The process of active transport requires energy to work against the concentration gradient. The required energy is provided by the cell which is accomplished from ATP.

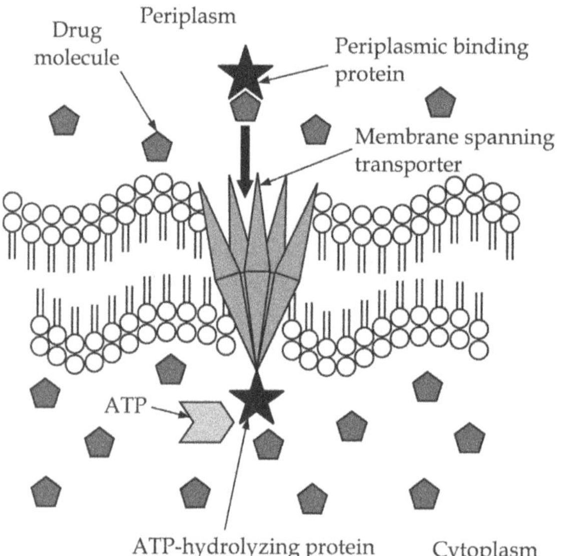

Figure 2.15 Active transport

2.6.4 Pinocytosis

Pinocytosis involves the engulfment of extracellular molecules and fluid by the cells. Initially the cell membrane fold inwards to make a pocket then the molecules or fluid to be transported are enclosed within the cellular pocket followed by fusion as a vesicle. This formed vesicle detaches from the membrane and travels towards the interior of the cell **(Figure 2.16)**. Pinocytosis plays a significant role in the transport of larger molecules such as protein drugs.

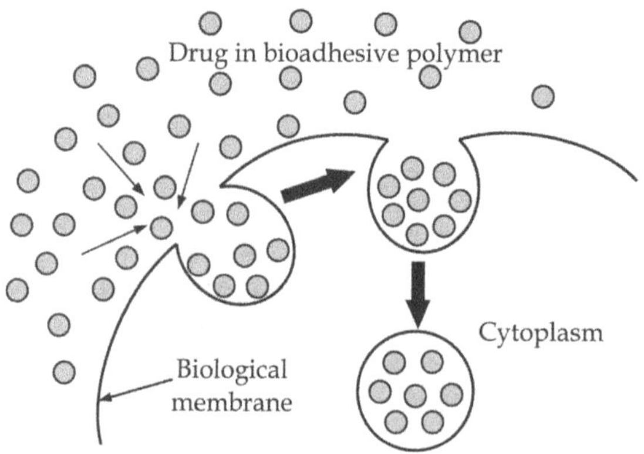

Figure 2.16 Pinocytosis

Bioadhesive Polymers

Bioadhesive polymers have been employing in numerous different dosage forms in efforts to accomplish systemic delivery of drugs through the different routes of delivery. Bioadhesive delivery systems are being investigated for the localization of the active agents to a particular location/site. Polymers have engaged in recreation role in designing such systems so as to amplify the residence time of the active agent at the preferred location. The ability of bioadhesive polymers to interact with biological/mucosal surfaces has been applied for drug administration by different routes. The adhering affinity towards the mucosal/biological surfaces lay down the basis for counting them as valuable excipients for drug delivery purpose. On the basis of ability to adhere mucosal/biological surfaces, these polymers can be categorized as:

1. Polymers transformed into sticky mass in contact of aqueous media to give bioadhesive effect.

2. Polymers which utilizes non-covalent interactions including electrostatic forces, hydrophobic, hydrogen bonding or other non-specific interactions to exert bioadhesive effect.

3. Polymers bind to specific receptors present on biological sites of interest.

All three polymer types can be used as carriers for the development of bioadhesive drug delivery systems. These polymers may perhaps be either natural such as gelatin, sodium alginate and guar gum or synthetic and semisynthetic such as hydroxy propyl methyl cellulose (HPMC), Carbopol 934 and Sodium carboxy methyl cellulose (Sodium CMC) **(Table 3.1)**. Also, different blends of two or more adhesive polymers may possibly be used as bioadhesives in drug delivery systems.

Over the years, a range of other polymers (e.g. sodium alginate, sodium carboxy methyl cellulose, guar gum, hydroxyl ethyl cellulose, karaya gum, methylcellulose, polyethylene glycol (PEG), retene and tragacanth) have been established to demonstrate bioadhesive characteristics. During the episode of 1980s poly-acrylic acid, hydroxyl propyl cellulose and sodium carboxy methyl cellulose were widely investigated for the development of formulations having bioadhesive properties. Since then the utilization of acrylate polymers for the development of bioadhesive formulations have amplified many-fold, various investigators have explored the bioadhesive properties of different polymers by means of varying molecular structural design. Following a lot of investigations, the researchers concluded that a polymer will show evidence of sufficient bioadhesive property if it can form strong intermolecular hydrogen bonding with the biological/mucosal layer, infiltration of the polymer into the mucus network or tissue fissures, effortless wetting of mucosal layer and high molecular weight of the polymer chain. Polymers used in bioadhesive delivery system may be of natural or synthetic source. In this segment we will briefly talk about some of the common classes of bioadhesive polymers.

Table 3.1 Examples of different bioadhesive polymers

CATEGORY	EXAMPLES
Cationic Polymers	Chitosan (Hydrogel polymers)
Anionic Polymers	Polyacrylic acid (Hydrophilic soluble polymer)
	Carbopol 934P, 971P, 980 (Hydrogel polymers)
	Polycarbophil (Hydrogel polymers)
	Poly methacrylic acid
	Sodium alginate
Non-Ionic Polymers	Methocel (HPMC) K100M, K15M, K4M
	Hydroxy ethyl cellulose (HEC)
	Hydroxy propyl cellulose (HPC)
	Polyoxy ethylene (POE)
Ion Exchange Resins	Cholestyramine (Duolite AP-143)
Miscellaneous	Sucralfate
	Gliadin

3.1 CATEGORIZATION OF BIOADHESIVE POLYMERS

3.1.1 Based on Origin

3.1.1.1 Synthetic mucoadhesive polymers

Cellulose derivatives

Poly-acrylic acid polymers

Poly-hydroxyl ethyl methyl acrylate

Poly-ethylene oxide

Poly-vinyl pyrrolidone

Poly-vinyl alcohol

3.1.1.2 Natural mucoadhesive polymers

Tragacanth

Sodium alginate

Karaya gum

Guar gum

Xanthan gum

Soluble starch

Gelatin

Pectin

Chitosan

3.1.2 Based on Nature

3.1.2.1 Hydrophilic polymers

The polymers of this class are soluble in water. Matrices developed in the company of these polymers swell when locate into an aqueous media with successive dissolution of the matrix. Due to the formation of viscous solutions in aqueous media, these polymers may also be incorporated as viscosity enhancers in bioadhesive formulations which exert their effect by restricting the drainage/flushing by biological fluids upon administration. Direct compression of these polymers with therapeutic agent is also effective for the development of solid bioadhesive dosage forms. The polyelectrolytes demonstrate greater bioadhesive property when judge against neutral polymers.

The ionic complexes present in ionic bioadhesive polymers may possibly contribute for the entrapment/complexation of drug as they may interact with opposite charge ionic groups on drug molecule. In designing and development of bioadhesive systems for drug delivery, anionic polyelectrolytes have been explored widely due to their proved ability to form strong hydrogen bonds when exposed to mucin glycoproteins present at mucosal surfaces. Anionic polymers like poly-acrylic acid and carboxy methyl cellulose have successfully employed for the development of such bioadhesive systems. Chitosan, a biodegradable cationic polyelectrolyte with superb *in-vivo* biocompatibility provides a breakthrough in the development of bioadhesive polymers. Chitosan and its several derivatives are dominantly incorporated and still under scanner to develop more effective biocompatible polymers to further accentuate the development of bioadhesive systems. Electrostatic interactions between chitosan and negatively charged mucin chains are the primary reason for the exhibition of bioadhesive property. Recently, a potent cardiac β-blocker levobetaxolol HCl was developed as bioadhesive complex with moderately neutralized poly-acrylic acid. This complexation technique can be utilized to formulate microcapsules by orifice-ionic gelation technique. An extended release bioadhesive system of gliclazide was also developed with a combination of sodium alginate, carbopol 934P, hydroxy propyl methyl cellulose and sodium carboxy methyl cellulose.

The utilization of several non-ionic polymers including methyl cellulose, poly vinyl pyrrolidone, poloxamer, poly vinyl alcohol, hydroxy propyl methyl cellulose etc., was also reported for bioadhesive delivery by different researchers.

3.1.2.2 Polysaccharides and its derivatives

Researches on bioadhesive systems for ocular administration highlighted the importance of polysaccharides and their derivatives. Different literatures report successful application of xanthan gum, guar gum, gellan gum, carrageenan hyaluronic acid, chitosan, methyl cellulose etc., for ocular bioadhesive delivery. In addition to film forming, cellulose based polymers also shows surface activity, which cause irritancy on ocular administration. That's why these polymers are selectively utilized for ocular administration, with keeping a check on minimal surface activity to confirm reduced ocular irritancy. Sodium carboxy methyl cellulose offers superior bioadhesive property in biological environment in comparison to other cellulose derivatives. Cellulose derivatives with cationic groups are reported to be utilized for sustained delivery of therapeutics in combination of several other anionic polymers.

3.1.2.3 Hydrogels

Hydrogels are formed by three dimensional cross-linking of polymer chains in order to develop a highly porous polymeric network. As indicated by the name, these porous gel materials entrap the water molecules within their porous configuration. High content of hydrophilic group bearing polymer chains i.e. hydroxyl, carboxyl and amino functional groups, within the polymeric network markedly supports them to hold the water molecules. As discussed earlier in bioadhesion hypotheses, the extent of polymer cross-linking affects the bioadhesive assets with a negative impact. The reason for reduced bioadhesive strength with an increase in cross-linking density is accounted for decline in swelling ability and reduced solubility parameters. A group of researchers working on bioadhesive delivery revealed these facts by performing thermal cross-linking of poly acrylic acid and methyl cellulose. Later on condensation reaction of sucrose and poly acrylic acid has been suggested to formulate densely cross-linked hydrogels with enhanced bioadhesive strength. Such condensation process results into an increase in polymer chain density within the per unit area which supports the bioadhesion process. With the aid of acrylates based bioadhesive delivery systems, bioactive peptides are successfully delivered to the upper region of small intestine without any degradation. Another classic attempt by Wood and Peppas give rise to a bioadhesive system which consists of ethylene glycol polymeric chains cross-linked with hydrogels of methacrylic acid further functionalized by wheat germ agglutinin. The specific binding ability of wheat germ agglutinin to the carbohydrate segments available over the intestinal mucosal surface results in enhanced residence time within the intestinal region.

The water holding ability of hydrogels is also utilized to improve the bioavailability of therapeutic agents with poor aqueous solubility. Chitosan and carbopol hydrogels based nanosuspension increased the bioavailability of buparvaquone when compared to simple nanosuspension of same drug. This enhancement in bioavailability was credited to bioadhesion as it makes the drug to spend more time in gastrointestinal region.

3.2 NOVEL BIOADHESIVE POLYMERS

Frequent efforts have been made in order to improve the adhesive properties of polymers. Counting from neutralization of ionic polymers, poly ethylene glycol embedded hydrogels, polymer conjugation, sustained hydration phenomenon etc., all of them provides better and specific binding to different epithelial layers. In the view of fact that all of these approaches supports bioadhesion by weak non-covalent bonds i.e. ionic bonds, Van der Waal's forces and hydrogen bonds, there is a chance of bioadhesion failure resulting in non-efficient localization of therapeutic agent at targeted biological site. That's the reason why *in-vitro/in-vivo* methods were developed to assure the performance of these systems and to minimize the incidences of therapeutic failure. However, the experiences of inefficient bioadhesion enforce the researchers to develop stronger bioadhesive polymers for drug delivery purpose.

In attempt to develop novel bioadhesive polymers, existing bioadhesive polymers have been modified, although several new materials are also developed. The chemical adaptation of well-established bioadhesive polymers by the use of derivatization with various reagents bearing sulfhydryl functions sources a remarkable improvement in the polymer's properties. Bioadhesiveness and cohesiveness are strongly enhanced. In contrast to well recognized bioadhesive polymers these novel polymers are proficient of forming covalent bonds. The human biological environment has a rich presence of disulfide bonds. These disulfide bonds are the soft targets for bioadhesive polymers to be exploited for covalent bonding to generate stronger bioadhesive strength in biological environment.

3.2.1 Lectins

Lectins belong to a group of structurally diverse proteins and glycoproteins which have the talent to reversibly attach with specific sugar/carbohydrate residues and are found in both animal and plant kingdom in addition to a variety of microorganisms. These are naturally occurring proteins that play a fundamental function in biological recognition phenomenon involving cells and proteins. Many lectins have been found to be toxic and immunogenic which may show the way to systemic anaphylaxis in susceptible individuals on subsequent exposure. The structure of lectins corresponds to structures of biologically available carbohydrate residues and sugars, this structural resemblance lead to the formation of bioadhesive bonding for selective cellular adhesions. These selective cellular adhesions may be useful for the development of target oriented bioadhesive systems.

Naturally occurring lectins have an upper hand in terms of lower toxicity and biodegradability and for that reason natural lectins, especially originated from legumes are on the focus of researchers to develop targeted bioadhesive systems. The lectins extracted from soybean, peanut, *Ulex europaeus I* and *Lens culinarius* are successfully reported for their potential to bind specifically with mucosal glycoproteins. Amongst existing lectins, utilization of wheat germ agglutinin has been on the rise due to its least immunogenic reactions, in addition to its proficiency of attachment to the intestinal and alveolar epithelium and for this reason could be used to design oral and aerosol delivery systems.

After preliminary mucosal cell-binding, lectins are capable of either remain on the cell surface or in the case of receptor mediated adhesion probably turn out to be internalized by the use of a process of endocytosis. Such systems possibly will offer duality of function in that lectin supported platforms may perhaps permit targeted specific attachment and as well propose a technique of controlled drug delivery of macromolecular pharmaceuticals using active cell mediated drug uptake. This observable fact has been accounted to be beneficial, specified that the mucus layer provides preliminary however entirely reversible binding site followed by allocation of lectin mediated drug delivery systems to the cell layer. According to the molecular configuration, three groups of lectins can be notable:

1. *Merolectins*: lectins containing only one carbohydrate recognizing region;
2. *Hololectins:* lectins with two or more carbohydrate recognizing regions;
3. *Chimerolectins:* Lectins with supplementary unrelated regions.

Lectins are able to enhance the adherence of microparticles to the intestinal epithelium and improve penetration of drugs. Polystyrene microparticles coated by tomato lectin were revealed to be specifically adhesive to enterocytes. The utilization of lectins in support of targeting drugs to tumor tissue is currently under intensive research as the human carcinoma cell lines show evidence of higher lectin binding competence than the regular human colonocytes.

3.2.2 Thiolated Polymers

A presumptive novel generation of bioadhesive polymers is thiolated polymers or nominated thiomers, which demonstrate thiol bearing side chains **(Figure 3.1)**. This is a unique category of multifunctional polymers which are customized existing polymers by adding thiol fraction. Based on thiol/disulfide switch over reactions and/or a simple oxidation progression disulfide bonds are produced between such polymers and cysteine-rich subregions of mucus glycoproteins building up the mucus gel coat. Thiomers mimic the normal mechanism of secreted mucus glycoproteins, which are moreover covalently attached to the mucus layer by the arrangement of disulfide bonds, the bridging structure most frequently come across in biological systems. Subsequently the cationic thiomers chitosan–cysteine, chitosan-thiobutylamidine as well as chitosan-thioglycolic acid and the anionic thiomers poly acrylic acid-cysteine, poly acrylic acid-cysteamine, carboxy methyl cellulose-cysteine and alginate-cysteine have been produced. Owing to the immobilization of thiol groups on bioadhesive polymers, their bioadhesive properties are enhanced up to 140 fold. The superior effectiveness of this novel generation of bioadhesive polymers in contrast to the corresponding unmodified bioadhesive polymers may perhaps be established by way of various *in-vivo* experiments on different mucosal membranes in different animal species along within humans.

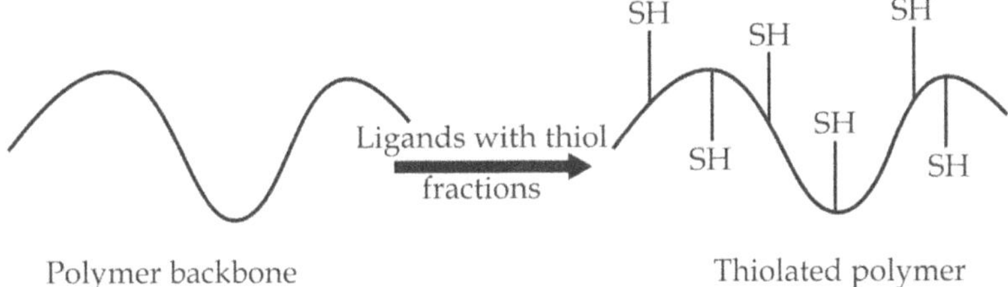

Figure 3.1 Thiolated polymers-thiomers

The polymeric skeleton of these hydrophilic macromolecules consists of open thiol groups. The existence of open thiol groups in the polymeric skeleton assists in the development of disulphide bonds with that of the cysteine-rich sub-regions available in mucin which are able to significantly improve the bioadhesive assets of the polymers e.g. poly acrylic acid and chitosan in addition to the paracellular uptake of the bioactive agents. Thiomers are capable of forming intra and inter chain disulphide bonds within the polymeric association leading to impressively enhanced cohesive properties and stability of drug delivery systems. When evaluated by thiol-disulfide exchange and oxidative methods, thiomers proved superior to all other polymers in terms of bioadhesive strength. This superior bioadhesive strength is owed to the involvement of covalent bonds between thiomers and mucosal glycoproteins. Thiomers have been revealed to interact with different natural/ synthetic polymers in order to provide a wide range of bioadhesive polymers for drug delivery. Several available thiomers encompasses poly acrylic acid-homocysteine, poly acrylic acid-cysteine, chitosan-thioethylamidine, chitosan-iminothiolane, chitosan-thioglycolic acid, poly methacrylic acid-cysteine, sodium carboxy methyl cellulose-cysteine and alginate-cysteine combinations.

The bioadhesive properties of thiomers in contrast to well recognized so far evaluated polymers were significantly enhanced irrespectively from the method of evaluation, due to the immobilization of thiol groups. In case of anionic bioadhesive polymers the poly-acrylic acid–cysteine conjugate appears to be a high-quality illustration in favor of this observation. Investigations demonstrate that the viscosity of poly-acrylic acid/ mucin mixtures straight forwardly shows a relationship among the interactions of the polymer with the mucus and as a result demonstrating the bioadhesive properties can be more than 10-fold enhanced. The similar thiomer showed in contrast to the corresponding unmodified polymer more than 2-fold and 20-fold improved bioadhesive properties in tensile investigations and by using the rotating cylinder technique, respectively. In addition, it could be revealed that the residence time of poly-acrylic acid microparticles on the small intestinal mucosa can be more than 3-fold extended by the immobilization of thiol groups. In case of cationic thiomers, on the other hand, the chitosan–thiobutylamidine conjugate appears to be a good example, as it has been evaluated by various bioadhesion test methods. It was demonstrated that a more than 100-fold increment in viscosity of chitosan-thiobutylamidine conjugate in contrast to unmodified chitosan. Furthermore in tensile studies and rotating cylinder experiments the bioadhesive properties of the thiolated transformation were 100-fold and 140-fold enhanced respectively.

In case of both acknowledged thiomers the molecular mass of the polymer chains had an immense impact on their bioadhesive properties. For the anionic as well as for the cationic thiomer the maximum bioadhesive properties were attained when they exhibited a medium molecular mass. For example poly-acrylic acid–cysteine, polymer conjugates with molecular mass of 450 kD were more bioadhesive than one with a molecular mass of 2 kD, 45 kD and 1000-3000 kD. Furthermore, tensile experiments carried out with thiolated chitosan with a molecular mass of 150 kD, 400 kD and 600 kD are evidenced for the relatively highest bioadhesive properties for the medium molecular mass thiomer. Utilizing a medium molecular mass chitosan-thiobutylamidine conjugate polymer consequently led to a more than 100-fold enhancement in bioadhesion in contrast to unmodified chitosan. In general, it could be observed in the majority executed bioadhesion experiments among thiomers, that the bioadhesive properties are proportional to the amounts of immobilized thiol groups. Additionally, the bioadhesive properties of thiomers showing signs of a relative low pH are always superior.

3.2.2.1 Cationic thiomers

Cationic thiomers are primarily based on chitosan. The primary amino group at the 2-position of the glucosamine subunit of this polymer is the crucial target in support of the immobilization of thiol groups. As sketched out in **Figure 3.2** sulfhydryl bearing agents can be covalently attached to this primary amino group by the formation of amide or amidine bonds. In case of the formation of amide bonds the carboxylic acid group of the ligands cysteine and thioglycolic acid reacts with the primary amino group of chitosan mediated for example by carbo-di-imides. An accidental oxidation of thiol groups during synthesis can be avoided by performing the reaction under inert surroundings. Otherwise synthesis can be accomplished at pH 5 as the concentration of thiolate-anions, representing the reactive form for oxidation of thiol groups is low and the formation of disulfide bonds can almost be excluded at this pH. Furthermore, by the addition of reducing agents such as dithiotreithol or borohydride after the synthesis disulfide bonds can be diminished. In case of the formation of amidine bonds 2-iminothiolane is used as coupling reagent. It offers the advantage of a simple one step coupling reaction. In addition, the thiol group of the reagent is protected towards oxidation due to its chemical structure. The amount of immobilized thiol groups in reduced and oxidized form can be determined via Ellman's reagent with and without previous quantitative reduction of disulfide bonds with borohydride.

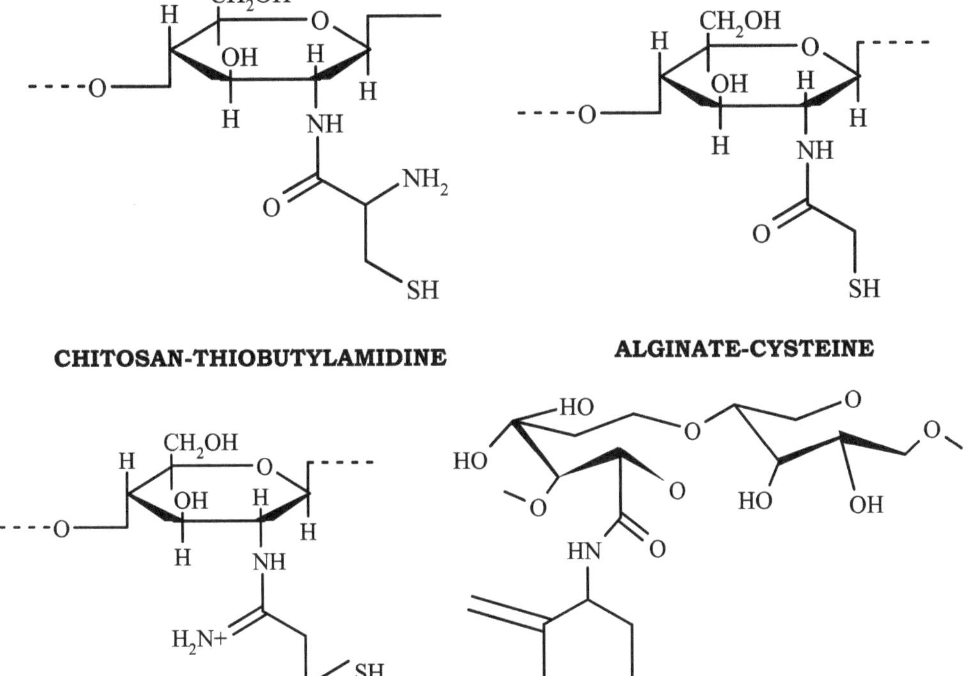

Figure 3.2 Structure of thiolated polymers

3.2.2.2 Anionic thiomers

All anionic thiolated polymers contain carboxylic acid groups as anionic substructures. Due to the presence of these carboxylic acid groups sulfhydryl moieties can be attached easily to such polymers by forming the amide bonds. The formation of amide bonds can be facilitated by carbo-di-imides. The chemical structure of some anionic thiolated polymers is presented in **Figure 3.2.** Thiol oxidation during synthesis can be avoided as described for the cationic polymers.

3.2.2.3 Explanations for the superior bioadhesion property of thiomers Formation of disulfide bonds

The disulfide bonds among thiomers and mucus layer formed either by thiol/disulfide exchange reactions or by simple oxidation of free thiol groups **(Figure 3.3)**. All mucosal glycoproteins or mucins contain cysteine-rich subdomains which provide the free thiol groups for the interaction. In comparison to non-covalent bonds disulfide bonds are not affected by factors such as ionic strength and pH. Rate and extent of disulfide bond formation be subjected to the concentration of thiolate anions representing the reactive form for thiol/disulfide exchange reactions and oxidation processes. The concentration of thiolate anions in turn depends on:

(a) *pKa value of thiol group*: The ionization of thiomer greatly affects the extent of thiolate anions. Thiol groups of the chitosan–thiobutylamidine conjugate **(Figure 3.2)**; for instance, exhibit a pKa value of 9.9, whereas the pKa value of the thiol groups of poly acrylate-cysteine conjugates is 8.35.

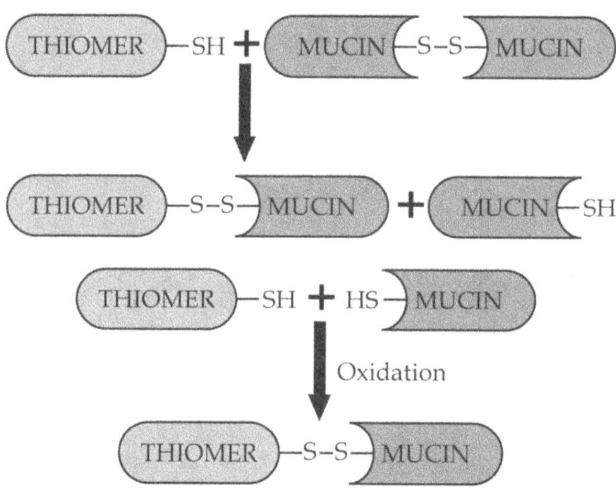

Figure 3.3 Mechanism of disulfide bond formation between thiomers and mucus glycoproteins (mucin)

(b) *The pH of the thiomer*: In contrast to non-ionic thiomers ionic thiomers are reactive in nature and possess high buffer capacity e.g. buffer capacity comparable to 25 M acetate buffer is shown by a matrix tablet composed of sodium poly-acrylate. The dense polymeric network of these polymers with excessively embedded charged moieties gives rise to a unique microenvironment at biological site. To a certain level the concentration of reactive thiol groups can be controlled by regulating the pH of polymer. The higher pH of polymer lead to more number of reactive thiol groups and vice versa.

(c) ***The pH of the surrounding medium***: The reactivity of thiol groups inside the polymeric network is primarily controlled by the pH of the thiomer, whereas the reactivity on the surface of the polymer is more controlled by the pH of the surrounding medium. As the mucus gel layer being close to the epithelium has a pH around 7, thiol groups penetrating into the mucus are always adequately reactive. The covalent bonding between thiomers and mucus gel layer has been evidenced recently. It was also revealed that mucin can be effectively bound to thiolated poly-acrylate, while it is not at all bound to unmodified poly-acrylate. Due to the addition of dithiothreitol, a disulfide bond breaker which immobilized mucin could be completely removed from the thiolated polymer.

(d) ***In-situ cross-linking process***: Another probable mechanism being accountable for the enhanced mucoadhesive properties of thiomers is based on their *in-situ* cross-linking behavior. During and after the interpenetration process disulfide bonds are formed within the thiomer itself which acts as additional anchors by binding up with mucus gel layer. It is similar to the mechanism on which the adhesive properties of most adhesive polymers are based on i.e. penetration of polymer followed by stabilization of the adhesive. In case of superglues, for instance, monomeric cyanoacrylates penetrate into raw surfaces followed by polymerization. Thiolated polymers exhibit *in-situ* gelling properties due to the oxidation of thiol groups at physiological pH-values and cause formation of inter and intramolecular disulfide bonds. For example sol-gel transition of thiolated chitosan was observed at pH 5.5 after 2 hr and highly cross-linked gels were formed. In parallel, formation of disulfide bonds is confirmed by significant decrease in the thiol group content of the polymers. The rheological properties of unmodified chitosan remained constant over the whole observation period. Rheological analysis of thiolated chitosans also demonstrated a strong relationship between the total extent of polymer-linked thiol groups and the increase in elasticity of formed gel. Higher elasticity was achieved in solutions of thiolated chitosan by immobilizing the more thiol groups on chitosan. This *in-situ* gelling property is particularly significant for liquid or semisolid vaginal, nasal and ocular formulations for the stabilization at site of application.

3.2.3 Bioadhesive Nanopolymers as Drug Carriers

The combination of bioadhesive polymers with nanoparticles increases the effectiveness of nanomedicine. Nanomedicine is defined as the use of nanometer-scale particles or systems to detect and treat diseases at the molecular level. Bioadhesive nanopolymers proved their efficiency to overcome the challenge of achieving bioavailability with topical drugs especially in ocular drug delivery system. The rationalization of particulate systems for the delivery of ophthalmic drugs is explained by the potential entrapment of particles in the ocular surface mucus layer and the interaction of bioadhesive polymer chains with mucin which consequently results into the increased precorneal resident time.

3.2.4 Alginate-Polyethylene Glycol Acrylate (Alginate-PEGAc)

As a novel member of bioadhesive materials community, alginate-polyethylene glycol acrylate (alginate-PEGAc) possesses bioadhesion strength with gelation ability. Structurally it composed of acrylated polyethylene glycol side chains supported by backbone of alginate moiety. Acrylated polyethylene glycol side chains provide bioadhesive properties and gelation ability owed to alginate portion. A strong bioadhesive bonding results as the mucus interpenetration ability of PEG's combines with addition reaction among the sulfide end present on mucosal glycoprotein chains and acrylate end present on bioadhesive polymer surface. It has multifunctional bioadhesive material for a variety of biotechnological and biomedical applications.

3.2.5 Poloxamers

The copolymers of poly ethylene oxide (PEO)-poly propylene oxide (PPO) are acknowledged as poloxamers which are non-ionic in nature **(Figure 3.4)**. Their multifunctional applications i.e. emulsifier, solubilizers, absorbance enhancer, surface active agent and dispersing agent are well established for pharmaceutical formulation development. Apart from the very good excipient properties, poloxamers are utilized for clinical and therapeutic purposes to cure and treat several physiological conditions. It has wide applications in DNA technology, brain injury, burns and ophthalmic formulations. Poloxamers are synthetic triblock copolymers represented by following formula:

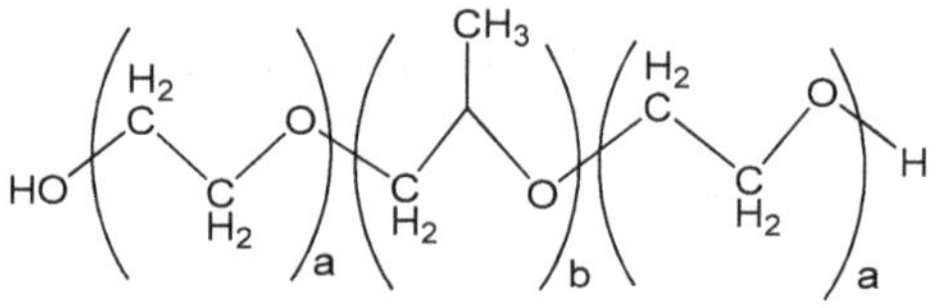

Figure 3.4 Structure of poloxamer

Poloxamer gels have been explored for *in-situ* gelation at the site of interest as they show phase transition from liquids to bioadhesive gels at body temperature. Two polymers from this category: poloxamer 188 and poloxamer 407, shows inverse thermosensitivity as they are soluble in aqueous solutions at low temperature but gets converted into gel at higher temperature.

A poloxamer 407 based *in-situ* gel was formulated as nanoemulsion in order to develop novel ophthalmic formulation of dorzolamide HCl. Better biological performance of optimized *in-situ* nanoemulsion containing triacetin, miranol C2M, poloxamer 188, poloxamer 407 and water in normotensive albino rabbits shows faster onset of action with prolonged residence time when compared to simple drug solution and marketed formulation. The success of this novel formulation ensures the effectiveness of poloxamers ability of *in-situ* gel formation resulting into prolonged residence time for enhancement of bioavailability.

In-situ thermoreversible mucoadhesive gel of an antibacterial agent, Moxifloxacin HCl is formulated by a combination of poloxamer 407 and poloxamer 188 with different mucoadhesive polymers such as Xanthan gum and Sodium alginate with a prediction to increased gel strength and bioadhesion force and thereby increased precorneal contact time and bioavailability of the drug. Formulations were found to be transparent, uniform in consistency and good spreadability within a pH range of 6.8 to 7.4. The drug release from the formulation with xantham gum was superior to the sodium alginate formulation.

Another thermoreversible bioadhesive formulation based on poloxamer was developed for rectal administration of mebeverine HCl. The effectiveness of formulation to control chronic irritable bowel syndrome suggested its reliable and safe for sustained release via rectal administration in addition to bypassing first-pass metabolism. Bioadhesive delivery confirms the immobility of dosage form in lower section of rectum to allow sufficient time for absorption.

In-situ gel-forming systems seem to be preferred in the development of ophthalmic drug delivery systems as they can be administered in the form of drop and create considerably less problems with vision. Moreover, they provide good sustained release properties. A good number of *in-situ* formulations triggered by pH, ion and temperature have been noticed in research literatures in last two decades. Each system has its own advantages and drawbacks. The choice of a particular hydrogel depends on its intrinsic properties and envisaged therapeutic use.

3.2.6 Pluronics and Combination

Pluronics have also been chemically combined with poly-acrylic acids to fabricate systems with superior adhesion and retention in the nasal cavity. Di-hydroxy phenyl alanine (DOPA), an amino acid found in mussel adhesive protein that is believed to contribute to the adhesion process, has also been combined with pluronics to enhance their adhesive properties.

3.2.7 Other Novel Bioadhesive Polymers

A more hydrophobic and plasticized polymer system was developed by incorporating ethyl hexyl acrylate into a copolymer with acrylic acid by Shojaei et al. The incorporation of ethyl hexyl acrylate diminish the hydration rate while allowing optimal interaction with the mucosal surface, and the mucoadhesive force was found to be superior with the copolymer than with poly-acrylic acid alone. Glyceryl monooleate/water liquid crystalline phases have also been found to be mucoadhesive to a wide range of mucosal surfaces, although the mechanism will differ somewhat from that of other mucoadhesives.

3.2.7.1 Bacterial bioadhesion

With more multifaceted bioadhesion mechanism several bacterial cells have been explored for their potential to be utilized in bioadhesive drug delivery systems. The phenomenon of their adhesion to biological surfaces depends on their fimbriae, a distinct attachment on its cell surface which anchors bacterial cell on biological surfaces. The specificity of bacterial adhesion towards different surfaces is also considered for targeted delivery. These extracellular fimbriae are responsible for transfer of toxic materials to the host cell and its long thread like polymeric protein binds to specific receptors of biological or other non-living surfaces. The presence of extracellular fimbriae symbolized the pathogenicity of bacterial cell. Interaction to specific receptors of mucosal surface is similar to lectins of plant origin and for that reason provides effective residence time with targeting ability. The specificity of *E. coli* stains for gastrointestinal epithelium has been explored for bioadhesive systems and as an attempt a fimbrial protein i.e. antigen K99 is combined with poly-acrylic acid which results in improved bioadhesive strength **(Figure. 3.5)**.

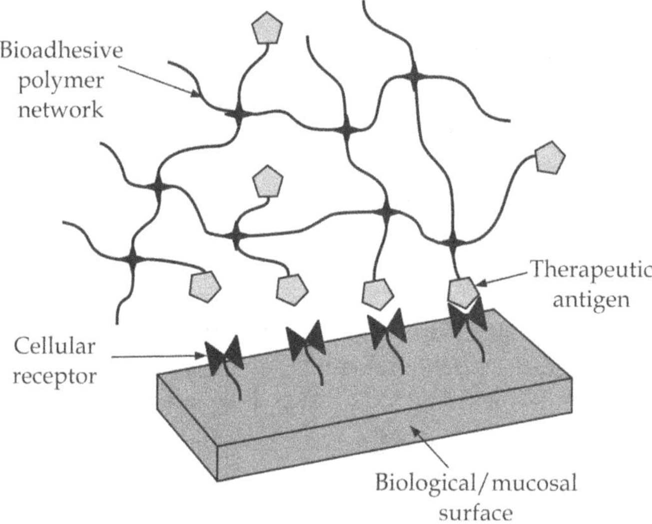

Figure 3.5 Bacterial adhesion: A diagram of covalently attached fimbrial protein (K99 from E. coli) to poly (acrylic acid) as a carrier system

Another attempt for the validation of bacterial bioadhesion involves a bacterial membrane protein 'invasin' from *Yersinia pseudotuberculosis* to develop nanospheres. The confocal laser microscopy of biological samples confirms cellular uptake of these invasin functionalized nanospheres.

3.2.7.2 Amino acid sequences for bioadhesion

Some of the amino acid sequences of mucosal surface respond well to interact with complementary structures. In pathological conditions these proteins show alterations in sequences which may be targeted by drug delivery systems. These specific adhesive interactions are resembled to lock and key theory between two complementary structures.

3.2.7.3 Antibodies for bioadhesion

Natural phenomenon of antibody production against foreign substance also has the potential to be utilized as bioadhesive interactions. With the expertise in antigen-antibody reactions these produced antibodies can be combined with selected molecules i.e. bioadhesive polymers to interact biologically. These types of highly specific bioadhesive polymers with antibodies as ligands can be utilized for drug targeting, especially to the tumor tissues.

3.3 SELECTION OF BIOADHESIVE POLYMER

A bioadhesive agent or polymer intended to promote the adhesion of the active pharmaceutical ingredient to the biological/mucosal surfaces can have some additional properties like swelling so as to accelerate the disintegration when comes in contact with the biological fluids (e.g. saliva). Various physical and chemical exchanges can influence the polymer/mucus adhesion **(Table 3.2)**; hence polymer should be cautiously selected on the basis of following properties:

(a) Polymer must have a high molecular weight up to 10,000 D or more to intensify the adhesiveness between the polymer and mucus.

(b) The chain length of polymers must be optimum i.e. long enough to encourage the interpenetration and not be too long that diffusion becomes a problem.

(c) High viscosity to increase the initial residence time at the desired site to allow the formation of interactive bonds between the bioadhesive polymer and biological surface.

(d) Degree of cross linking is also important as it influences chain mobility and dissolution. Highly cross linked polymers swell in aqueous surroundings and retain their structure. Swelling favors controlled release of the drug and increases the polymer/mucus interpenetration. But as the cross linking increases, the chain mobility decreases which consequences into diminished bioadhesive strength.

(e) Spatial conformation is also accountable to bioadhesive potency of polymers. Several active groups, predominantly responsible for the bioadhesive interactions may possibly shielded due to the conformational arrangements which results into decreased bioadhesive potency of the polymer.

(f) Polymer chains must be flexible enough to promote the interpenetration of the polymer within the mucus network.

(g) An optimum concentration of the polymer is required to generate sufficient bioadhesive strength. However, it depends on the dosage form. For solid dosage form the adhesive strength increases with increase in the polymer concentration. But in case of semisolid dosage forms an optimum concentration is essential beyond which the adhesive strength decreases.

(h) Charge and degree of ionization: The effect of polymer charge on bioadhesion was evidently revealed by Bernkop-Schnurch and Freudl. They attached various chemical entities to chitosan and the bioadhesive strength was evaluated. Cationic chitosan HCl showed outstanding adhesiveness when compared to the control. The attachment of EDTA, an anionic group improves the bioadhesive strength significantly. DTPA/chitosan system exhibited inferior bioadhesive strength in comparison to other substituted forms of chitosan due to low charge. Hence, the bioadhesive strength can be attributed as anion>cation>non-ionic.

(i) Optimum hydration of bioadhesive polymer is required to exert its bioadhesive property. Excessive hydration of polymer network is detrimental to bioadhesive strength due to formation of slippery mucilage.

(j) At very high pH values, positively charged polymers like chitosan develop polyelectrolyte complexes with mucus and exhibit strong bioadhesive forces.

(k) High applied strength and initial contact time are directly proportional to the bioadhesive strength of polymer.

(l) It should be non-toxic, economic, biocompatible and preferably biodegradable.

Table 3.2 Key attributes of polymers which contribute to bioadhesion

- Sufficient quantity of hydrogen bonding functional groups (−OH and −COOH)
- High molecular weight and chain flexibility.
- Anionic surface charges.
- Adequate surface tension to promote spreading into the mucus layer.
- Surface anchored groups with affinity to form bridges between polymer and mucin.

3.4 CHARACTERISTICS OF IDEAL BIOADHESIVE POLYMER TO BE USED IN DRUG DELIVERY SYSTEM

The characteristics of a bioadhesive polymer matrix include the instant adherence to the biological layer without any alteration in the physical property of the delivery matrix, minimum interference to the release of the active agent, biodegradable with no toxic byproducts, inhibit the enzymes present at the delivery site and augment the penetration of the active agent (if the active agent is intended to be absorbed from the delivery site). The characteristics of an ideal polymer are as follows:

- The polymer and its degradation products should be non-toxic and non-absorbable from the site of action.

- It should be non-irritant to the applied biological surfaces.

- It should preferably form strong non-covalent bonds with the mucin-epithelial cell surfaces.

- It should adhere quickly to soft tissue and should possess some site specificity.

- It should permit hassle-free incorporation of the drug and offer no hindrance to its release.

- The polymer must not decompose on storage or during shelf life of the dosage form.

- Economic production cost, so that the prepared dosage form remains competitive.

- The polymer should not possess interference in drug analysis.

Recent works in the field of bioadhesive polymers revolutionized the development of delivery systems based on these polymers. Involvement of most common bridging structure of biological systems i.e. disulfide bond for enhancement of bioadhesive strength of polymeric carriers proved a milestone. The superiority of thiolated polymers in terms of bioadhesive strength at mucus-polymer interface is credited to successful utilization of disulfide bonds as they are supposed to interact with mucosal glycoproteins at subdomains rich in cysteine.

3.5 SOME OF THE IMPORTANT AND FREQUENTLY USED BIOADHESIVE POLYMERS

3.5.1 Chitosan

Nonproprietary names: BP: Chitosan hydrochloride

PhEur: Chitosan hydrochloride

Synonyms: 2-Amino-2-deoxy-(1,4)-b-D-glucopyranan; chitosanihydrochloridum;

Deacetylated chitin; deacetylchitin; b-1,4-poly-D-glucosamine; poly-D-glucosamine; poly-(1,4-b-D-glucopyranosamine).

Chemical name: Poly-b-(1, 4)-2-Amino-2-deoxy-D-glucose

CAS registry number: [9012-76-4]

Empirical formula and molecular weight: Chitosan is polysaccharide consists of copolymers of glucosamine and N-acetyl glucosamine and produced by partial deacetylation of chitin. The prediction of exact chemical composition of chitosan is difficult as the degree of deacetylation and depolymerization varies at different stages. The composition of chitosan varies from one manufacturer to another which depends on degree of deacetylation. In other terms, soluble amine salts resulted from deacetylation of chitin are known as chitosan. In order to obtain soluble form of chitosan the degree of deacetylation must be greater than 80-85%. The molecular weight of different grades of commercially available chitosan is ranging from 10,000-10,00.000 D with a varying degree of deacetylation **(Figure 3.6)**.

Structural formula

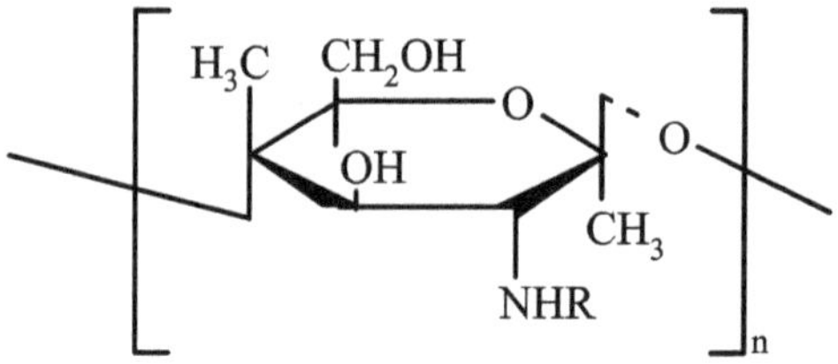

Figure 3.6 Structure of chitosan

Functional category: Biodegradable bioadhesive polymer, binder, coating material, viscosity modifier, film forming material, disintegrant, mucosal permeation enhancer.

Applications in pharmaceutical formulation or technology: In the course of last two decades, chitosan has been used as a safe excipient in drug formulations. Due to its bioadhesive property, it can adhere to hard and soft tissues and has been used in dentistry, orthopedics and ophthalmology and in surgical procedures. It adheres to epithelial tissues and to the mucus coat present on the surface of the tissues. Clinical tests of chitosan has been carried out in order to promote chitosan based biomaterials do not report any inflammatory or allergic reactions following implantation, injection, topical application or ingestion in the human body.

Chitosan is currently proposed to be one of the most promising polymers in wound dressing development. One of the most important features of chitosan based wound dressing is its bioadhesion to the wounded site. Chitosan is biodegradable, with hemostatic, bacteriostatic and wound healing properties; therefore, it's potential for wound and burns dressing offers advantage on conventional dressings.

Chitosan marks its presence in cosmetic formulations in addition to its reported uses in pharmaceutical dosage forms. This natural bioadhesive polymer is still under scanner of formulation developers to exploit it for several other applications. The effectiveness and compatibility of chitosan for bioadhesive applications in drug delivery systems has been reported in a number of studies. Different literatures reports its suitability for mucoadhesive formulations, rapid release formulations, colonic delivery, controlled release formulations, gene delivery and enhancement of peptide delivery. Wide spread applications of chitosan in different formulations i.e. tablets, films, patches, microparticles, nanoparticles, nanoemulsions, beads, gels, liposomes etc., increases its reputation in novel drug delivery systems. In addition the ease of manufacturing of chitosan based formulations is comparable to conventional techniques i.e. direct compression, granulation, coacervation, spray drying, ionotropic gelation, heat coagulation, solvent evaporation etc., with no or minor improvisations.

Description: Commercially chitosan is available as odorless white to creamy-white powder or flakes. Its cotton resembling appearance is owed to fibers, formed during precipitation process.

Typical properties: The affinity of chitosan towards the negatively charged surfaces e.g. chelates metal ions is owed to high density of cationic amine residues at pH $\leq$ 6.5. This linear polyelectrolyte has reactive amino and hydroxyl groups which are available for salt formation or chemical interactions. The high density of amino groups supports chemical interactions with anionic groups present on biological surfaces or other substances. These polyelectrolyte and polymeric carbohydrate nature of chitosan results in altered physicochemical properties of so formed complexes. Due to the primary aliphatic nature of amino groups, chitosan positively supports typical reaction of amines e.g. N-acylation and Schiff reactions. The length of polymeric chain, density of charged groups and their distribution throughout the polymeric network markedly influences the functional properties of chitosan. The pharmaceutical applications of chitosan depend upon its molecular weight, degree of deacetylation, salt form and pH of site of application/absorption.

Acidity/alkalinity: The pH of 1% w/v aqueous solution ranges 4.0-6.0. pH = 4.0-6.0 (1% w/v aqueous solution)

Density: 1.35-1.40 g/cm^3 at room temperature.

Glass transition temperature: 203 °C

Moisture content: Atmospheric moisture adsorbs on chitosan surface and its extent depends on storage conditions i.e. initial moisture content, relative humidity and temperature.

Particle size distribution: < 30 mm

Solubility: Chitosan is practically insoluble in ethanol (95%), organic solvents, and neutral or alkali solutions of pH above 6.5. It is sparingly soluble in water but readily soluble in almost all dilute or concentrated organic acid solutions. It shows limited solubility in mineral inorganic acids except sulfuric and phosphoric acids. The solubility of chitosan salts i.e. chloride or glutamate is depends on the degree of deacetylation. Addition of other salts also affects its solubility as higher ionic strength lowers the solubility due to salting-out effect which causes precipitation of chitosan. In solution form the amine groups of polymeric network become protonated and build up a strong positive charge. It exists in an extended conformation in solutions due to the repulsive forces between glucosamine entities and adjacent deacylated divisions. Electrolyte addition reduces these repulsive forces in solution form and conformation transforms into a more random and coiled conformation.

Viscosity (dynamic): Different viscosity grades of chitosan are available in commercial market. In acidic environment it works as a superb viscosity enhancer due to its high molecular weight and unbranched linear structure. At increased shear rates it shows a decrease in viscosity and act as a pseudo-plastic stuff. In solutions its viscosity is directly proportional to the degree of deacetylation and concentration while inversely proportional to temperature.

Stability and storage conditions: Chitosan powder is a stable material at room temperature, although, it is hygroscopic after drying. Chitosan should be stored in a tightly closed container in a cool, dry place. The PhEur 6.5 specifies that chitosan should be stored at a temperature of 2-8 °C.

Incompatibilities: Chitosan is incompatible with strong oxidizing agents.

Method of manufacture: Commercially chitosan is manufactured from shells of crustaceans such as shrimps and crabs by chemical treatment process. The basic chemical treatment with alkali and acid removes proteins and minerals e.g. calcium phosphate and calcium carbonate, respectively. The shells are grounded prior to chemical treatment to increase the surface area for the better accessibility of regents. Deproteinization is done by treating the grounded shells with an aqueous solution of 3-5% sodium hydroxide. After neutralization, decalcification is done by the treatment with an aqueous solution of 3-5% hydrochloric acid and chitin is precipitated at room temperature. The precipitated chitin is dried and stored for further processing of deacetylation. For N-deacetylation chitin is treated with 40-45% aqueous sodium hydroxide at elevated temperature of 110 °C and precipitated crude chitin is washed with water. This crude chitin is dissolved in 2% acetic acid and insoluble impurities are removed. Then the acidic solution containing chitosan is neutralized with aqueous solution of sodium hydroxide and purified chitosan is collected as white precipitate which is processed for grounding to get fine uniform granules or powder. The animals from which chitosan is derived must fulfill the requirements for the health of animals suitable for human consumption to the satisfaction of the competent authority. The method of production must consider inactivation or removal of any contamination by viruses or other infectious agents.

Safety: The safety of chitosan as an excipient in pharmaceutical dosage forms has been investigated and reported in several literatures. It is generally reported to be non-irritant and non-toxic for human use. The cosmetic formulations with chitosan as an excipient are also reported. The LD50 of this biodegradable polymer in mouse for oral route is >16 g/kg.

Handling precautions: Normal precautions appropriate to the circumstances and quantity of material handled. Chitosan is combustible; open flames should be avoided. Chitosan is temperature-sensitive and should not be heated above 200 °C. Airborne chitosan dust may explode in the presence of a source of ignition, depending on its moisture content and particle size. Water, dry chemicals, carbon dioxide, sand or foam fire-fighting media should be used. Chitosan may cause skin or eye irritation. It may be harmful if absorbed through the skin or if inhaled, and may be irritating to mucous membranes and the upper respiratory tract. Eye and skin protection and protective clothing are recommended; wash thoroughly after handling. Prolonged or repeated exposure (inhalation) should be avoided by handling in a well-ventilated area and wearing a respirator.

Regulatory status: The regulatory status of chitosan in pharmaceutical formulations is still debatable but in some countries it is registered as a food supplement.

Comments: Chitosan derivatives are easily obtained under mild conditions and can be considered as substituted glucens.

3.5.2 Gelatin

Nonproprietary names: BP: Gelatin
   JP: Gelatin
   PhEur: Gelatin
   USP-NF: Gelatin

Synonyms: Byco; Cryogel; E441; Gelatina; Gelatine; Instagel; Kolatin; Solugel; Vitagel.

Chemical name and CAS registry number: Gelatin [9000-70-8]

Empirical formula and molecular weight: Gelatin is a generic term for a mixture of purified protein fractions. The protein fractions consist almost entirely of amino acids joined together by amide linkages to form linear polymers, varying in molecular weight from 20000-200000 D.

Functional category: Coating agent; film-forming agent; gelling agent; suspending agent; tablet binder; viscosity-increasing agent.

Applications in pharmaceutical formulation or technology: Gelatin is a biodegradable polymer utilized for many implantable systems in addition to other pharmaceutical dosage forms. The most common use in soft and hard gelatin capsule shells still claims the highest consumption. Advances in bioadhesive polymer science in past few decades restrict the utilization of adhesives based on gelatin and several of them are replaced by other developed synthetic bioadhesive polymers. But the biodegradability property of this natural polymer is still in the focus of pharmaceutical scientists for the development of novel drug delivery systems. The supremacy of gelatin as a tackifying agent has been utilized in manufacturing of decals, glass laminates, gummed tapes and packaging ribbons. Gelatin is used as a substrate for cell adhesion and growth. Cross-linking of gelatin makes it more stable and harder at higher temperatures. Cross-linked gelatin was used in a drug delivery system, on biomedical films and for coatings on arterial grafts.

An effort has been made to introduce free dangling aldehyde groups in order to produce a powerful bioadhesive gelatin film. The attempt involved the treatment of gelatin films with 0.5M glutaraldehyde at 60 °C for an addition of free aldehyde groups up to 150 μmol/g. The strength of bioadhesive bonding between biological tissues and these modified gelatin films was directly proportional to the aldehyde content of the film. The superiority of these modified gelatin films over normal gelatin films in terms of bioadhesive strength can be clearly evidenced, as modified gelatin films shows high bonding strength of 250 gf/cm^2 in comparison to 40 gf/cm^2 of normal/unmodified gelatin films.

An *in-situ* tissue adhesive was also developed which is based on enzymatic cross linking of gelatin hydrogels. Different gelatin derivatives with varying phenolic content were prepared by conjugation of tyramine and hydroxyphenyl propionic acid with gelatin skeleton. Out of these developed derivatives of gelatin two derivatives i.e. gelatin–hydroxyphenyl propionic acid-tyramine and gelatin-hydroxyphenyl propionic acid with maximum phenolic content of 395.7 μmol/g and 146.6 μmol/g respectively, were selected for the preparation of hydrogels. Hydrogels were prepared in presence of hydrogen peroxide by horseradish peroxidase mediated reactions which markedly affects the properties of hydrogels. Mechanical strength, rate of degradation and gelation time of hydrogels can be tailored by altering the concentrations of horseradish peroxidase and hydrogen peroxide. To some extent rate and degree of cross linking is also controlled by changing the concentration of horseradish peroxidase and hydrogen peroxide. Moreover, the mechanical strength of hydrogels is increased with an increase in phenolic content.

Gelatin has also shown its therapeutic effect in wound dressings and plasma replacement therapy. However, aphylactoid reactions restricted its utilization for plasma replacement therapy. Absorbable gelatin is used for the preparation of sterile films for various routes i.e. ophthalmic films, sterile powder sponges, sterile compressed sponges and simple sterile sponges. The haemostatic properties of gelatin sponges have successfully employed for wound dressing materials. Its widespread use in food products and photographic emulsions is well known from a long time.

Description: Gelatin appears as a brittle solid with light amber to faint yellow color. It is an odorless and tasteless material. Gelatin is commercially available in different forms e.g. coarse powder, flakes, granules and translucent sheets.

Typical properties: The properties of gelatin depend on its source and grade and vary significantly from each other.

Acidity/alkalinity: A 1% w/v aqueous solution of different grades of gelatin shows following pH ranges at 25 °C:

Type A shows pH in the range of 3.8-5.5;

Type B shows pH in the range of 5.0-7.5.

Density: Type A – 1.32 g/cm^3;

Type A – 1.28 g/cm^3.

Isoelectric point: Type A – 7.0-9.0;

Type B – 4.7-5.4.

Moisture content: Ranges between 9-11%.

Solubility: Gelatin is soluble in glycerin, alkalis and acids. However precipitation of gelatin is observed in strong acidic and alkaline solutions. It is practically insoluble in methanol, acetone, ether, chloroform and ethanol (95%). In aqueous media gelatin swells due to water absorption and form a soft mass. It presents a water absorption capacity to an extent of 5-10 times of its own weight. Its aqueous solubility is influenced by temperature as it is soluble in water at temperatures above 40 °C and form a colloidal solution which transforms into gel form on cooling to 35-40 °C. This heat reversible sol-gel transformation revealed the thixotropic potential of gelatin. The transition temperature range is very narrow which can be tailored by the addition of glycerin.

Stability and storage conditions: Gelatin is stable in dry form at room temperature. In cool conditions it is stable as aqueous solutions for long periods but there is a risk of bacterial degradation. At high temperature i.e. about 50 °C depolymerization of gelatin is observed in aqueous solution which causes diminution in gel strength on resettling. The depolymerization reactions proceed rapidly at temperature above 65 °C and gel strength may be decreased to half of its initial level if heated for 1 hour at 80 °C. The rate and extent of depolymerization is inversely proportional to the molecular weight of gelatin i.e. low molecular weight gelatin depolymerized more rapidly in comparison to high molecular weight grades. Airtight containers should be used for the bulk storage of gelatin in cool, dry and well ventilated conditions.

Incompatibilities: Gelatin reacts with both acids and bases which confirms its amphoteric characteristic. As a natural protein, it also shows the characteristic reactions of proteins e.g. proteolytic hydrolysis into amino acid components. In gel form preservation/preservatives are required to prevent degradation leading to liquefaction. Its reaction with ether, tannic acid, mercury salts, chloroform and alcohols results into precipitation of gelatin. Gelatin is also reactive with electrolytes, metal ions, aldehydes, aldehydic sugars, plasticizers, strong oxidizing agents, surfactants, preservatives and other cationic/anionic polymers. However, several of these reactions are favorable to manufacture other forms of gelatin for different dosage forms e.g. gelatin and plasticizer i.e. glycerin interaction is utilized to manufacture soft gelatin capsule and suppositories etc. Its reaction with formaldehyde results in enhanced resistance in gastric environment.

Method of manufacture: Natural presence of gelatin in collagen rich animal tissues i.e. sinew, skin and bone is exploited for the commercial extraction of gelatin. Direct extraction of gelatin from animal tissues using boiling water as a solvent is difficult but extraction can be easily performed by pretreatment of animal tissues with either acid or alkali. When pretreatment is done by acid, obtained gelatin is called as Type A gelatin and if pretreatment is done by alkali, obtained gelatin is called as Type B gelatin. To achieve high yields, acid pretreatment is utilized for the extraction of gelatin from demineralized bones, sinew and skins of calf, fish, pig etc. The raw material is cut into small pieces and superficial fat is removed by washing for several hours with cold water. Then this washed raw material is treated with mineral acid solutions, generally hydrochloric acid or sulphuric acid of pH 1-3 at 15-20 °C for approximately 24 hours in order to achieve maximum swelling. After swelling the excess of acid is removed by washing with water and pH is maintained at 3.5-4.0 for pig and fish skin and 2.0-3.5 for all other tissues, before this material is subjected to hot-water extraction. For maximum yield of gelatin, a batch process is applied for hydrolytic extraction of animal tissues using successive portions of hot water at progressively higher temperatures of 50-75 °C. After extraction gelatin solution is subjected to filtration through previously sterilized cellulose pads and concentrated to about 20-25% w/v before sterilization by exposing at 138 °C for 4 seconds. Then the concentrate solution of gelatin is transformed into gel by chilling and kept in temperature controlled ovens for air drying. The powdered gelatin of desired particle size is obtained by grounding the dried gelatin. The alkali pretreatment process is generally utilized with cattle skins and demineralized bones. In this process raw material is kept in 2-5% calcium hydroxide at 14-18 °C for 2-4 months. Then the excess of alkali is removed by washing with cold water for about 24 hours and the resulted slurry is neutralized by acidic solutions of hydrochloric acid, sulphuric acid or phosphoric acid. This neutralized slurry is subjected to extraction process similar to acid pretreatment process but in contrast the pH is maintained at 5.0-6.5. For gelatin manufacturing, all the raw materials are tested for the presence of transmissible spongiform encephalopathies (TSEs) vectors which must be removed before processing to ensure the TSE infectivity free grades of gelatin for pharmaceutical use.

Safety: The safety of gelatin incorporation in pharmaceutical formulations for oral and parenteral administration is well accepted. For oral formulations gelatin is considered as non-toxic and non-irritant ingredient. However, some incidents of local irritation are reported e.g. adhesion of gelatin capsules to esophageal lining gives rise to irritation. In case of parental formulations hypersensitivity reactions with serious anaphylactoid reactions are considered as potential restriction for gelatin. The potential risk of BSE/TSE (Bovine spongiform encephalopathy/Transmissible spongiform encephalopathy) infections is also associated with the incorporation of gelatin in pharmaceutical formulations. However, the extent of these contaminations is very low and can be controlled by strict quality control measures. LD_{50} value of 5 g/kg is reported for oral administration of gelatin in rats.

Handling precautions: Generally, no special precautions are required and depend on the quantity and condition of material to be handled. Gloves and eye protection is recommended to avoid direct contact. Handling environment for gelatin should be well ventilated and stored away from heat and ignition sources. As the gelatin aids ignition, its residues should be evaporated appropriately i.e. under a fuming hood.

Regulatory status: Gelatin is listed in GRAS (Generally Recognized As Safe) materials and accepted as an inactive ingredient for inhalations, parenterals, syrups, tablets, capsules, pastilles solutions and dental preparations by FDA. It is also licensed for medicinal use in Europe, Japan and UK and listed as acceptable non-medicinal ingredient by Canadian regulatory authorities. Preparation of microcapsules of vitamin A by gelatin-acacia complex coacervation and sustained release alginate-gelatin beads of pindolol has been reported. A specification for gelatin is also mentioned in Food Chemicals Codex (FCC).

Comments: Pharmacopoeial discussion group selected the gelatin as a material for harmonization. The past history of potential transmission of TSE vectors from raw bovine materials into gelatin warns regulatory authorities to mention the measures for safe use of gelatin in pharmaceutical products especially in case of gelatin obtained from bovine sources. The best method to avoid such contamination which is also practiced by European countries is to control the geographical source of animals to be utilized for gelatin manufacturing in parallel to strict control over method of production. The absence of BSE infectious vectors should be confirmed by scientific geographical data showing the locations with BSE infectivity. If bones are used as raw material for the production of gelatin keep a check on source country to avoid the source material from countries listed under Geographical BSE Risk (GBR) I and II. However, bones from GBR III countries can be accepted after confirmation of complete vertebrae removal. In case of hides as starting material for gelatin production which is regarded as a safer source in comparison to bones, recommended precautions should be practiced to avoid cross contamination from probable contaminated materials. Different grades of gelatin are usually classified on the basis of gel strength which is expressed in terms of 'bloom strength'. Bloom strength is defined as weight in grams applied to a plunger of 12.7 mm diameter under controlled conditions to produce an exact 4 mm deep depression in a matured 6.66% w/w aqueous gelatin gel. The commercially available grades of gelatin differ in molecular weight, particle size, bloom strength and other properties.

3.5.3 Sodium Alginate

Nonproprietary names: BP: Sodium alginate

PhEur: Sodium alginate

USP-NF: Sodium alginate

Synonyms: Algin; alginic acid; Alginatosodico; Kelcosol; Keltone; Natriialginas; Protanal; Sodium polymannuronate.

Chemical name and CAS registry number: Sodium alginate [9005-38-3]

Composition: Sodium alginate is generally available as sodium salt of alginic acid which is a mixture of polyuronic acids and composed of D-mannuronic acid and L-guluronic acid residues.

Functional category: Viscosity enhancer; stabilizer, binder; disintegrant for tablet and capsules; suspending agent.

Applications: Sodium alginate is successfully employed in different pharmaceutical formulations meant for oral and topical administration to perform different functions. Its binding and disintegrant properties can be utilized for tablet formulations. It is also used as a filler/diluent for capsules. As a polymer its sustained release behavior has been utilized in oral sustained release systems and it also delays the drug dissolution in several dosage forms i.e. tablets, capsules and suspensions. The effects of particle size, viscosity and chemical composition of sodium alginate on drug release from matrix tablets have been observed. In topical formulations, sodium alginate is widely used as a thickening and suspending agent. Recently, a possibility of aqueous microencapsulation has been revealed with sodium alginate in contrast to conventional microencapsulation techniques which mostly utilizes organic solvents. Nanotechnological techniques also open the prospect of sodium alginate nanoparticles for the delivery of different drugs. Its bioadhesive properties are also been investigated for the interaction with mucosal surfaces to explore the possibilities of mucoadhesive drug delivery. Work in the field of bioadhesive formulations i.e. buccal tablets, hydrogels, vaginal tablets confirms the effectiveness of this polymer. The esophageal bioadhesion of sodium alginate suspensions may provide a barrier against gastric reflux or site-specific delivery of therapeutic agents. Some other novel systems for therapeutic delivery via different routes are also developed e.g. ophthalmic and oral *in-situ* gels, mucoadhesive microspheres for intranasal delivery and a device to deliver bone growth factors. Possibilities for the delivery of proteins and peptides have also been explored through alginate hydrogels. In addition, sodium alginate microspheres have been used in the preparation of a foot-mouth disease DNA vaccine, and in an oral vaccine for Helicobacter pylori; chitosan nanoparticles coated with sodium alginate may have applications in mucosal vaccine delivery systems. It also shows therapeutic efficacy in the management of gastro-esophageal reflux when combined with H_2-receptor antagonists and as a haemostatic agent in surgical dressings. The incorporation of sodium alginate in dressings for exuding wounds improves the gelling properties which supports the wound healing. In combination with chitosan it is used for the preparation of sponges which can be effectively applied as wound dressings and matrices for tissue engineering. Lyophilized wound healing wafers composed of sodium alginate have been found to exhibit large reductions in viscosity following gamma irradiation. Sodium alginate is also used in cosmetics and food products.

Description: Sodium alginate appears as a tasteless white to yellowish brown powder having no odor.

Typical properties

Acidity/alkalinity: 1% w/v aqueous solution of sodium alginate shows a pH value of 7.2.

Solubility: Sodium alginate forms a viscous colloidal solution when dissolved in water. It is practically insoluble in ether, ethanol, chloroform and other organic solvents but shows some solubility in aqueous mixture of ethanol with a concentration lower than 30% of ethanol. It is also practically insoluble in acidic solutions of pH less than 3.

Viscosity (dynamic): Commercially available grades of sodium alginate show a variable viscosity in aqueous solutions. In order to establish a standard, generally the viscosity of 1% w/v solution of sodium alginate is ranged between 20-400 mPas. The aqueous solubility of sodium alginate is markedly influenced by pH, temperature, concentration and presence of metal ions. At pH values of above 10 its solubility decreases.

Stability and storage conditions: Sodium alginate should be stored carefully as it is hygroscopic in nature. To keep it stable it should be stored at cool temperature with low relative humidity. Alginic acid is precipitated from the aqueous solution of pH below 3. However, pH between 4-10 is considered most suitable for the stabilization of aqueous sodium alginate solutions. Metal containers should be avoided for the storage of sodium alginate. This polymer is also susceptible for microbial degradation resulting into alterations in viscosity. To avoid microbial contamination, its solutions are sterilized by filtration though 0.45 µm filter or by ethylene oxide. At temperatures above 70 °C sodium alginate solutions undergoes depolymerization reactions which are detrimental to viscosity. Autoclaving is avoided as it may decrease the viscosity. Irradiation with gamma rays is prohibited for the sterilization of alginate solutions as it is detrimental to the viscosity. Preparations meant for external application can be protected from microbial degradation by incorporating 0.1% chloroxylenol, 0.1% chlorocresol or parabens in the formulations. Benzoic acid may also be used in case of acidic preparations. Air tight containers must be used for bulk storage of sodium alginate and kept in a cool and dry place.

Incompatibilities: Sodium alginate reacts with crystal violet, phenyl mercuric acetate, phenyl mercuric nitrate, different calcium salts, acridine derivatives and heavy metals. It is also incompatible with ethanolic solutions with concentrations higher than 5%. The effect of electrolyte addition depends on concentration of electrolyte. In low concentrations they increase the viscosity while higher concentration results in salting out of sodium alginate e.g. at concentration higher than 4% sodium chloride salting out of sodium alginate occurs.

Method of manufacture: Sodium alginate is sodium salt of alginic acid. For commercial production of sodium alginate, first alginic acid is extracted from brown sea weeds and then extracted alginic acid is neutralized by the addition of sodium bicarbonate to yield sodium alginate.

***Safety*:** Sodium alginate is established as a non-toxic and non-irritant to be utilized in pharmaceutical formulations, food products and cosmetic formulations. It is effectively employed in the formulation of tablets, wound dressings and several other topical preparations. Its safety in humans is proven by different studies e.g. in a study five healthy male volunteers were kept on a daily dose of 175 mg/kg sodium alginate for 7 days then dose was increased to 200 mg/kg for further 16 days. None of the volunteer shows any significant adverse effect during and after the study period. WHO has not provided any guidelines on safe amount of alginic acid or alginate salts for daily intake as they does not show any hazard to health with the concentrations present in food products. However, excessive oral ingestion for long terms may be harmful. The persons involved in alginate production should be provided with masks to avoid inhalation of alginate dust which may cause irritation leading to industrial hazard like asthma. However, several reports claims that the incidence of asthmatic cases is associated with individuals who were exposed to seaweed dust and pure alginate dust do not cause such risk. Different LD_{50} values are reported for sodium alginate via different routes of administration in several animal models:

- LD_{50} for cats via intraperitoneal (i.p) route: 0.25 g/kg
- LD_{50} for rats via oral route: > 5 g/kg
- LD_{50} for rats via i.v route: 1 g/kg
- LD_{50} for mouse via i.v route: 0.2 g/kg
- LD_{50} for rabbits via i.v route: 0.1 g/kg

***Handling precautions*:** Generally, no special precautions are required and depend on the quantity and condition of material to be handled. Gloves, masks and eye protection are recommended to avoid direct contact/inhalation which may cause irritation. Handling environment for sodium alginate should be well ventilated.

***Regulatory status*:** Sodium alginate is listed in GRAS (Generally Recognized As Safe) materials and accepted as an inactive ingredient for oral suspensions and tablets by FDA. It is also licensed in UK as an excipient for non-parenteral formulations e.g. capsules, modified release tablets, enteric-coated tablets and lozenges. It also makes an entry in Canadian list of acceptable non-medicinal ingredients.

***Related substances*:** Alginic acid; calcium alginate; potassium alginate; propylene glycol alginate.

***Comments*:** The commercially available grades of sodium alginate provide solutions with different viscosities. Sodium alginate may be mixed with dispersing agents e.g. propylene glycol, ethanol, sucrose, glycerol etc., for the formulation of dispersions. Different derivatives of sodium alginate are also available as its salts i.e. magnesium alginate, ammonium alginate, potassium alginate and calcium alginate which can also be utilized for pharmaceutical purposes.

3.5.4 Albumin

Nonproprietary names: BP: Albumin solution

PhEur: Human albumin solution

USP: Albumin human

Synonyms: Alba; albuconn; albuminar; human albumin solution; albumisol; albuspan; albutein; human serum albumin; normal human serum albumin; octalbin; plasbumin; plasma albumin; proserum.

Chemical name: Serum albumin

Empirical formula and molecular weight: The molecular weight of human serum albumin is about 66500 and it occurs as a single polypeptide chain with 585 amino acids. Characteristically it contains 17 cysteine residues, 6 methionine residues and a single tryptophan residue. It also contains the charged amino acid residues of glutamic acid, lysine, aspartic acid and arginine 23 with an extent of 61, 59, 36 and 23, respectively.

Structural formula: The primary structure of human albumin is a single polypeptide chain made up of 585 amino acids with seven disulfide bridges. A secondary structure of human serum albumin is also exists that is about 55% a-helix. The remaining 45% is supposed to be divided among turns, disordered and b-structures. It is the only major plasma protein having no carbohydrate constituents and this fact is supported by the assay of crystalline albumin which claims less than one sugar residue per albumin molecule.

Functional category: Stabilizer; therapeutic agent.

Applications: In parenteral formulations of proteins and enzymes, albumin is incorporated as an excipient and primarily work as a stabilizer. Several researchers utilized it for the preparation of microcapsules and microspheres for investigational purpose to develop effective and biodegradable drug delivery systems. Generally, albumin concentrations in the range of 1-5% are used for the stabilization of protein formulations. However, it is effective as a stabilizer even in low concentration of 0.003%. For pharmaceutical purpose, albumin has also employed as a co-solvent in parenteral formulations and as a cryo-protectant in lyophilization process. It also inhibits the adsorption of other proteins to surface. For the treatment of severe acute albumin deficiency it is used as a therapeutic agent. Its therapeutic advantage is also utilized as parenteral solutions for plasma volume replacement. However, therapeutic effectiveness of albumin in such pathological conditions for critically ill patients is still debatable.

Description: According to USP human serum albumin is a sterile non-pyrogenic preparation of serum albumin which is obtained from healthy human donors. Different strength of human serum albumin i.e. 4, 5, 20 and 25 g are available as 100 ml solutions which contains not less than 96% albumin as total protein content. These albumin preparations do not contain any antimicrobial agent or preservative but sodium acetyl tryptophanate with or without sodium caprylate may be added as a stabilizer. Similarly, in

PhEur (European Pharmacopoeia) albumin solution is defined as aqueous protein solution obtained from plasma of healthy humans. These albumin preparations are available in concentrated strength of 150-250 g/L or in isotonic strength of 35-50 g/L with not less 95% albumin as total protein content. Similar to USP preparations no antimicrobial agent or preservative is incorporated. For protection from heat, a stabilizing agent e.g. N-acetyl tryptophan or sodium caprylate (sodium octanoate) or their combination may be incorporated in these preparations. Solid albumin powder, lumps or scales have a brownish appearance with amorphous nature while aqueous solutions of albumin appear slightly viscous and their color ranges from colorless to amber with respect to their concentrations.

Typical properties

Acidity/alkalinity: A 1% w/v solution of albumin in 0.9% w/v sodium chloride solution shows pH value ranging from 6.7-7.3 at 20 °C.

Osmolarity: The aqueous solutions of albumin in concentrations ranging from 4-5% w/v are considered iso-osmotic with human serum.

Solubility: Albumin is freely soluble in water and salt solutions of low concentration. Its high solubility in aqueous medium is owed to prominent net charge of peptide content. Aqueous solutions of albumin up to a concentration of 40% w/v can be readily prepared at pH 7.4. The seven disulfide bridges in peptide chain of albumin contribute to its chemical and spatial conformation. The net electrostatic charge of albumin is about -17 units at physiological pH.

Stability and storage conditions: Similar to other proteins albumin is also susceptible to chemical degradation and denaturation when exposed to high salt concentrations, enzymes, heat, extreme pH environments, organic solvents and other chemicals. To store albumin solutions in stable form they should be kept in light resistant containers and stored at temperatures mentioned on label, preferably at 2-25 °C.

Method of manufacture: Albumin for medicinal use is prepared by fractionation of source materials e.g. placenta, serum, plasma or blood of healthy human volunteers. Before processing all source materials must be tested in order to confirm the absence of infectious materials i.e. HIV, hepatitis B surface antigen etc. Albumin solution are generally administered through intravenous route therefore aseptic conditions are maintained during its production. The final solutions are passed through the filters which are able to retain bacterial contamination and the filtered solution distributed to pre-sterile containers and sealed under aseptic conditions. The final containers are heated at controlled temperature of 60 °C for not less than 10 hours followed by incubation at 30-32 °C for not less than 14 days or at 20-25 °C for not less than 28 days. These final containers are visually examined for any microbial contamination before final labeling.

Safety: Albumin is natural biological protein present in humans with an extent of more than 60% of total plasma proteins. Its status as a biological component, makes ground for consideration as an essentially non-toxic and non-irritant material to be incorporated as an excipient in pharmaceutical formulations. Rare cases of adverse reactions i.e. chills, hyper salivary secretion, febrile reactions, nausea and vomiting were reported with albumin infusion. Incidence of allergic reactions including anaphylactic shock may be experienced. In several cases urticaria and skin rashes have been reported. For dialysis purpose, albumin solutions with less than 200 mg/L aluminum content should be used. For patients with severe anemia or cardiac failure, albumin infusions are contraindicated. It shows the LD_{50} values of greater than 12.5 g/kg in both monkey and rat models after i.v administration.

Handling precautions: Handled with similar precautions appropriate for other biological products derived from blood.

Regulatory status: Albumin is accepted as an inactive ingredient for oral tablets, film coatings, i.v injections, i.v infusions and subcutaneous injectables by FDA. It is also licensed in UK as a parenteral product and also included in Canadian list of acceptable non-medicinal ingredients.

Related substances: Bovine serum albumin is also available commercially as an alternative to human serum albumin.

Comments: The osmolarity of a 100 mL aqueous albumin solution containing 25 g of serum albumin is equivalent to the osmolarity of 500 ml normal human plasma.

Of late, scientists are trying to improve the bioavailability of therapeutic agents by tailoring the properties of the delivery systems as an alternative of designing new agents. Bioadhesive polymers offer improved residence time for better absorption from the delivery site which is accountable for the enhanced bioavailability of delivered therapeutic agents. The several sites where bioadhesive polymers have been effectively employed include buccal cavity, nasal cavity, rectal lumen, vaginal lumen and gastrointestinal tract. Development of novel bioadhesive delivery systems is being undertaken in an attempt to understand the different mechanism of bioadhesion and upgraded permeation of therapeutic agents. Several potential bioadhesive systems are under clinical trials which may possibly introduce soon into the market. Hydrophilic, high molecular weight, anionic molecules like carbomers are the most extensively explored and accepted polymers for bioadhesion. Recently the emphasis has been on the novel second generation polymers like thiolated polymers, lectins and lecithins.

Bioadhesive Drug Delivery System

Researches in the field of bioadhesive materials provide a good empirical framework for the concept of bioadhesive drug delivery systems. But as a young field, there are no well-defined guidelines for the development of this technology. The control of residence time of a dosage form permits to develop new delivery systems that also come with a unique set of design considerations. Newly developed bioadhesive systems were considered as new biomaterials and initial phase of development emphasized on their material properties and biocompatibility studies.

The primary objective for new biomaterials is explained by the Greek terms *'primum non nocere'* meaning 'do no harm', to the human body, either locally or systemically. This constraint of biocompatibility has also been appropriately described as "the quality of not having toxic or injurious effects on biological systems". Beyond this, much of the design considerations for bioadhesive systems are dictated by application and human biology.

To understand the distinct benefits of intelligent bioadhesive delivery systems in drug delivery it is necessary to overview the existing goals, properties and applications of these delivery systems in the field. While not being guidelines per se, there are several desirable qualities for bioadhesive systems. These include:

1. Extended residence time and circulation
2. Targeting
3. Biodegradation

As these objectives are explained below, along with approaches to achieve them, it is noteworthy to consider that they may perhaps be described independently and may not employ to all applications. For example, the implication of 'extended circulation' could be vastly different subjected to whether a treatment regime is chronic vs. acute or systemic vs. targeted. Considerable amount of scientific literature published in last decade is focused on bioadhesive drug delivery. To a certain extent, this signifies the status of current research in drug delivery for effective therapeutics.

Extended Circulation

The foremost challenge in the process of competent therapeutic system development is to provide an extended period to maintain sustained level of active compound or for targeting to a specific site. Incorporation of bioadhesive materials in the formulation of dosage forms is one of the several approaches which are utilized to increase the residence time of dosage form at specific absorption site.

Targeting

All therapeutic agents have adverse/toxic effects in addition to their therapeutic effects. At systemic front whole body is exposed to these adverse/toxic effects due to the fast circulation throughout the body. For some drugs the adverse/toxic effects are so critical that they impede or rule out clinical effectiveness. This can be explicated by doxorubicin a remarkably effective anticancer agent but yield significant risk for congestive heart failure on systemic administration. The primary objective of bioadhesive delivery system is to cater selectivity and specificity to control the toxicity exposure to other parts. Utilization of biodegradable or non-biodegradable bioadhesive polymers assisted the pharmaceutical dosage forms to achieve this target. Active tissue targeting involves those bioadhesive polymers which encompass biological as well as physicochemical specificity. It generally involves the coating or surface conjugation of polymers with ligands for specific cell surface receptors. Novel targeting systems for tumors have been developed by the assistance of bioadhesive polymers with notable achievements. For evident motives, most active *in-vivo* targeting has been focused towards tumor tissue or macrophages of the reticulo endothilial system (RES). Both of these can be targeted passively by customizing bioadhesive nano-carriers. The low pH environment of tumor, exacerbated and aggravated tissue can also be exercised for targeting by the exploitation of pH-triggered bioadhesive polymers.

Biodegradation

A crucial factor for the design of novel bioadhesive systems is ensuring that they can be eliminated after the exhaustion of therapeutic agent. This involves the elimination from the body and as well as the environment. Occupational and environmental health issues presented by non-degradable materials have spawned the field of nano-toxicology. A review of these environmental health issues is out of the scope of this book but important enough that readers should consult these factors for more information.

These health issues related to the use of bioadhesive systems can be neglected by making sure that the systems do not remain in the circulation for longer period than needed. The lack of information regarding the effects of chronic accumulation of bioadhesive systems in the body possesses a significant obstacle to regulatory approval. Be aware of the fact that the bioadhesive systems which are administered intravenously sooner or later penetrate into macrophages, where they will be degraded by lysosomes. If these bioadhesive materials do not degrade naturally or serve as substrates for lysosomal enzymes it is possible that they will cause a kind of lysosomal storage disease (LSD). LSD's are often progressive, and those that involve the RES consequences into a pathologically enlarged liver and spleen. Micro and nanosize debris from long term biomedical implants are also known to cause inflammation and granulomas. Exogenous micro and nanoparticulates have been demonstrated to accumulate in the body and correlate with liver, kidney and colon pathology. Ballou and coworkers recently proved that a single injection of quantum dots remained in the lymph nodes of mice for over two years. This is positively fascinating for post-treatment follow-up imaging, but the long term effects are doubtful. Some recent investigations indicate that the control over size and charge effectively aided the elimination of bioadhesive systems from the body.

From a toxicological and regulatory viewpoint, bioadhesive systems with natural polymers are more attractive due to their degradative capacity in comparison to non-degradable polymers owing to their ill-defined means for elimination. Nel and coworkers revealed that non-degradable, aminated polystyrene nanoparticles show evidence of more oxidative stress on macrophages when compared to titanium oxide or carbon black nanoparticles. The safest bioadhesive systems may be those that can undergo the same kind of controlled breakdown. This may be the reason that the first nanoparticle approved for clinical use, Abraxane®, is primarily formulated by albumin. The span and necessity for biodegradation be subject to the condition in which a bioadhesive system is administered.

4.1 TARGETS FOR BIOADHESIVE FORMULATIONS

Bioadhesive or mucoadhesive formulations have been targeted to various anatomical sites to aid drug delivery and absorption. These anatomical sites are lined with mucous membranes which protect the underlined cells from damage. Drug delivery to these anatomical regions is discussed below:

- Ocular bioadhesive delivery
- Nasal bioadhesive delivery
- Oral bioadhesive delivery
  - Oral cavity
    - Sublingual bioadhesive delivery
    - Buccal bioadhesive delivery
- Transdermal bioadhesive delivery
- Vaginal bioadhesive delivery
- Rectal bioadhesive delivery

4.1.1 Ocular Bioadhesive Delivery

Ocular drug delivery is one of the most interesting and challenging site for the deliverance of therapeutics. The anatomy, physiology and biochemistry of the eye make this organ highly resistant to external materials **(Figure 4.1)**. A substantial problem is to by-pass the protective barriers of the eye devoid of permanent tissue destruction for the effective therapy of pathological conditions. Development of newer, more sensitive techniques and intelligent polymers are accountable for the systems with high therapeutic efficacy for ophthalmic use. Conventional ophthalmic solution, suspension and ointment dosage forms no longer found suitable for optimal therapy.

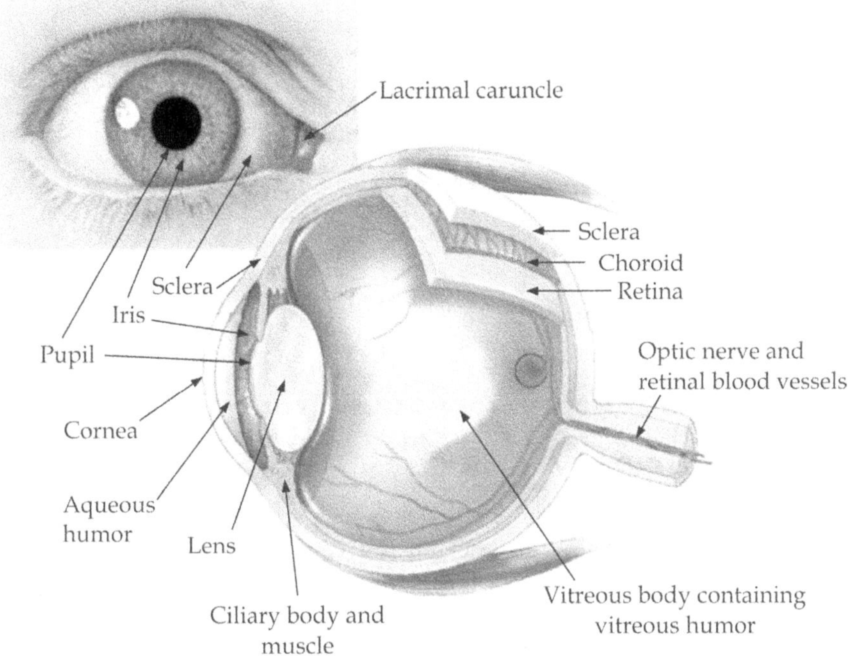

Figure 4.1 Anatomical features of eye globe (right eye)

The objective of pharmacotherapeutics is to treat a disease in a consistent and predictable fashion. According to a hypothesis there is a correlation among the concentration of a drug at its proposed site of action and the resultant pharmacological effect. The exclusive goal of designing a bioadhesive system is to accomplish an optimal concentration of therapeutic agent at the site of absorption/action for appropriate time span. Ocular disposition and elimination of a therapeutic agent is dependent upon its physicochemical properties as well as the relevant ocular anatomy and physiology. Therefore, successful designing of a bioadhesive delivery system requires a collective understanding of the drug molecule and the obstacles proposed by the ocular route.

Ocular absorption

The ocular absorption from the dose administration site (precorneal area) is quite complex. The usual progression of events involves drug instillation, dilution in tear fluid, diffusion through mucin layer, corneal penetration (epithelium, stroma and endothelium) and transfer from cornea to aqueous humor **(Figure 4.2)**. Nasolacrimal drainage or systemic absorption via the conjunctiva operates to carry drug away from the eye and limit the time allowed for the absorption process.

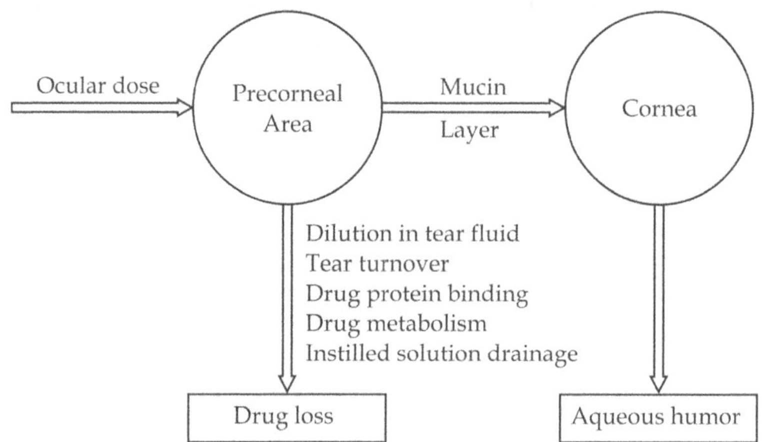

Figure 4.2 Schematic representation of ocular absorption

Obstacles in ocular delivery

Ocular tissues are protected from exogenous noxious elements of surroundings or systemic circulation by a variety of mechanisms, especially, tear excretion persistently cleansing its surface, an impervious surface epithelium and a transportation arrangement consistently clearing the retina to protect it from potential agents able to bother visual process. Conversely, the same protective mechanisms may cause sub-therapeutic drug levels at the intended site. On the other side the structure of the eye globe itself poses difficulties in drug delivery, where several of its internal structures are isolated from the blood and the outside surface of the eye. A major challenge in the development of ocular formulations is to circumvent these structural obstacles and protective mechanisms to exert desired therapeutic outcome.

Physiological barriers to the diffusion and productive absorption of topically applied ophthalmic drugs exist in the precorneal and corneal spaces **(Table 4.1)**. Precorneal barriers include solution drainage, lacrimation and tear dilution, tear turnover and conjunctival absorption. To achieve effective therapeutic levels, dosage form must be stay in contact for sufficient time to allow proper absorption. Local bioavailability of ophthalmic drugs is greatly limited due to the drainage of applied dosage form from precorneal area which causes significant loss of active drug. Generally, instilled dose resides for approximately 5 minutes and then flushed off from the precorneal area naturally in the view of fact that as per normal physiological phenomenon, fluid volume of cul-de-sac reduced to 7-10 μl on its own. A standard ophthalmic dropper delivers 30 μl, most of which is promptly lost owing to nasolacrimal drainage immediately after administration leading to systemic absorption across the nasal mucosa or the gastrointestinal tract. Systemic loss from topically employed drugs after ocular administration also takes place as conjunctival absorption and owing to comparatively large surface area of conjunctiva this loss is considerable.

Table 4.1 Anatomical and physiological factors for ophthalmic delivery

Factor	Denomination
Tear volume (μl)	7-30
Tear turnover rate (μl/min)	0.5-2.2
Spontaneous blinking rate	6-15 times/min
Lacrimal puncta	2
pH of lacrimal fluids	7.3-7.7
Milliosmolarity of tears	305
Corneal thickness (mm)	0.52
Corneal diameter (mm)	12
Corneal surface area (cm^2)	1.04
Ratio of conjunctival and corneal surface	17
Aqueous humor volume (ml)	0.1-0.25
Aqueous humor turnover rate (μl/min)	2-3

Tear turnover accomplishes the drug solution removal from the conjunctival cul-de-sac. Normal tear turnover rate in human is about 16% per minute, which can also be stimulated by various factors. All these factors collectively complicate the topical application of ophthalmic solutions to the cul-de-sac and make them extremely inefficient. Enzymatic metabolism possibly will account for further loss, which can take place in the precorneal space and/or in the cornea.

Some pathological conditions of the eye

Infected or inflamed areas within the anterior as well as the posterior segments of the eye are the operational sites for the therapeutic agents like antibiotics, antivirals and steroids. Iris ciliary body contains receptors for the mydriatics and miotics. A mass of diverse tissues may perhaps present its specific challenge to the formulator of ophthalmic delivery systems. Hence, the therapeutic agents necessitate targeting to various sites within the eye globe. Several common pathological conditions related to eye are discussed below.

Conjunctivitis: It is an infection triggered by bacteria, viruses or allergens and results in inflammation of the conjunctivae, mucous membranes covering the whites of eye and interior of the eyelids. The signs and symptoms expressed by the patient will be subjected to the type of conjunctivitis. Usually characterized by redness of eyes, roughness, itchy eyes and presence of a sticky or watery infectious discharge.

Dry eye: This happens when there is inadequate lacrimal fluid production which is essential for the proper lubrication of eyes. The manifestation of dry eye increases with age and is therefore become more common in geriatrics. Clinically dry eyes are characterized by itchiness, grittiness and painful burning sensation in eyes.

Glaucoma: This disorder is characterized by increased ocular pressure and grounds for excessive production of aqueous humor (the fluid that fills the eye globes). This coagulates stress on optic nerves and compresses the blood vessels in eye globe. The resultant consequences include abnormal vision and total blindness.

Ocular bioadhesive formulations

Several ocular bioadhesive formulations have been marketed to cure different pathological conditions relating to eye **(Table 4.2)**. All these formulations are able to produce an extended or sustained release of drugs into the eye owing to increased residence of formulation due to bioadhesion. Ocular formulations containing bioadhesive polymers attach to mucin on the conjunctival surface by means of non-covalent bonding. The bioadhesive polymers remain in contact with mucosal surface of eye until mucin replaces itself or until the pressure of blinking detaches/remove the formulation from the eye.

Table 4.2 Marketed ophthalmic bioadhesive products

Product	Polymer	Indication
Hypotears®	Poly vinyl alcohol	Dry eye
SnoTears®	Poly vinyl alcohol	Dry eye
GelTears®	Carbomers 980	Dry eye
Viscotears®	Carbomers 980	Dry eye
Pilogel®	Poly acrylic acid	Glaucoma

4.1.2   Nasal Bioadhesive Delivery

In both humans and animals, key functions of the nasal cavity are breathing and olfaction. Additionally, resonance of generated sounds, cleaning of inhaled air, mucociliary clearance, immunological events, heating and humidification of the inspired air prior to access the lungs are also valuable utilities of the nasal cavity. Hairs in the nasal vestibule or mucus layer overlaying the surface of nasal cavities entrap inhaled particles or microorganisms. Furthermore, the nasal mucosa has the capability to facilitate the metabolism of endogenous stuffs into composites that can easily be eliminated from the body.

The nasal cavity has a complicated structure **(Figure 4.3)** and turn out to be inflammed during pathological circumstances such as the common cold, nasal allergies and flu. Therapeutic agents such as antihistaminic and steroids are administered intranasally as drops or sprays to treat pathological conditions distressing the nose. However, nasal mucociliary clearance has an effect on the retention of dosage form and as a result alters the nasal bioavailability. By the process of mucociliary clearance the mucus layer is propelled in a direction from the anterior towards the posterior part of the nasal cavity and protects the respiratory tract from damage caused by inhaled stuffs containing dirt particles and medications. The mucus secretion offers immune protection against inhaled bacteria and viruses. It also performs a number of physiological functions such as (a) It covers the mucosa for physical and enzymatic protection, (b) It has water-holding capacity, (c) It exhibits surface electrical activity, (d) It assures efficient heat transfer, (e) It acts as adhesive and transports particulate matter towards the nasopharynx.

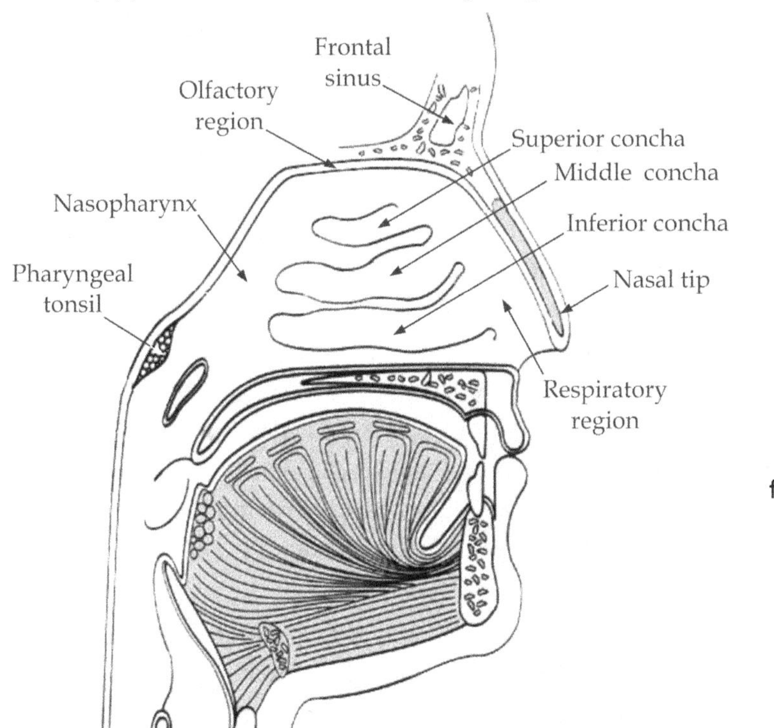

Figure 4.3 Anatomical features of human nose

The nasal cavity is separated into two halves by the nasal septum and spreads posteriorly upto nasopharynx, while the utmost anterior part of the nasal cavity, the nasal vestibule, opens to the face by means of nostrils. The three main regions of nasal cavity are nasal vestibule, olfactory region and respiratory region. The core nasal airway having the narrow passages usually has 1-3 mm wide and these narrow structures are valuable to carry out its main functions.

Nasal absorption

The initial step in the absorption of drug from the nasal cavity is passage through the mucus layer. Small uncharged particles easily pass through this layer. However, large or charged particles may find it more difficult to cross. Mucin, the major protein in the mucus has the potential of binding with solutes therefore hinders the diffusion. Subsequent to passage through the mucus, there are several

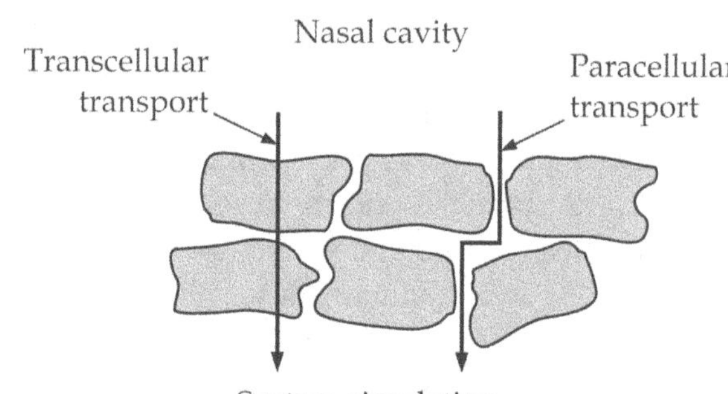

Figure 4.4 Paracellular and transcellular transport through nasal mucosa

mechanisms for drug absorption through the nasal mucosa. These include transcellular or simple diffusion across the membrane, paracellular transport via movement between cell and transcytosis by vesicle carriers. Several mechanisms for drug absorption from the nasal mucosa have been proposed but the following two mechanisms have been considered important **(Figure 4.4)**:

(a) *Paracellular mechanism***:** The nasal route is limited to the drugs with molecular weight lower than 1000 daltons, as the drugs with higher molecular weight shows poor nasal bioavailability. Paracellular process governs drug transport passively with a slower rate. This mechanism utilizes aqueous channels exist between the cells to transport the drugs for intranasal absorption. The molecular weight of nasally administered hydrophilic drugs correlates with intranasal absorption through an inverse log-log correlation.

(b) *Transcellular mechanism***:** In contrast to paracellular mechanism; this mechanism utilizes lipoidal channels i.e. across the cells and preferred for lipophilic compounds. The rate of transport depends on the lipophilicity of administered drugs. By this process drug crosses the cell membranes by active transport via carrier-mediated channels or through the tight junctions e.g. chitosan, a natural bioadhesive and biodegradable polymer alters the opening of tight junctions of epithelial membranes and enhancement in bioavailability was observed.

Possible fate of drug after nasal administration

After nasal administration a drug may enter into the systemic circulation, may permeate to the brain directly or in some cases may follow both pathways. In general there are three routes for the transport of drug from the nasal cavity **(Figure 4.5)**. These routes include:

(a)   Entry into the systemic circulation directly from the nasal mucosa

(b)   Entry into the olfactory bulb via axonal transport along the neurons

(c)   Direct entry into the brain via trigeminal nerves

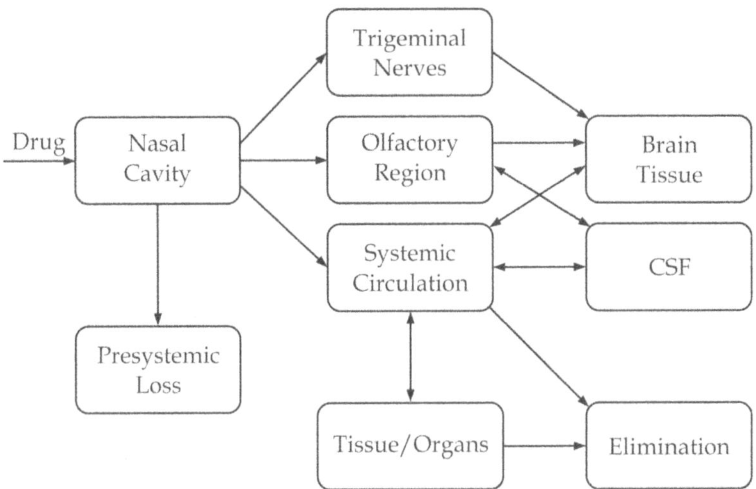

Figure 4.5 Possible routes for drug transport from nasal cavity

Obstacles in nasal delivery

The major obstacles to drug absorption from nasal cavity are presystemic metabolism/loss (mucociliary clearance, enzymatic degradation and mucin interaction) and limited residence time in the cavity. These factors and their impact on nasal absorption are discussed below:

Mucociliary clearance

The collective action of the mucus layer and cilia is called mucociliary clearance. This is a valuable, non-specific physiological defense process of the respiratory tract for protection against noxious inhaled materials. Mucus traps the foreign materials like particles of dust, bacteria and drug substances and transports them towards the nasopharynx at a speed of 5-8 mm/min, where it is swallowed. In this manner particles trapped in the mucus layer are transported with it and thereby effectively cleared from the nasal cavity. The routine mucociliary transit time has reported to be 12-15 min in humans. The nasal mucosal membrane is a physical barrier and mucociliary clearance is a progressive barrier to drug absorption across the nasal epithelium.

According to well-known fact, time of contact is directly proportional to the extent of absorption and mucociliary clearance clears the inhaled substances form the nasal cavity. It is concluded that mucociliary clearance inversely affects the drug absorption from nasal cavity. By the utilization of bioadhesive polymers the process of mucociliary clearance is slowed down to a certain extent which eventually extend the residence time of formulation and hence resulted into enhanced nasal bioavailability.

Protective barriers

The mucus layer lining the nasal mucosa is the first protective barrier faced by any inhaled material. Uncharged substances with small molecular weight can easily pass through this layer in comparison to larger or charged materials. Mucin, the major protein in the mucus has the potential of binding with solutes therefore hinders the diffusion. Additionally, structural changes in the mucus layer are possible as a result of physiological environmental changes such as pH, temperature etc.

Enzymatic barrier

The nasal mucosa encompasses many enzymes such as cytochrome-P450 dependent monooxygenase, carboxyl esterase and amino peptidase. The function of the enzymatic barrier is to protect the lower respiratory airways from toxic agents. Even though nasal route is devoid of hepatic first-pass metabolism to some extent, the nasal mucosa provides a pseudo-first-pass effect. In addition, there is a choice of barriers in nasal membrane for the protection from microorganisms, allergens and irritating substances from the environment that must be overcome by drugs before they can be absorbed from the nasal mucosal surface.

Nasal bioadhesive formulations

Incorporation of bioadhesive polymers in formulations intended for the nasal administration assist them to combat with mucociliary clearance. Zhou and Donovan studied the effect of bioadhesive polymers on mucociliary clearance and concluded the inverse relationship between them as all the bioadhesive polymers in study demonstrated decrease in mucociliary clearance. In their study methyl cellulose exhibited the maximum reduction in mucociliary clearance whereas carbopol 934P showed the lowest reduction in mucociliary clearance in rats. Some examples of the marketed bioadhesive formulation for intranasal delivery of therapeutic agents are enlisted below **(Table 4.3)**.

Table 4.3 Marketed intranasal bioadhesive products

Product	Polymer	Indication
Rhinocort®	Hydroxy propyl cellulose	Nasal allergy
Beconase®	Carboxy methyl cellulose Microcrystalline cellulose	Hay fever
Nasacort®	Microcrystalline cellulose	Nasal allergy

4.1.3 Oral Bioadhesive Delivery

The cheeks, hard and soft palates and tongue collectively represent the oral cavity/mouth **(Figure 4.6)**. It also encompasses highly permeable sublingual mucosa underneath the tongue. This section considers both local and systemic delivery of drugs and discussion about drug delivery systems that are applied to a variety of sites of the oral cavity including the gingiva, buccal, sublingual and periodontal pocket. It is an entrance of the digestive system and performs many substantial operations such as chewing, speaking and taste recognition. Microbial infections and inflammatory diseases such as ulcers impair some of these functions. For the treatment of these local infections and inflammatory diseases the major challenge is posed by the saliva which instantly transports the medications towards the gastric region. Bioadhesion approaches are quite effective for the formulation of medications to be retained in oral cavity.

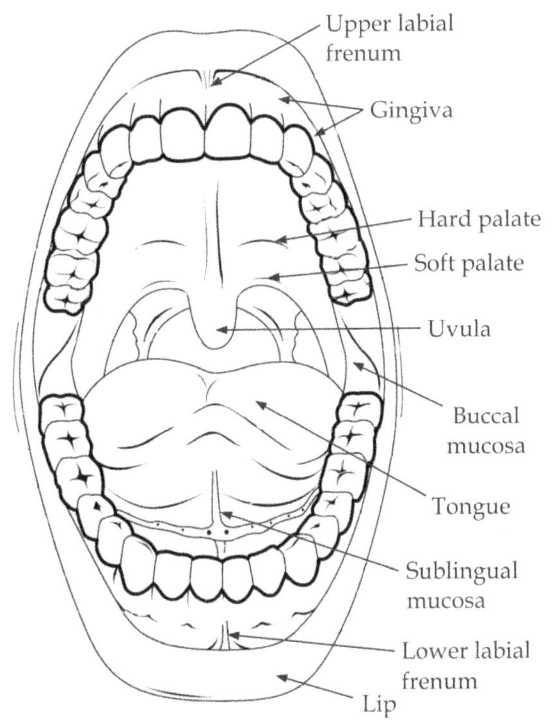

Figure 4.6 The oral cavity

4.1.3.1 Sublingual bioadhesive delivery

The sublingual mucosa sited underneath the tongue, surrounds the salivary gland which contains mucin as a chief constituent in its secretion. Sublingual region is highly permeable and have rapid absorption rate for several drugs owing to its exceptionally rich vasculature. The sublingual route is convenient, accessible and generally well accepted by patients for the delivery of therapeutic agents. Different dosage forms like tablets, powders, solutions and aerosols are utilized for the administration of medications via sublingual route. This route is specifically appropriate for the drugs which are susceptible to enzymatic degradation, first-pass metabolism or degraded in harsh gastric environment. For the effective absorption from sublingual region it is prerequisite to hold the dosage form in the sublingual region as long as the drug is able to go into solution with saliva. This objective is fulfilled by the incorporation of bioadhesive polymers.

4.1.3.2 Buccal bioadhesive delivery

The buccal mucosa corresponds to inner lining of the lips and cheeks. The epithelium layer of buccal mucosa is approximately 40-50 cells thick and the epithelial cells of superficial layers are smoother when compared to the basal layers. The buccal mucosa is less permeable than sublingual mucosa and lacking the ability to retain dosage forms for sufficient time at the site of absorption. The employment of bioadhesive polymers in buccal drug delivery systems facilitates dosage forms for better retention capability by spreading it over the absorption site.

Pathological conditions affecting the oral cavity

***Mouth ulcers*:** A mouth ulcer can be defined as a breach or disruption in the mucous membrane that lines the interior surface of the oral cavity. The majority of peoples experience minor aphthous ulcers (MAU). These ulcers are circular, shallow and greyish white in colour with intense pain. They are small in size and generally appear in small zone.

***Oral thrush*:** This fungal infection of oral cavity is caused by *Candida albicans*. The patients with diabetes, recent antibiotic therapy and inhaled corticosteroids are more prone to this fungal infection. Oral thrush is characterized by soft creamy-white patches. These abrasions are painful and can appear at any part of the oral cavity.

***Gingivitis*:** Inflammation of gums is articulated as gingivitis. It is triggered by plaque (a bacterial layer) buildup over teeth line. Due to the gingivitis the gums become reddish in colour, swollen and bleed easily even on facing slight stress such as brushing of teeth.

Oral bioadhesive formulations

Oral bioadhesive formulations are applied topically to deliver drugs within the oral cavity which act by adhering to oral mucosal surface and exert their therapeutic effects locally to heal the pathological conditions related to oral cavity. To treat the local infections and pathological conditions of oral cavity and also for systemic effect several formulations are marketed which contains bioadhesive polymers to increase their residence time for effective healing **(Table 4.4)**.

Table 4.4 Marketed oral bioadhesive products

Product	Polymer	Indication
Corlan®	Acacia	Mouth ulcers
Bonjela®	Hypromellose 4500	Mouth ulcers
Daktarin®	Pregelatinized potato starch	Oral thrush
Corsodyl®	Hydroxy propyl cellulose	Gingivitis
Buccastem®	Poly vinyl pyrrolidone Xanthan gum	Nausea Vomiting Vertigo
Suscard®	Hydroxy propyl methyl cellulose	Angina

4.1.4 Dermal and Transdermal Bioadhesive Delivery

In spite of several similarities there are some fundamental differences among dermal and transdermal delivery of therapeutic agents. Systemic absorption of active agent is a prerequisite objective for transdermal delivery in contrast to the dermal delivery where systemic absorption is not required and probably unwanted. In case of dermal delivery the barrier properties of skin are generally impaired as the dosage form is applied for the treatment of diseased conditions such as wounds, allergies etc., whereas transdermal deliverance faced the intact skin for the drug delivery. Due to the difference in barrier properties higher drug amounts will reach the underlying tissues after dermal delivery but as the diseased state is treated the permeation of drug becomes more and more difficult and lower concentrations will be reached.

Transdermal absorption

The sequence of the events involved in the absorption of medicaments through skin is summarized in **Figure 4.7.** The exact mechanisms of drug permeation through stratum corneum (SC) are still ambiguous but there are considerable facts supporting intercellular channels as the route of permeation. The intercellular channels have a complicated positioning of lipids that are arranged in well-organized manner as bilayer arrays. To exert its therapeutic effect a drug has to encounters a series of lipophilic and hydrophilic domains confining in these sequential and repeated bilayers. The various routes of drug penetration through the skin are illustrated in **Figure 4.8.**

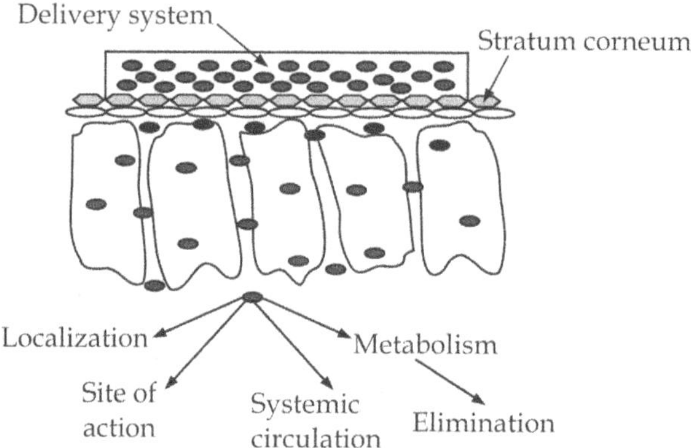

Figure 4.7 Schematic representation of transdermal absorption

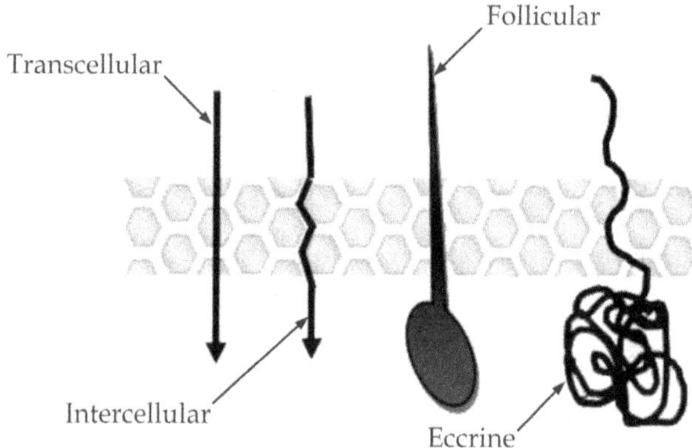

Figure 4.8 Schematic representation of various routes of drug penetration through the skin

Obstacles in transdermal delivery

The prevalent obstacle to deliver the drug by transdermal delivery is its own protective nature owing to the different layers of the skin **(Figure 4.9)**. The outstanding barrier property of the skin is being a feature of outermost layer, the SC. This characteristic membrane is merely 20 μm thick but has evolved as a layer that counteracts against the excessive loss of water and restricts the access of foreign stuffs which come into contact. To overcome this obstacle several approaches like iontophoresis and sonophoresis are introduced for breaching SC with the aid of electric current and ultrasound respectively, are utilized. Microneedles are also developed to puncture the skin to permit delivery of therapeutic agents to sensitively controlled depths. But all these approaches need residence of delivery system at the site of application for the whole duration of therapy. Here the bioadhesive polymers come into the play.

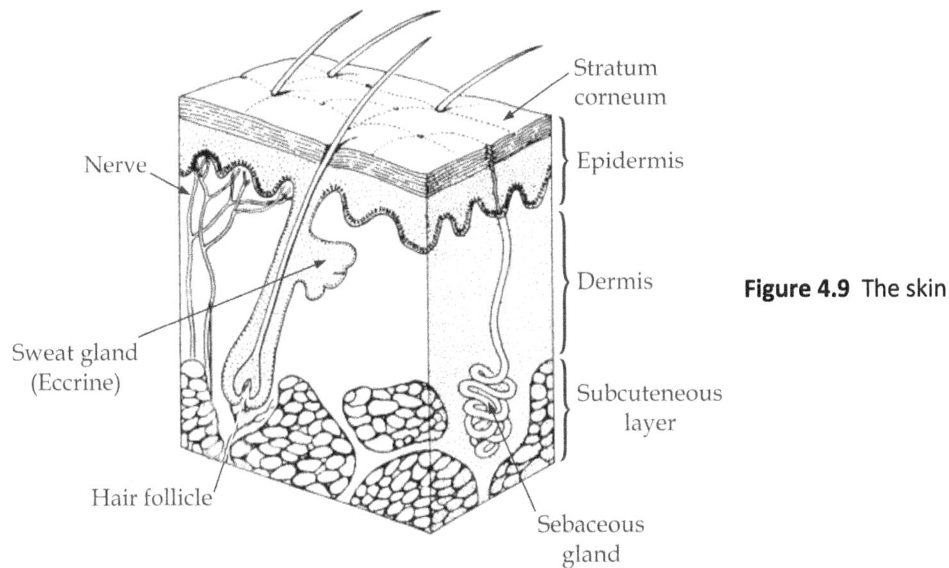

Figure 4.9 The skin

Substantial efforts are spent by the formulation scientists on the appropriate formulation or device development for the deliverance of enough medication such that there is sufficient time of residence at its site of application. The recent advances and development in the field of bioadhesive polymers have solved this problem as these polymers have properties that are incompatible with easy transfer of active agents through the skin.

Transdermal bioadhesive formulations

Transdermal drug delivery is the deliverance of therapeutic agents through intact skin at controlled rates in order to maximize therapeutic efficacy. Bioadhesive transdermal therapeutic systems are designed to enhance the bioavailability, superior comfort, ease of application, reduced dosing frequency and controlled delivery. The bioadhesive property of drug delivery systems for transdermal therapy is beneficial in the view of following purposes:

- Protection from physical contact/exposure especially in case of wounds, rashes and other inflammations

- Local/systemic delivery of therapeutic agents

A wide range of bioadhesive dosage forms is available in the market for transdermal application e.g. powders, patches, lotions, creams, ointments, solutions etc **(Figure 4.10 and Table 4.5)**. Patches for transdermal application are devices with an arrangement to sustain/modify the release of incorporated drug as per therapeutic requirement along with firm attachment over the skin surface. These patches must adhere to the skin firmly without any irritation and should be easily removable after drug release with no or minimal effort.

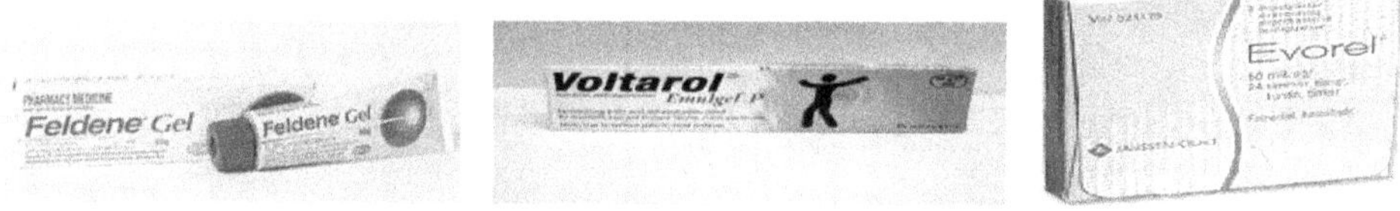

Figure 4.10 Topical bioadhesive formulations

Table 4.5 Marketed transdermal bioadhesive products

Drug	Product	Company	Indication
Granisetron	Sancuso	Prostraken (Europe)	Chemotherapy induced nausea
Ravastigmine	Ravastach	Osaka (Japan)	Dementia
Methyl salicylate and Menthol	Solonaps	Hismitu Pharm (Japan)	Arthritis pain
Nicotine	Nicoderm Habitrol ProStep	GlaxoSmithKline (Philadelphia, PA) Novartis Consumer Health (Parsippany, NJ) Elan (Gainesville, GA)	Smoking cessation
Lidocaine/Epinephrine	Iontocaine	Iomed (Salt Lake City, UT)	Local dermal analgesia
Scopolamine	Transderm-Scop	Novartis Consumer Health (Parsippany, NJ)	Motion sickness

Bioadhesive transdermal therapeutic systems improve bioavailability by providing more prolonged residence time through a patch resembling a small adhesive bandage that is placed on the surface of intact skin. Their design varies according to drug delivery requirements, but generally a backing film, a drug reservoir, a rate-controlling polymer membrane and an adhesive are incorporated.

4.1.5 Vaginal Bioadhesive Delivery

Vagina is the lower portion of the female reproductive tract. It is a muscular tube lined with mucous membrane which is covered with a layer of stratified squamous epithelium with an underlying layer of connective tissue. The vagina is an extremely flexible, somewhat S-shaped fibro-muscular expandable tube positioned between the rectum, which is situated posterior to it, and the urethra and bladder, which is situated anterior to it **(Figure 4.11)**. It stretches out from the lower part of the uterine cervix to the exterior portion of the vulva known as the labia minor. The anterior wall of vagina is more or less

6-7 cm in length, whereas the posterior wall is marginally longer (about 7.5–8.5 cm) owing to the intrusion of the cervix.

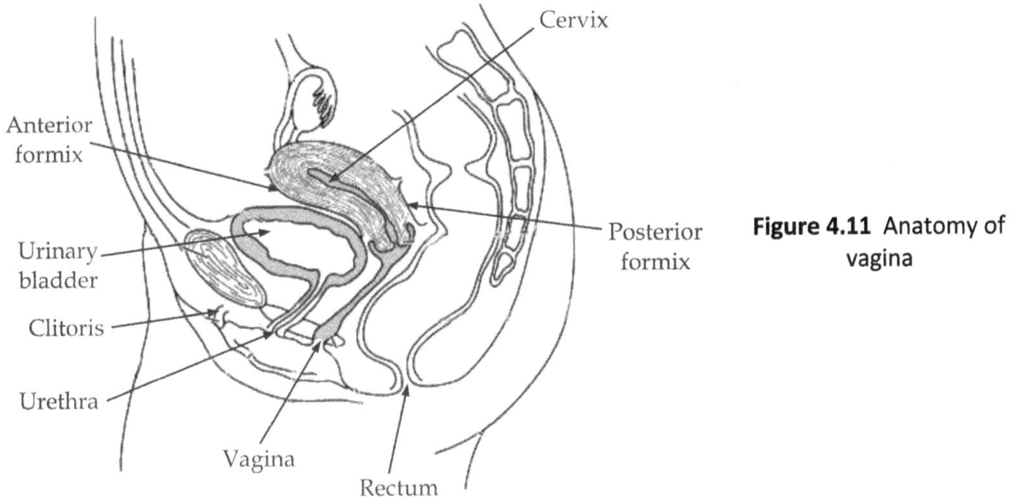

Figure 4.11 Anatomy of vagina

From ancient times, a wide range of therapeutic substances have been administered via vaginal route, predominantly for contraceptive medications/devices or for the treatment of local infections. The *Kahun Papyrus*, an ancient Egyptian treatise on gynaecology, the use of a vaginal suppository containing crocodile dung blended with honey and sodium carbonate, as a contraceptive method. The *Papyrus of Ebers*, another ancient Egyptian document on medicine, recommends the vaginal insertion of acacia tips containing gum arabic which liberates lactic acid in the aqueous environment to maintain the vaginal pH. This approach is somewhat similar in concept to existing intravaginal pessaries of lactic acid to restore or maintain the natural, slightly acidic pH of the vagina. More surprisingly, in the nineteenth century, vaginal route is utilized for the purpose of abortion, suicide and homicide by administering arsenic and other poisons. Thus, the systemic absorption after vaginal administration is well proven. However, this belief was well recognized after the publication of important investigation by David Macht in 1918, on the systemic absorption of alkaloids, inorganic salts, esters and antiseptics after vaginal delivery. A major benefit of intravaginal drug delivery is the avoidance of hepatic first-pass metabolism. For example, intravaginal delivery of hormonal compounds, which are susceptible to extensive first-pass metabolism, is successfully done with significantly lower dose compared to oral delivery to attain therapeutic blood levels.

Intravaginal absorption

The substantial absorption potential of the vaginal mucosa is now considerably accredited. Formerly understood rather inactive and impervious to foreign agents, the intravaginal absorption of various compounds has now been reported with prominent evidences. The number of human clinical trials on the systemic delivery of contraceptives, estrogenic and progestogenic compounds evidenced the current importance of vaginal route for drug delivery purposes. Recently, this route attracted the scientific community for the delivery of therapeutically active peptides and proteins.

Systemic drug absorption across the vaginal epithelium involves drug release from the delivery system, drug dissolution in vaginal fluid and penetration through the mucosal surface. Local intravaginal delivery follows drug release, dissolution and distribution throughout the vaginal mucosa. The vaginal absorption of drugs or other exogenous materials is influenced by the condition of epithelial layer, nature of delivery system and physicochemical properties of penetrant. The intended pharmacological action, thickness of mucosal layer, existence of cervical mucus and exclusive cytoplasmic receptors may also be critical. Drug absorption is also altered by variations in thickness of vaginal wall owing to menstruation cycle/pregnancy and postmenopausal transformations in the vaginal epithelium layer and intravaginal pH.

The diffusion pathways across vaginal epithelial layer are fundamentally analogous to other epithelial layers and are well exemplified by the "fluid mosaic hypothesis" as a lipid strip intermingled with aqueous apertures. The sequence of events in vaginal drug delivery depends partially on the nature of delivery system i.e. whether it is solid or semisolid, swellable or erodible, soluble or insoluble, immediate or controlled release.

The intravaginal bioavailability can be improved by the incorporation of penetration enhancers. These normally act on tight junctions of epithelial layer to support intercellular penetration that may be particularly significant for vaginal absorption of high molecular weight therapeutic peptides and proteins. In general, the permeability of vaginal epithelium is superior to rectal, buccal or transdermal routes but subordinate to the nasal and pulmonary routes.

Obstacles in vaginal delivery

Anatomical and physiological factors directly influence the design of intravaginal drug delivery systems. The major obstacle in the development of intravaginal systems is the physiological changes associated to its functions (conception and birth), menstruation cycle and postmenopausal changes. Eventually its physiology changes throughout the female life cycle. For drug delivery purpose it is a potential route with exceptionally fluctuating environment. Thus, the design of intravaginal drug delivery systems must take account of vaginal anatomy and physiological changes.

Vaginal walls are composed of four typical layers **(Figure 4.12)**. The stratified mucosal layer, submucosal layer, muscularis layer and tunica adventitia layer. The substantial barrier for drug absorption stratified mucosal layer, which is composed of an epithelium and an underlying lamina propria, with varying thickness of epithelial cells (200–300 µm) owing to fluctuations in estrogen levels in the course of menstrual cycle. For that reason, the degree of estrogenization of vaginal epithelium has crucial consequences for drug permeation across it.

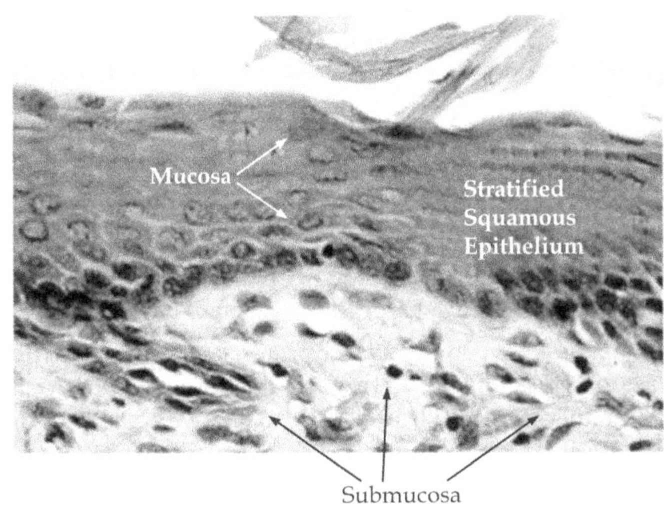

Figure 4.12 Histology of the vaginal mucosa

Epithelium layers of vagina consist of living cells that renew continuously as they are stimulated by hormonal action and intracellular communication. The characteristic constant loss and renewal of epithelial cells also poses obstacle for drug delivery. Vaginal fluid, chiefly composed of transudate that passes through the vaginal wall from blood vessels, constantly flushes the surface of epithelial layer. Vulval secretions from sebaceous and sweat glands with minor contributions from Bartholin's and Skene's glands also mixed with vaginal fluid. Vaginal fluid may additionally contain some enzymes, enzyme inhibitors, amino acids, proteins, alcohols, carbohydrates, hydroxy ketones and aromatic compounds. The overall volume of vaginal fluid further increases at the time of ovulation due to excessive cervical secretions. Accordingly, there is an increase in pH, fibrosity and mucin content with a decrease in the viscosity, cellularity and albumin concentration which potentially affects the drug absorption.

Enzymes present in vaginal fluid also influence the absorption of drugs. For example, enzymatic degradation of polypeptides results into lower vaginal absorption of these drugs. The basal layer of the vaginal epithelium has a high activity of enzymes found in the citric acid cycle, in fatty acid metabolism and in 17-ketosteroidogenesis, e.g. succinic dehydrogenase, diaphorase, acid phosphatase, β-glucuronidase and phosphoamidase. The outer cell layers of the vagina contain β-glucuronidase, acid phosphatase and smaller quantities of α-naphthylesterase, diaphorase, phosphoamidase and succinic dehydrogenase. Basal cell layers contain β-glucuronidase, succinic dehydrogenase, diaphorase, small amounts of acid phosphatase and α-naphthylesterase. Levels of alkaline phosphatase, lactate dehydrogenase, amino-peptidase and esterase activity are all high in the follicular phase of the menstrual cycle, but fall immediately prior to ovulation. Infective diseases obviously affect the levels and varieties of enzymes found in vaginal fluid.

Common pathological conditions affecting the vagina

The glycogen present in vaginal epithelium causes break down of enzymes and bacteria into acids such as lactic acid which maintains the vaginal pH between 4 and 5. This pH range is desirable as it makes the vagina unfriendly to pathogenic agents. Reduction in the levels of vaginal glycogen content results into increased vaginal pH and make it more vulnerable for infections. Some common vaginal infections are discussed below:

- *Vaginitis*: It has many causes which includes infection with *Trichomonas vaginalis*, dietary deficiency or poor hygiene. Vaginitis is clinically characterized by the inflammation of vagina with watery discharge, odour, irritation or itching.

- *Bacterial vaginosis*: This infection is predominantly caused by *Gardnerella vaginalis*, although other bacteria present in the vagina also contribute to the cause. The infection develops due to the overgrowth of these bacteria. About 50% of patients will have a thin white discharge with a strong fishy odour.

- *Candidiasis (Thrush)*: It is a common yeast infection caused by *Candida albicans*. This infection is clinically characterized by a white cheesy discharge with itching and irritation in the vagina.

- *Trichomoniasis*: It is a sexually transmitted infection caused by *Trichomonas vaginalis*. The clinical symptoms include vaginal itching with a frothy greenish-yellow discharge and foul-smelling.

Vaginal bioadhesive formulations

Bioadhesive polymers can extend the residence time of drug and control the rate of drug release from intravaginal delivery systems. The epithelium which constructs vaginal surface does not forms a true mucosal epithelium as it is devoid of secretory goblet cells. But due to the covering of cervical mucus from vaginal fluid it is considered as a mucosal surface. The mucoadhesive formulations applied to this body cavity may generally contain moisturizing agent with one or more active drugs. The role of incorporated moisturizing agents is to control vaginal dryness.

Hydrogels of weakly cross linked polymers which swell when exposed to aqueous environment are combined with mucoadhesive ability to develop bioadhesive systems for vaginal administration. Hydrogels also provides an advantage in terms of ease of spreading and increases the patient compliance. The properties which make it suitable for intravaginal delivery include ability to form intimate contact with vaginal mucosa and localization of therapeutic agent to a specific site leading to extended residence time for better absorption.

Poly-acrylic acids and poly-cationic materials like chitosan are preferably utilized to prepare hydrogels for vaginal application. A scintigraphic study for vaginal administration of dosage forms in postmenopausal women reveals the major issues associated with intravaginal application of hydrogels such as spreading and retention followed by formation of sticky mass which alters the natural viscosity of vaginal mucus.

Six healthy postmenopausal female volunteers were selected for the study which involves evaluation of radiolabled pessaries and a commercial polycarbophil based gel for spreading and clearance for a period of 6 hours by gamma scintigraphy. There is a very slight intra-subject variation in clearance of both formulations in five volunteers out of the six. Both of the formulations dispersed the content up to the cervix in all subjects. However, the comparison of clearance revealed considerable inter-subject variability. In majority of volunteers the applied dosage forms does not resides for significant duration which limits the bioavailability of delivered therapeutic agents. The development of bioadhesive systems for vaginal administration may increase the residence time and may prove beneficial for:

- Delivery of contraceptives in addition to anti-infectives e.g. anti-fungal agents to cope with local infections. A variety of dosage forms i.e. tablets, creams and gels are found to be suitable for vaginal administration.
- For effective treatment protocols, targeting of specific mucosal sites which limits the spreading of dosage form to other areas.
- Enhancement of retention time due to the mucoadhesive interactions between mucosal surface and bioadhesive polymer.

Table 4.6 enlists some of the marketed bioadhesive formulations for different therapeutic objectives.

Table 4.6 Marketed vaginal bioadhesive products

Product	Polymer	Indication
Aci-Jel®	Acacia, Tragacanth	Maintains vaginal pH
Crinone®	Carbomer	Progesterone deficiency
Estring®	Silicone Polymers	Oestrogen deficiency
Gynol-II®	Carboxy methyl cellulose	Spermicidal Contraceptive
Zidoval®	Carbomer	Bacterial vaginosis

4.1.6 Rectal Bioadhesive Delivery

The most distal part or terminus of gastrointestinal tract is known as rectum **(Figure 4.13)**. It may prove an effective route of administration for the drugs with severe side effects in gastrointestinal region. In the case of patients who have difficulty in swallowing i.e. pediatric patients, unconscious patients or patients with mouth injuries, this route may be used as an effective alternate for the administration of therapeutic agents. Additionally, in contrast to oral route this route bypasses the hepatic metabolism of administered drug. These advantages of rectal administration have been considered for the development of bioadhesive suppositories for the treatment of several local diseases e.g. rectal cancer and haemorrhoids.

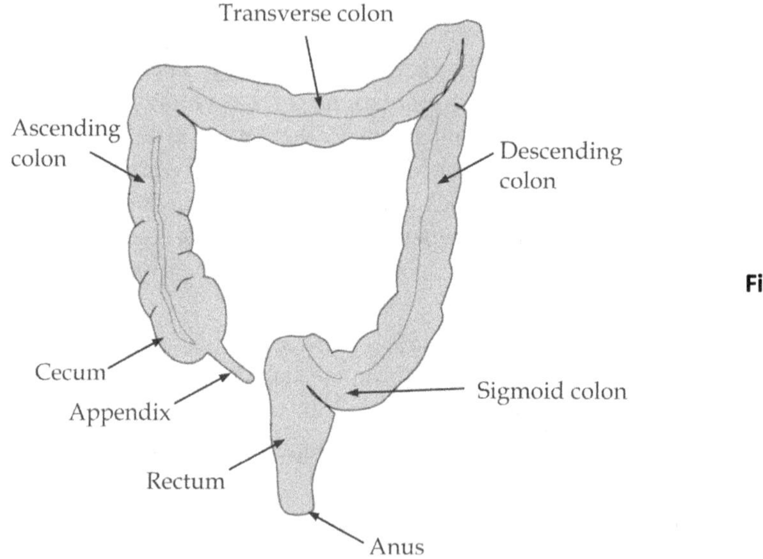

Figure 4.13 The Rectum

Baume, a French pharmacist utilized cocoa butter as a vehicle for suppositories in way back to 18th century and seeds the development tree for dosage forms to be utilized for rectal administration. Later on during and after the Second World War, a great variety of vehicles of fatty nature were developed to be utilized for rectal dosage forms. Several non-fatty vehicles are also available and become worthy to prepare different dosage forms such as soft-shell capsules, ointments and microenemas for rectal drug delivery.

This route can be exploited for local as well as systemic delivery of different therapeutic agents. For local action ointments and suppositories are commonly adopted to deliver drugs for relief in pain and itching caused by haemorrhoids. Such formulations generally contain local anaesthetics, antipruritics, antiseptics, vasoconstrictors and astringents. Melting or softening of suppositories in ampulla-recti supports the spreading of dosage form through rectum and hence partly passed the target i.e. anus.

Retention enemas can be beneficial for the delivery of corticosteroids alone or in combination of antibiotics to exert their effect locally, as for the treatment of colitis. Retention enemas or soap-gelled glycerine suppositories are also evaluated successfully for laxative purpose. For constipation patients, suppositories which release carbon dioxide to accelerate defecation process after rectal administration are developed. Recently two new formulations are added to this category i.e. soft-shell gelatin capsules and microenemas. For the ease of application microenemas are marketed in plastic container with detachable applicator tubes e.g. Reticole. After attachment of applicator tube simple compression is applied on container to administer the dosage form into rectal cavity. This system of container with applicator tube allows the administration of both aqueous and oily solutions for local or systemic effect. Paraffin or oil filled capsules are used to deliver systemic drugs by this route. The most common dosage form for therapeutic delivery via rectal route is suppositories made up of fatty materials. Semi-synthetic vehicles comprising suspensions of hydrophilic substances in cocoa butter are also common. These vehicles are generally prepared by esterification of glycerine with saturated fatty acids isolated from hydrolyzed vegetable fats or hydrogenation of vegetable oils such as coconut oil.

All these vehicles differ from each other in terms of hydroxyl number. To prevent batch-to batch variations switching of vehicles from one to other is avoided essentially however, the actual significance of this is still in doubt. The aqueous glycerinated gelatin vehicles are an exception which only utilized in formulations for topical treatments. Occasionally, macrogels are utilized for lipophilic drugs like chloral hydrate.

Rectal absorption

The mechanism of drug absorption form rectal region is quite similar to that from other gastrointestinal region. But the differences in anatomy and physiology of both regions accounts for variability in absorption kinetics irrespective of specific membrane properties. The transport of drug across the rectal surface is mainly governed by passive diffusion process. The absorption from this site is greatly influenced by partition coefficient and solubility properties of the incorporated drugs. Rectal region has a rich blood circulation for systemic absorption as the lower rectum veins directly drains into general circulation and the veins from middle and upper parts drains via vena porta. A clear boundary is lacking between these regions due to the presence of several anastomoses. The extent of absorption from these regions is mainly governed by pH partition theory. Ionized or unionized form of drugs also affects the absorption; drugs that are in unionized form at physiological pH of 7.5-8.0 of this region are preferred for rectal administration. However, several reports claim the limited absorption of completely ionized drugs after rectal administration e.g. quaternary ammonium compounds are absorbed upto a extent of < 10% when administered rectally.

The mechanism of drug release depends on the properties of drug and vehicle used. Hydrophilic vehicles are preferred for rectal dosage forms but drugs with poor aqueous solubility such as indomethacin are also incorporated with the aid of polyethylene glycol. These systems release the incorporated drug as they come in the contact of rectal fluid. The rate limiting factors for absorption include diffusion rate in aqueous rectal content or membrane transport and partitioning behaviour of drug between biological membranes and rectal contents. A more rapid *in-vitro* release of indomethacin was reported from hydrophilic vehicles when compared to that from fatty vehicles. Similar to *in-vitro* release the *in-vivo* absorption of indomethacin from hydrophilic vehicles was also rapid but in somewhat lesser extent. Particle size may also act as a rate-limiting step where drug is incorporated as a suspension in aqueous vehicles.

Several therapeutic agents show good binding efficiency towards polyethylene glycols. This property of polyethylene glycols is utilized for the preparation of microenemas. As mentioned earlier, fatty vehicles are preferred over hydrophilic vehicle but such dosage forms are rarely used, particularly for the delivery of suspensions of highly water soluble drugs. From these systems drug releases principally by two mechanisms:

- Suspended drug particles are exposed to aqueous rectal fluid for the initiation of dissolution.
- Vehicle itself dissolves the suspended drug particles and releases them through diffusion process.

A model has been developed for suspension ointments, and in some instances, this model has been applied to suspension suppositories. Since suppositories melt fairly rapidly after insertion, a rather thin layer of a medium-viscosity suspension is formed. Assuming that the particles spread homogeneously with the vehicle, not all conditions under which the model operates are met. The particles will not remain distributed homogenously throughout the vehicle, but will reach an equilibrium position in the vehicle/rectal fluid interface. This is because the viscosity of the melted suppository permits particles to settle. This is reflected in the observed rate of release from suppositories, which is far more rapid than predicted. Therefore, a release mechanism composed of three steps may be inferred. These steps are: approach of the suspended drug particles toward the interface between the melted vehicle and the aqueous rectal fluid, transport through that interface, and dissolution in the aqueous rectal fluid.

This transport process (the first step) may take place through two different driving forces. First, sedimentation is possible as soon as the viscosity is lowered during the melting process. This will be more important as the spreading area is smaller, and therefore the layer thickness of the melted mass remains larger. Second, the pressure waves occurring in the rectum may induce particle motion in the melted mass and thus collision with the interface, in which the particles will reach equilibrium. Both processes would predict an influence of viscosity of the melted mass and also of the particle size of the drug. This latter observation is in contrast with the Higuchi ointment treatment, where no such influence is predicted. Also, particle concentration could be a factor, as it influences the viscosity of a melted mass. Particles will cross the interface (the second step), depending on their surface properties, in relation to the same properties of both liquid phases.

The dissolution process (the third step) is clearly an intrinsic property of the drug substance and can be derived by using the appropriate equations. There is one factor, however, that has to be considered (i.e. the surface exposed to the dissolving rectal fluid). The situation at the interface is not comparable to the one in which a particle dissolves in a stirred medium. The flow of liquid is negligible, and the particle continuously adjusts its position to maintain its equilibrium position as dictated by the surface forces. It is also relevant to know if one of the steps is rate-limiting and if so, which one is rate-limiting step. Experiments have been performed in a model system consisting of different substances suspended in paraffin, as the fatty vehicle substitute, and water. For a highly soluble substance, the second and third steps are rapid and the release rate is limited by the first step, at least in the thickness layer used (1 cm).

Rectal bioadhesive formulations

Bioadhesive polymers are incorporated into rectal suppositories to prolong the retention of the active drug in the rectum. Prolonged retention in the rectum increases the chances of reaching a therapeutic outcome.

- *Anacal*® is an ointment for rectal administration to manage the symptoms allied with haemorroids. In this marketed rectal formulation polyethylene high polymer 1500 is incorporated as bioadhesive constituent.
- *Germoloids*®, another bioadhesive ointment available for rectal administration contains propylene glycol as polymer. It is indicated for the relief of haemorroids associated pain, itching, swelling and irritation.
- *Preparation H*® Suppositories help shrink the haemorrhoidal tissue which is swollen by irritation. It contains the polymer polyethylene glycol.

4.2 TYPES OF BIOADHESIVE FORMULATIONS

The choice of bioadhesive formulation for different regions depends on the physiological functions and action to be achieved i.e. local or systemic effect. **Table 4.7** gives a general idea of formulations employed for different body sites.

Table 4.7 Formulation systems for various body sites

Body site	Systems
Eye	Mucoadhesive eye drops / inserts
Nasal cavity	Nasal drug delivery systems
Oral cavity	Dental gels / buccal systems
Skin	Patches, tapes, dressings
Vagina	Local vaginal delivery systems
Rectum	Local/systemic rectal delivery systems

4.2.1 Solid Bioadhesive Formulations

4.2.1.1 Mucoadhesive tablets

For systemic delivery, oral route is always a preferable route for the administration of therapeutic agents. For the development of dosage forms for new drug entities, oral route is generally considered as first possibility due its superiority on other routes in terms of cost effectiveness, patient compliance and convenient administration. This route also offers the applicability of a wide range of pharmaceutical dosage forms including tablets, capsules, gels, microspheres etc., for the treatment of target pathological conditions.

As a dosage form, mucoadhesive tablets are preferentially utilized for oral delivery successfully but recently some works in the field of vaginal delivery demonstrate its limited effectiveness for this route of administration. This dosage form can be tailored as per target mucosal surface to achieve optimum adherence according to specific requirement of the disease under consideration. Mucoadhesive tablets are capable to provide sustained release, controlled release or delayed release patterns of drug release at different specific sites of human body. The suitability for incorporation of a wide range of therapeutic agents including proteins, peptides and genes makes it more worthy. Many investigational studies reveal their prospect for local action in stomach as gastroretentive system. Several bioadhesive polymers e.g., polyacrylates, polyphosphazenes, HPMC, carbopol and its derivatives etc., are currently employed to prepare mucoadhesive tablets for different mucosal sites. Further advancement in bioadhesive polymer science expand the scope of mucoadhesive tablets.

Current growth of mucoadhesive polymers is substantially significant but some milestones are still unturned i.e., lack of universally acceptable methods for standardization and evaluation of bioadhesive polymers and developed systems for therapeutic delivery. Development of site directed bioadhesive polymers is also a challenge for polymer scientists. In order to develop newer bioadhesive polymers, attempts are focused on several properties i.e., biocompatibility, biodegradability, targeting of specific mucosal cells and capability to act as enzyme inhibitor for successful delivery of peptides and proteins. However, numeral efforts are centered on evaluation of bioadhesive dosage forms and put forward some novel techniques to evaluate the strength of mucoadhesive bonding between mucoadhesive tablets and some specific cellular surfaces. To exhaust the full potential of this cutting edge technology for the development of drug delivery systems to target different biological sites and to overcome the hurdles related to evaluation parameters, a multidisciplinary approach is required.

Dry formulations such as tablets are able to form strong interactions with mucosal surfaces by attracting water from the mucosal surface. The controlled release mucoadhesive tablet are designed to increase the residence time of the drug in the stomach and release for extended period of time in order to; increase bioavailability of the drug, reduce the dosing frequency and improve patient compliance. An example is Buccastem® which is used in the treatment of nausea, vomiting and vertigo. It is administered to the buccal mucosa (inside of the cheeks).

For the formulation of oral mucoadhesive tablet various polymer used like Hydroxy propyl ethyl cellulose K15M, Hydroxy propyl methylcellulose K4M, Carbopol 974P, used as hydrophilic matrix forming mucoadhesive polymer in varying concentration along with Magnesium stearate, talc and lactose as filler. Tablets were subjected to various evaluation parameters such as drug content, hardness, weight variation, friability, mucoadhesive strength, swelling index and *in-vitro* drug release study.

4.2.1.2 Inserts

Bioadhesive inserts are popular as novel biomedical devices to control the drug release. They enhance the drug effectiveness by constant maintenance of drug concentration within the therapeutic window i.e. between the minimum effective concentration and maximum safe concentration. These systems also inhibits the drug dilution in body fluids of other parts, as its inherent bioadhesive property supports localization and targeting of drugs to specific biological sites. This approach ultimately increases the patient compliance as medication can be continued for longer durations with lesser dosing frequency.

Several bioadhesive ocular inserts are marketed as ophthalmic gels and drops e.g. Pilogel® is indicated for glaucoma patients to relieve the raised ocular pressure. It contains carbomer 940 as bioadhesive polymer to combat with instant flush from eye and to increase the residence time for efficient drug absorption.

4.2.1.3 Lozenges

The ease of administration makes lozenges a good carrier for medicinal agents especially for local pathological conditions e.g. inflammation related to mouth ulcers. The highly vascular buccal mucosa can also be a potential target for lozenges. Generally, lozenges may contain local anesthetics and antibiotics to treat topical inflammatory conditions of oral cavity. However, their potential for controlled drug delivery is also revealed by various investigational researches.

4.2.2 Semi-Solid Bioadhesive Formulations

4.2.2.1 Gels

The inherent gel forming property of several bioadhesive polymers is successfully employed to prepare bioadhesive gels for medicinal use. Some bioadhesive polymer i.e. polyacrylic acid have the ability to adhere mucosal surfaces in biological environment. These bioadhesive gels make a very close contact with mucosal surfaces by cross linking and releases the incorporated medicament rapidly. These bioadhesive gels may employ to target different mucosal surfaces including oral, ocular, vaginal, rectal and nasal mucosa.

4.2.3 Liquid Bioadhesive Formulations

4.2.3.1 Viscous liquids

Higher viscosity of liquids markedly influences their residence time on the biological surfaces. Addition of bioadhesive polymers increases the viscosity which supports their higher residence time in combination with bioadhesive interactions. These viscous liquids containing bioadhesive polymers can be used as a protective for mucosal membranes to prevent from irritation and damages. Carboxymethyl cellulose may be used to prepare such viscous liquids and can also be utilized for the delivery of therapeutic agents to specific biological sites. For example, carbomer solution is used as artificial tears for the treatment of dry eyes.

4.2.3.2 Gel-forming liquids

A particular term '*in-situ* gels' is frequently used for such formulations. These formulations or *in-situ* gels are administered as liquids but transforms into gels in response to biological conditions such as pH or temperature change. Such formulations are utilized for controlled release of medications through nasal, vaginal, ocular or oral administration.

4.2.4 Novel Bioadhesive Drug Delivery Systems

4.2.4.1 Bioadhesive films/patches

Bioadhesive films/patches are commonly used for wound dressing. These flexible bioadhesive films can also be used for direct drug delivery in local pathological conditions related to mucosal surfaces or other systemic diseases. Due to their flexibility a close contact between the film and mucosal/biological surface is established which leads to accurate dose delivery for absorption from target biological site. For example, a bioadhesive film Zilactin® for the treatment of mouth ulcers and cold sores is available in market.

Solvent casting technique is most commonly used for the preparation of bioadhesive buccal films. The materials which generally preferred for these bioadhesive films include aluminium, teflon, glass and mercury. Incorporation of mercury for these delivery systems results into superior outcomes. In case of buccal and dental diseases these bioadhesive formulations are emerged as a novel therapeutic tool with several advantages over conventional dosage forms.

4.2.4.2 Bioadhesive micro/nanopatches

In today's era no field is untouched by the applications of nanotechnology. Drug delivery systems are also developed on nano-scale size range with the aid of wide range of available polymers. Nano-scale structures made up of solid synthetic polymeric materials; provide a coherent separate phase in a bulk carrier form. Their hydrophobic and amorphous nature with typical glassy appearance or rigid cross linked structures with stand alone integrity which is lacked by dendrimers or self-assembled systems; makes them favorable systems for the delivery of therapeutic agents. With the advancements in nanotechnological methods; it is possible to prepare these amorphous polymeric nanoparticles having a much broader size range. Techniques for the preparation of nano-structures such as emulsification and micro-fabrication are capable to fabricate nano-structures in the size range of 1 nm to hundreds of micron with different shapes like bars, cones, spheres, arrows etc.

Mucoadhesive Nanoparticles

The controllable degradation kinetics of biodegradable bioadhesive polymers put them in center of attraction of researchers; to be utilized for drug delivery applications. The well-known polyesters of polyhydroxy alkanonates class e.g., poly glycolic acid (PGA), poly lactic acid (PLA) and their co-polymer PLGA has a long history of biomedical applications. The first use of PLA as a bone prosthesis material was reported by Kulkarni and co-workers in 1966 and PGA based sutures DEXONR for clinical applications were first marketed in 1970's.

Phase separation, water-oil-water (w/o/w) emulsification and spray drying are the common techniques employed for the fabrication of PLGA nanoparticles. Incorporation of drugs with both low and high molecular weight is possible with these techniques. These techniques are also associated with common drawback; requirement of organic solvents for polymer solubilization which may lead to significant loss in the biological activity of incorporated biopharmaceuticals.

The release of active drug from these nanoparticles can be easily controlled as per requirement of therapy by varying the crystallinity and ratio of lactide/glycolide content of polymer. To assist the aqueous dispersal; polymer surface can be coated or modified by grafting steric stabilizers. Biospecific ligands are also utilized for surface modification. Currently, seven different PLGA based multiparticulate systems for the delivery of low molecular weight drugs are available for clinical use. A novel formulation for single administration was also tested for the destruction of prostate tumors in a mouse model. The current approval of PLGA by regulatory authorities for several biomedical products attracts the scientific community to utilize it for the development of nanotechnology based biomedical devices.

Some novel biodegradable polymers are in investigational phase which are composed of poly (β-amino esters), poly caprolactone, polyanhydrides, poly (glycerol sebacate) and various other co-polymers. The hydrolysis of back bone chain of polyanhydrides and polyesters causes their degradation in biological environment. Another degradation mechanism for biodegradable polymers involve cleavable side chains, this mechanism is successfully utilized to develop poly (alkyl cyano acrylated) (PACA) based nano-carriers. Rapid polymerization of PACA based polymers is observed in the presence of a weak base. The polymerization of PACA results into a hydrophobic solid which on side chains hydrolysis yields water soluble poly (cyano-acrylic acid) and corresponding alkyl alcohol. This phenomenon is accelerated in biological conditions with presence of pancreatic secretions, esterases in serum and lysosomes. Their biocompatibility is significantly affected by the length of alkyl chain. However, PACA based bioadhesive polymers were withdrawn from the market due to toxicity of low molecular weight alcoholic degradation products i.e. methanol, lead etc.

Mucoadhesive microparticles/microspheres

Due to their binding efficiency with mucosal surfaces; mucoadhesive microparticles are proven quite effective for drug delivery to stomach and other sites of gastrointestinal tract. These microparticles with bioadhesive property adhere to the mucosal surface and release the incorporated therapeutic agent at a slower rate or might be used as a direct targeting tool for different parts of gastrointestinal mucosa.

Mucoadhesive microcapsules

Mucoadhesive microcapsules are similar to mucoadhesive microparticles except that microcapsules are hollow spherical particles whereas microparticles are rigid particles. These hollow particles can be used for therapeutic delivery via oral, vaginal or rectal administration for the treatment of various local pathological conditions as well as for systemic delivery. As a multiparticulate system they reduced the incidence of dose dumping. They also offer a number of benefits such as controlled or sustained release, incorporation of a wide range of therapeutic agents and better patient compliance.

4.2.4.3 Mucoadhesive nanogels and microgels

*Hy*drogels, as the terms itself suggests they are cross-linked polymeric network which absorb water in large amounts and transforms into swollen gels. Due to their inherent mechanical properties, hydration capability and unique structural network several hydrogels resembles the natural tissues. Hydrogels are established as potential biomaterials for drug delivery, biosensing devices, tissue engineering and several other biomedical purposes. They are highly biocompatible with human biological environment and may control the drug release as per the requirements.

When fabricated in nano size range, hydrogels or nanogels offer some additional benefits over other nano-sized drug delivery systems. The interconnected hydrophilic polymer chains provides extra space for absorbed water molecules similar to dendrimers but with a more freedom to select the size range. Due to the cross linked polymeric network they are more stable in comparison to other nano-carriers. They can be easily modified by incorporation of pendant groups, ligands or other functionality into the polymer backbone, cross linked network or on the polymeric surface. To achieve controlled or targeted delivery drug can be conjugated or entrapped within the polymeric network. With the aid of different fabrication techniques e.g., emulsion polymerization, micro/nanofabrication, self-assembly and precipitation/dispersion polymerization; size and shape of nanogel and microgels can be easily managed in a controlled manner. Generally, hydrophilic monomers are used for gel formation which permits the proceeding of reaction without phase separation and hence restricts the employment of organic solvents. The avoidance of organic solvents results in less intense environment for biological molecules.

In-situ gel formation around the whole cells is also possible by initiating polymerization at site of application. For that cross linking can be achieved during or after polymerization process and provoked *in-situ* by physical, biological or chemical stimulants. Advancement in polymer therapeutic allows the utilization of drug conjugates with synthetic polymer chains for clinical purpose. Therapeutic superiority of these conjugates over unconjugated drug makes them favorable for biomedical use. However, their use for intravenous delivery is limited as they are cleared by RES due to their small size ranging from 6-15 nm.

With available techniques, the size of drug conjugates can be tailored according to therapeutic needs and can be formulated as nanogels for prolonged circulation. These highly cross linked polymeric networks are able to incorporate more amounts of drugs in comparison to systems without cross linking. They can act as high affinity receptors similar to antibodies or cell surface receptors by tailoring its three dimensional structure during polymerization process. The development of several molecularly imprinted nanogels and microgels for drug delivery has been reported. Incorporation of hydrophobic drug is also possible with the introduction of amphiphilic macromers which creates hydrophobic regions within the polymeric network. An amphillic nanogel based on pluronic macromers is developed by Hubbell and co-workers for the delivery of hydrophobic drugs with low molecular weight. Nanogels containing macromolecules composed of interpenetrating PEI chains were also developed and successfully employed for brain targeting, nucleoside delivery and as transfection agents.

pH-Responsive nanogels and microgels

Some physical, biological or chemical factors also affect the polymeric network of hydrogels which significantly responds in terms of shape and volume enhancement. These factors may include light, heat, pH, electrolyte concentration or other specific bio-signals e.g. glucose concentration. These factors can be utilized as a stimulus for the development of hydrogel based delivery systems which are also known as 'intelligent' or 'stimuli responsive' hydrogels. The variation in pH of different biological sites can be easily utilized for the development of such pH-responsive intelligent systems. An ionizable pendant group is incorporated within the polymeric network which sensitively responds to pH variation. Ionization of this pendant group causes transition in polymeric network and converts into a swollen mass. Buffering capacity of incorporated ionizable pendant group decides the pH at which this transition occurs. To selectively control the swelling of these pH-responsive hydrogels either acidic or basic pendant groups can be incorporated during synthesis. Incorporation of acidic pendant group e.g. carboxylate exhibit maximum swelling of hydrogel in pH range above pKa of corresponding acid and the phenomenon is known as upper critical swelling pH phenomenon (UCSpH). For example, a system is developed by grafting methacrylic acid pendant group with pKa ≈ 4.5 into a co-polymer network P(MAA-g-EG). After oral administration this grafted system remains de-swelled at pH ranges 2-4 of stomach as the acidic groups are in protonated state. But at higher pH of small intestine i.e. pH 6-7, acidic groups ionizes leading to swelling of polymeric network. When basic pendant group e.g. primary, secondary or tertiary amine is incorporated into the polymeric network, the phenomenon is known as lower critical swelling pH phenomenon (LCSpH).

The first instance of pH-responsive microgels for biomedical purpose was reported for oral administration of bio-macromolecules. Bio-macromolecules e.g. proteins are degraded in stomach after oral administration due to acidic and proteolytic environment. Poly (ethylene glycol) grafted poly (methacrylic acid) [P(MAA-*g*-PEG)] microgels were developed by Peppas and co-workers to overcome this obstacle for oral delivery of bio-macromolecules. The microgels with basic pendant group avoid gastric degradation of incorporated molecules by pH-dependant complexation and release them when exposed to higher pH environment of small intestine. P(MAA-*g*-PEG) microgels also enhances the permeation of proteins through intestinal mucosa without any toxic effect. However, the mechanism for permeation enhancing action is still ambiguous but possibly owed to alteration in intercellular junctions of intestinal mucosa. Bioadhesive agents e.g. wheat germ agglutinin further increases the effectiveness of microgels by forming more intimate contact between microgels and intestinal mucosa.

The particle size of hydrogels markedly influences the enhancement in intestinal permeation. Insulin-loaded smaller microgels of <43 nm diameter depleted the blood glucose concentration more effectively in comparison to larger microgels of >180 nm. P(MAA-*g*-PEG) nanogels were also prepared to protectively encapsulate the insulin by precipitation/dispersion polymerization technique. But the *in-vivo* performance of these nanogels for insulin permeation was poor when compared to microgel formulations. pH-responsive hydrogels may also utilized to target other pH dependant biological sites i.e. interstitium of tumors and inflammed tissues. To target these sites pH-responsive hydrogels adopt unique mechanism of triggered volume swelling. To achieve high concentration of therapeutic/imaging agent at diseased tissue location, the swelling of microgels or nanogels can be triggered by an acid. The acid triggered swelling can also be applied for physical occlusion of tumor vasculature; in that case hydrogel act as a synthetic anti-angiogenic agent. Endosomal escape by pH-triggered phenomenon is also possible with the aid of carriers based on polyacidic/polybasic hydrogels. A study by Wilson and co-workers showed that as the size of alkyl group increased, acidic poly alkyl acrylates substantially increases the endosomal escape. This increase in endosomal escape can be attributed to enhanced interaction between the endosomal membrane and polymeric chains at lower pH values leading to endosomolysis. The protonation of acidic groups of polymeric chains increases the hydrophobicity and they become more endosomolytic. This approach was utilized by Das and co-workers for designing of polyacidic microgels to achieve intracellular delivery of chemotherapeutic agents.

Undoubtedly, uncrosslinked polybasic compounds that act as proton sponges are commonly utilized as polymers for such applications. There is a need of extensive investigation for the employment of polybasic nanogels for such biomedical application. At low pH, the intracellular delivery of a nanogel may result into capitalization of increased physical size and enhanced osmotic pressure for cytosolic delivery. Several recent investigations support the significance of this application. Application of pH-responsive microgels and nanogels for other biomedical purposes will possibly explore in future.

4.2.4.4 Self-assembled nano-carriers

Self-assembling of amphiphilic block co-polymers may result into the formation of liposomes, polymersomes and micelles. The driving force required for self-assembly phenomenon is emerged as free energy due to mixing of amphiphilic polymer and water which is maintained exclusively by supramolecular forces. Aqueous micelles are biphasic systems composed of sequential surfactant chains arranged in a manner that hydrophilic portions facing outward and lipophilic portions facing inward. Due to the formation of lipophilic pocket in the core these aqueous micelles are particularly attractive as a carrier for the delivery of lipophilic drug molecules. At concentrations above critical micellar concentration (CMC), a surfactant form micelles spontaneously. The utilization of micelles for drug delivery is associated with a risk of micelle dilution to below CMC concentration during administration. To overcome this obstacle some highly stable synthetic surfactants have been developed with CMC values below 10^{-6} M. Cross linking of cores further increased the stability of micelles. The size and shape of micelles is influenced by relative sizes of hydrophilic and hydrophobic blocks present on the polymer chain. Generally, micelles are spherical in shape but presence of longer hydrophobic blocks may give rise to other shapes like lamellae, rods etc. The diameter of spherical micelles may range between 10-80 nm. By manipulating the composition of di-block amphiphiles, Discher and co-workers developed a highly stable cylindrical structures termed as filo-micelles. The unique size and surface PEGylation of these developed filo-micelles blocks the macrophage recognition and they will remain in systemic circulation up to a period of one week. The hydrophobic core was utilized for the delivery of paclitaxel to tumor cells. The clinical success of nano-sized liposomes in the field of drug delivery is well known. These are self-assembled bilayer lipid vesicles of amphipathic compounds from natural or synthetic origin. They are first investigated for drug delivery in 1965. They can incorporate both hydrophilic and hydrophobic moieties for therapeutic delivery. Aqueous core and space between the bilayer is suitable for hydrophilic drug while hydrophobic drugs are incorporated by directly dissolving them in constituent lipids. Double chain amphiphiles e.g. glycolipids or phospholipids are commonly used for the preparation of liposomes. Unilamellar liposomes of size range 85-100 nm are proved most successful for intravenous administration of therapeutic agents. The liposomes for intravenous delivery are generally stabilized sterically by incorporation of poly (ethylene glycol) chains. Ortho Biotech (a Johnson & Johnson subsidiary company), get the approval of first liposomal product Doxil^R which are PEGylated liposomes of doxorubicin. At present this product is clinically approved for treatment of breast cancer and AIDS associated Kaposi's sarcoma. The clinical effectiveness of Doxil^R may be possibly due to passive accumulation of doxorubicin in the tumor tissue which is owed to EPR effect.

Biologically liposomes resemble the natural lipoidal bilayers which construct the cellular membranes. Similarly to biological cell membranes they can be stabilized with the help of cholesterol. However, they do not possess dense surface covering of highly sulfated proteoglycans and stability of cytoskeleton bound transmembrane proteins which are common in the membranes of animal cells. They posses best stability in aqueous environment but similar to cells, also fairly stable in suspension form. Loss in drug loading capacity and lysis of liposomes is observed when processed for freeze drying and freeze-thaw cycles. Liposomes are sensitive to temperature and pH fluctuations and possess a limited long term stability up to 6 months. Complementary activation and cardiopulmonary distress is also reported by several research groups with the use of simple and surface PEGylated liposomes which are possibly due to high cholesterol content incorporated for the stability of liposomes. Other vesicular carriers e.g. polymersomes, or mesoscopic synthetic polymer vesicles resembles liposomes very closely which also possess bilayer shell of diblock amphiphilic co-polymers with an aqueous core. In these vesicles polymer chains are typically larger in comparison to lipids utilized for liposomes formulation. Due to these extra large polymeric chains a 'hyper thick' hydrophobic compartment is formed. This extra thick membrane results in decreased permeability and increased viscosity. They are successfully evaluated to deliver active targeting agents *in-vivo*. Polymersomes are only quasi-stable however their integrity can be increased by free radical polymerization as reported by Discher and co-workers in their work related to polymeric nanoshells.

5 Evaluation of Bioadhesive Formulations

Bioadhesive formulations are subjected to the routine evaluation tests according to the type of formulation such as weight variation, thickness, friability, hardness, content uniformity, *in-vitro* release, tensile strength, film endurance, hygroscopicity, viscosity, effect of aging etc. They should also to be evaluated specifically for their bioadhesive properties. The measurement of bioadhesive properties is somewhat difficult as they possess highly variable results according to the factors considered for the designing of evaluation methods. The available methods of evaluation and the specific property to be evaluated itself cause variation in results. Most of the available evaluation techniques are based on measurement of stress-strain curves at low amplitudes which creates confusion, whether work of adhesion or force of adhesion is measured leading to variation in results. The area under stress-strain curve represent work of adhesion which is measured in terms of energy required for complete breakage of adhesive bonds between mucosal surface and bioadhesive formulation. The highest point of stress-strain curve refers to force of adhesion or maximum adhesion strength which is measured in terms of force required for the separation of probe from substrate. Some methods for the measurement of tangential shear are also reported.

Ranging from simple to complex, different models are developed to describe the phenomenon of bioadhesion and its evaluation **(Table 5.1)**. Majority of these models evaluate the bioadhesive properties on the basis of:

- Transport/motility of bioadhesive formulation in biological environment
- Physical contact at the application site
- Surface probing
- Polymer film formation at interface.

Table 5.1 Bioadhesion models for biological systems listed in order of increasing complexity

Model 1	Viscoelastic adhesive/smooth, inflexible, impermeable substrate(s).
Model 2	Viscoelastic adhesive/rough or flexible or permeable or anisotropic substrate, or adhesive has specific chemical interactions with substrate.
Model 3	Viscoelastic adhesive/rough or flexible or permeable or anisotropic substrate, or adhesive has specific chemical interactions with substrate; with mass transfer between phases (adhesive & substrate).
Model 4	Anisotropic adhesive; rough or flexible or permeable or anisotropic substrate or adhesive has specific chemical interactions with substrate.
Model 5	Anisotropic adhesive which changes with time/rough or flexible or permeable or anisotropic substrate or adhesive has specific chemical interactions with substrate.
Model 6	Anisotropic adhesive which changes with time/rough or flexible or permeable or anisotropic substrate or adhesive has specific chemical interactions with substrate; with mass transfer between phases.
Model 7	Anisotropic adhesive which changes with time/rough and/or flexible and/or permeable and/or anisotropic substrate, and/or adhesive have specific chemical interactions with substrate; with mass transfer between phases.
Model 8	Anisotropic adhesive which changes with time/rough and flexible and permeable or anisotropic substrate and adhesive has specific chemical interactions with substrate; with mass transfer between phases; substrate also changes with time.

Note: Model 1 is used to predict bioadhesion by advanced bioadhesive materials. Model 8 is typically used for a bioadhesive tablet dosage form, while Model 3 is typically used for syrup, ocular or oral suspension dosage model *in-vivo*.

The complications associated with biological systems add difficulties for *in-vitro* modeling of bioadhesion for measurement methods. As a matter of fact, in acidic conditions bioadhesive forces are greatest, therefore biological pH conditions plays an important role during the evaluation studies. With the variation in test materials and models, some other factors e.g. ionic strength of test solution markedly influence the evaluation of bioadhesive properties. For that reason the presence of divalent ions such as calcium is closely monitored. Physiological mucus turnover process further complicates the *in-vitro-in-vivo* correlations, as it is hindered during *in-vitro* evaluation. In the view of above facts, one can conclude that accurate measurement of bioadhesive properties is very difficult. Bioadhesive properties are so sensitive that simplest system consisting slab of impermeable substrate and bioadhesive formulation is unable to quantify them accurately.

Most of the currently available *in-vitro* methods for the evaluation of bioadhesive drug delivery systems do not differentiate that whether they measure adhesion forces between delivery system and substrate or cohesion forces of delivery system itself. A method for the measurement of bioadhesive properties utilizes Texture Analyzer instrument. This adjustable instrument can be programmed for the measurement of various hold times, it actually measures compression or extension forces and all the measurement data is displayed on a computer connected interface.

This simple model can also be implemented for the measurement of work of adhesion in terms of tacking. The relationship between tack (work of adhesion) and peak adhesive strength corresponds to distance over which bioadhesive forces are active. At low pressures, tack declines with an increase in peak adhesive strength while at higher pressures an increase in tack was observed with a decrease in peak adhesive strength.

For the evaluation of bioadhesive properties, generally models are fabricated according to drug delivery system to be evaluated. However, several probes and test jigs are available commercially for the evaluation of some specific bioadhesive formulation. These systems may also be customized as per the requirements of evaluation parameters for particular bioadhesive system.

5.1 EVALUATION OF BIOADHESIVE PROPERTIES

Several *in-vitro* and *in-vivo* test methods are developed to measure adhesion strength in order to quantify bioadhesive properties **(Table 5.2)**. Most of the developed *in-vitro/ex-vivo* methods are based on integrated chip system for the measurement of shear strength and tensile strength. Whereas to evaluate the bioadhesive properties in actual *in-vivo* conditions various imaging techniques are utilized. Various other *in-vitro* and *in-vivo* methods are used for testing the efficacy of the bioadhesive nature of a polymer matrix.

Table 5.2 *In-vitro* and *in-vivo* methods for the evaluation of bioadhesive properties

In-vitro/ex-vivo methods	*In-vivo* methods
• Methods determining tensile strength • Methods determining shear stress • Adhesion weight method • Fluorescent probe method • Flow channel method • Mechanical spectroscopic method • Falling liquid film method • Colloidal gold staining method • Viscometer method • Thumb method • Adhesion number • Electrical conductance • Swelling properties • *In-vitro* drug release studies Muco-retentability studies	• Radioisotopic methods • Gamma scintigraphy • Pharmacoscintigraphy • Electron paramagnetic resonance (EPR) oximetry • X-ray studies • Isolated loop technique

5.1.1 Tensile Strength Measurement

Several methods are utilized for the determination of tensile strength of bioadhesive formulations:

- Bioadhesion can be measured by determination the adhesive strength between the polymer and substrate. The maximum adhesive strength at the contact surface area can be determined by measuring the maximum force required to detach one surface from the other. The device used to measure this detachment force generally consists of a plate suspended from a microbalance that is coated with the polymer under investigation. The polymer-coated plate is then slowly dipped until it is in contact with the membrane model. The force required to remove the polymer-coated plate can then be compared (Andrews, Laverty & Jones, 2008:10). **Figure 5.1** is an illustration of an apparatus used in the measurement of tensile forces.

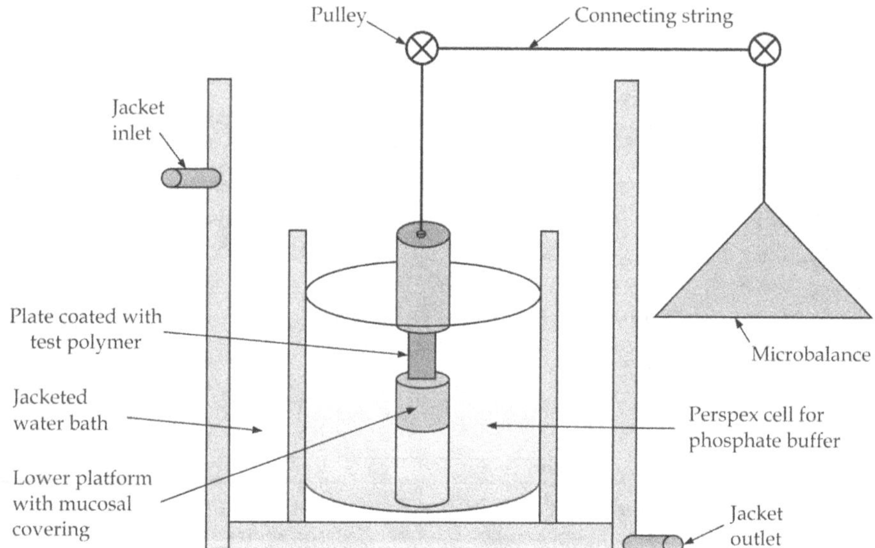

Figure 5.1 Schematic representation of tensile strength measurement

- *In-vitro* tensile strength can also evaluated by dipping a filter paper in 8% mucin/physiological solutions dispersion. Thereafter, the mucin/physiological solutions coated filter paper is placed in contact with the hydrated polymeric samples (in physiological solutions) for a definite period of time, followed by the determination of the maximum force required to detach the filter-paper and polymer surfaces after the bioadhesive bonding. Similarly, *ex-vivo* experimentations are also done with the exception that the mucin/physiological solutions coated filter-paper is replaced with excised mucosal tissues (e.g. buccal mucosa, intestinal mucosa, vaginal mucosa, skin).

- The tensile strength can also be determined by incubating the hydrated polymer matrix surface kept in contact with a viscoelastic 30% (w/w) mucin/physiological solutions in water with the subsequent determination of the maximum detachment force required to separate the polymer matrix and mucin/physiological solutions surfaces after the adhesion.

- Wash-off test may also be used to determine the bioadhesive property of delivery systems. In the test, the biological tissue is attached onto a glass slide with the help of a double-sided cyanoacrylate tape. Thereafter, the delivery system is put on the surface of the tissue (exposed mucosal surface) with the subsequent vertical attachment of the system into the USP tablet disintegrator apparatus, which contains 1 L of physiological solution maintained at 37 °C. The operation of the equipment gives an up-and-down movement to the tissue-delivery matrix system. In this method, the time for the complete detachment of the delivery system from the biological layer is determined.

- For the relative measurement of bioadhesive nature of powder polymer samples modified Du Nouy tensiometer may be used.

5.1.2 Shear Strength Measurement

In the shear strength measurement methods the force required to slide the polymer matrix over the biological tissue layer is determined. To measure bioadhesive forces with shear strength measurement methods, one side of the surface holding bioadhesive material should be elongated in order to provide enough distance for the detachment of test disc applied for shear studies. The pulley system plays significant role in detection of adhesion force with varying degrees and contributes toward measured adhesion force in terms of frictional forces. This hindrance hampers the accurate measurement of adhesion force with methods based on shear strength analysis. **Figure 5.2** demonstrates model equipment for the measurement of tensile strength and shear forces.

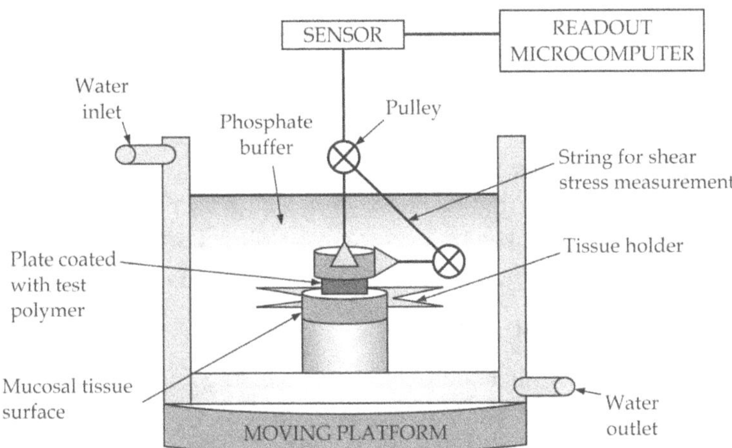

Figure 5.2 Schematic illustration of bio-adhesion apparatus showing arrangement for tensile and shear strength measurement

- Shear stress can also be measured by an alternative setup arrangement **(Figure 5.3)**. Two smooth, polished plexi-glass blocks are selected one block was fixed with a strong adhesive on a glass plate, which is fixed on a leveled table. To the upper block thread is tied and the thread is passed down through a pulley. The length of the thread from pulley to pan is 12 cm. At the end of the thread a pan of weight 17 g is attached into which the weights can be added. Different solutions of polymers under evaluation are prepared in aqueous medium with a concentration of 3% w/v. An appropriate volume of test polymer solution is kept on the center of lower/fixed block; generally a single drop of test solution is used. The second movable block is placed over the test solution and a 100 g weight is applied in order to achieve uniform spreading of test solution between the two blocks.

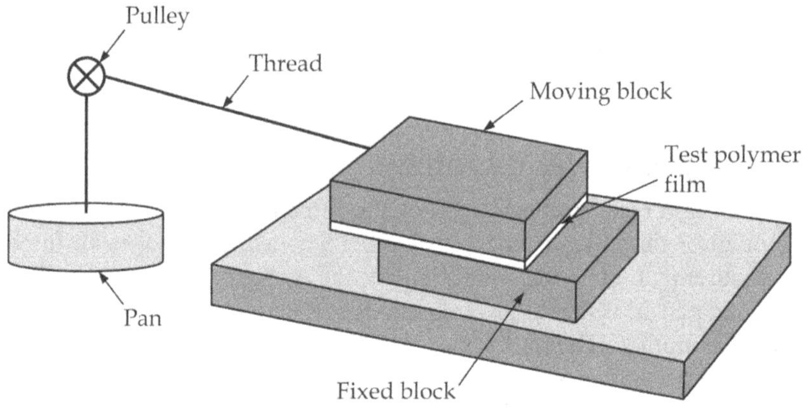

Figure 5.3 Setup for shear stress measurement

Then the blocks are kept for settlement for several fixed time intervals e.g. 5, 10, 15 and 30 minutes. After that weights are added to pan which works against the adhesive forces to move the upper block. The weights just sufficient to pull the upper block or to make it slide over the base block represent the adhesion strength, i.e,. the shear stress required.

- One more shear tester has been developed which measures the force required to separate two polymer coated glass slides joined by a thin film of natural or synthetic mucous. The results of this technique correlate well with *in-vivo* test results.

5.1.3 Rheological Measurements

Several researchers suggested that the study of the rheological profile of polymer–mucus/biological fluids mixtures provides an acceptable *in-vitro* model representative of the *in-vivo* behavior of a bioadhesive polymer. The bioadhesive potential of polymer candidates can therefore be determined by comparing binary polymer blends rheologically. The bioadhesive polymer mixtures exhibited synergistic rheological interactions, the causes of which were attributed to bond formation between the polymer and mucus culminating in an increase in total system structure. **Figure 5.4** outlines the basic principle of rheological testing.

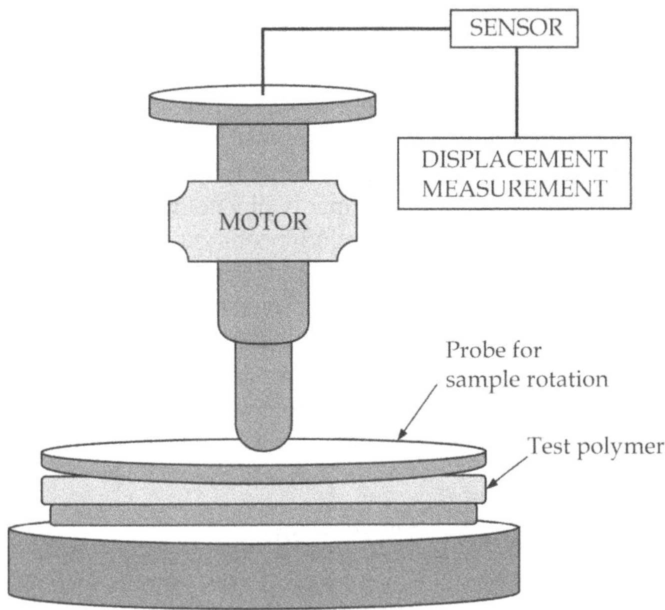

Figure 5.4 Schematic representation of rheological measurement

5.1.4 Florescence Probes

These probes are based on the comparative measurement of change in fluorescence before and after bioadhesion phenomenon. Pyrene is used as a fluorescent probe to label lipid bilayers of cultured cells. The bioadhesive interactions between test polymer and cultured cells results as change in fluorescence intensity. This change in fluorescence intensity is owed to surface compression which is compared quantitatively with control cells i.e. cells without bioadhesive interactions. The degree of adhesion can be measured in terms of change in fluorescence intensity which is directly proportional to the extent of polymer binding. For the assessment of effects of polymer charge, charge sign and density on bioadhesive interactions, a second probe can also be utilized. Park and Robinson used this technique to study the bioadhesive interactions of various polymers with cultured human conjunctiva cells.

A similar technique was designed by Batchelor and co-workers for the evaluation of bioadhesive properties of alginate solutions by exposing them to porcine oesophageal tissue. Alginate solutions of known rheological profile were labeled with fluorescent marker and applied over porcine oesophageal tissue. After 30 minutes, the mucosal surface was washed and residual fluorescence was measured. The results showed that 20% of initial dose was remained over the mucosal surface.

5.1.5 Refractive Index BIACORE® System

The BIACORE® instrument measures an optical phenomenon called surface plasmon resonance (SPR) integrated chip (IC) systems. SPR response is a measurement of the refractive index, which varies with the solute content in a solution that contacts a sensor chip. The method involves immobilization of the polymer (powder) on to the surface of the IC with the subsequent passage of the mucin/physiological solutions over the same. This results in the interaction of the mucin/physiological solutions with that of the polymer surface. When the analyte (mucin particle) binds to the ligand molecule (polymer) on the sensor chip surface, the solute concentration and the refractive index on that surface change, increasing the SPR response; when they dissociate, the SPR response will decrease. Quantitative measurements of the binding interaction between the chip surface and one or more molecules depend on the immobilization of target molecules that are in contact with the sensor surface.

5.1.6 Detachment Force Measurement

This process is used for solid bioadhesive dosage forms (tablets, pellets etc.) to measure *in-vitro* bioadhesive capability of distinct range of polymers. It is a reformed technique expanded by Mrti Marvola to evaluate the tendency of bioadhesive materials to adhere to the biological surfaces. The assembly consist a single organ bath, a stand, glass rod, a pan for keeping beaker and a reservoir for addition of water into beaker. In this method, freshly removed intestine of sheep/porcine after slaughter is kept in Tyrode solution (composition: sodium chloride-0.134 g/L, sodium bicarbonate-1.0 g/L, sodium dihydrogen phosphate – 0.05g/L and glucose-1.0 g/L). During the experiment the solution is aerated with pure oxygen and kept at 37 °C. 6-7 cm long segments of sheep/porcine intestine are used for the study. The lower end of the intestine segment is tied off and then tied to the aerator tube and the upper end is tied around a glass tube of diameter 15 mm.

The volume of water required to remove the tablet from the piece of intestine signifies the detachment force required to pull the tablet against the adhesive strength of polymer. The detachment force in Newton is calculated by the following equation:

$$\text{Detachment force (F)} = 0.00981 \times W/2$$

where, W is the volume of water.

The following characteristics can be studied from the experiment:

- Detachment force and effect of contact time on bioadhesive forces.
- Bioadhesive strength of different polymers and the effect of polymer concentration on detachment force.

5.1.7 Wilhelmly Plate Technique

This technique has traditionally been used for dynamic contact angle measurement and involves a microbalance or tensiometer. A glass slide is coated with the polymer of interest and then dipped into a beaker of synthetic or natural mucous **(Figure 5.5)**. The surface tension, contact angle and adhesive force can be measured using inbuilt software.

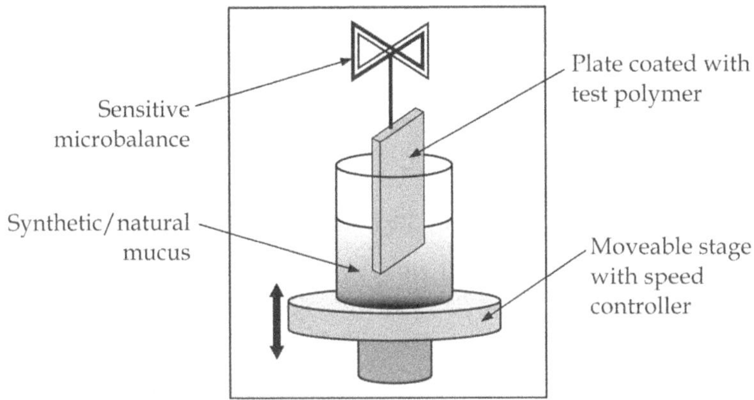

Figure 5.5 Wilhelmly plate technique

5.1.8 Other *In-vitro* Tests

5.1.8.1 Thumb test

It is a qualitative test for the determination of peel adhesive strength of polymer under evaluation. The strength of bioadhesion is measured in terms of difficulty experienced in pulling the thumb from adhesive with respect to applied pressure and contact time. Due to only qualitative measurement, this test does not provide conclusive results but provides useful information regarding detachment force required to remove the system after therapy.

5.1.8.2 Adhesion number

To calculate the adhesion number, test particles are applied over a substrate surface and washed after several fixed time intervals. The remaining particles were quantified as the ratio of particles remained attached to substrate surface after washing to the total number of particle applied initially. Adhesion number is generally expressed as percentage.

$$\text{Adhesion number} = \frac{\text{Number of particles remained}}{\text{Total number of particles applied}} \times 100$$

5.1.8.3 Falling liquid film method

It is an *in-situ* technique for quantitative measurement of bioadhesiveness of microspheres. In this method the percentage of particles which get retained on a mucosal tissue, spread on a plastic slide in an inclined position, when a suspension of the microspheres is allowed to flow down the tissue. The quantification can be done by the aid of coulter-current method.

5.1.8.4 Electrical conductance

A modified rotational viscometer can be used to determine electrical conductance of various semi-solid mucoadhesive ointments. It has been found that electrical conductance is low in the presence of an adhesive material.

5.1.8.5 Novel electromagnetic force transducer technique

It is a remote sensing instrument that utilizes a calibrated electromagnet to detach a magnetically loaded polymer from a tissue. It measures the adhesive force by monitoring the magnetic force required to exactly oppose bioadhesive force.

Another imaging technique was developed by Kockisch and colleagues. Here investigators developed a semi quantitative image analysis based on the technique for the *in-vitro* and *in-vivo* detections of polymers with an affinity for the biological/mucosal surfaces.

5.1.9 *In-vivo* Evaluation of Bioadhesive Properties

In-vivo bioadhesive studies are less commonly seen in the literature than *in-vitro* testing. This may be due to cost, biochemical factors, tedious handling, time constraints as well as ethical considerations. It is however, vital if the true bioadhesive potential of a system has to be determined.

5.1.9.1 Radioisotopic method

As the name indicates this method involves the utilization of radioisotopes which are used to label bioadhesive formulations under investigation. After proper labeling with specific radioisotope the test formulation is administered to a suitable animal/human model followed by quantification of radioactivity, at regular time intervals in regions where test formulation is supposed to adhere. The intensity of radioactivity decides bioadhesiveness of test formulation i.e. higher radioactivity represents the better bioadhesive properties. The transit of various radio labeled polyacrylic acid beads through the rat gastrointestinal tract has been studied. In order to study the transit overtime, the beads were fed to the rats at various time intervals. The rats were then systematically dissected and radioactivity is measured in the tissues of interest by suitable method. The requirement for the sacrifice of the subject resulted in ethical concerns.

5.2 EVALUATION OF BIOADHESIVE PROPERTIES OF MULTIPARTICULATE SYSTEMS

5.2.1 *In-vitro* Characterization of Cellular Interaction

For the analysis of multiparticulate systems (nanoparticles, microspheres) cell integration various techniques **(Table 5.3)** based on the nature of the multiparticulate systems and the cells are utilized. Some general methods and instrumentation used for cytomic study are discussed in this section.

5.2.1.1 Flow cytometry

This technique is utilized for the liquid samples only which involve the principles of light excitation, light scattering and emission of fluorochrome molecules. Flow cytometry provides specific data based on multiple parameters from the particles and cells under investigation with a restrictive size range of 0.5-40 μm. The particles/cells under investigation are hydrodynamically focused in a casing of phosphate-buffered saline (PBS) and intercepted to a optimally focused light source. The commonly used light sources in flow cytometry are lasers

After intercepting the light source, particles/cells scatter light leading to excitation of fluorochromes to a higher energy level and this extra energy is released as a light photon. Specific spectral properties of this released energy are unique for different fluorochromes. Optical detectors transform the emitted and scattered light into electrical pulses. At intersection point of cells and light source, confocal lenses are focused to pick up the collimated light. These confocal lenses direct the picked collimated light towards detectors. Before reaching the detectors this collimated light is passed through optical filters which separates it into colored fractions e.g. an optical filter of 525 nm allow only 'green' light to reach the detectors.

To maintain the specificity and accuracy, photomultiplier tubes (PMTs) are generally utilized as detectors for flow cytometry analysis. These PMTs transforms the detected light into electrical pulses which are further processed by a series of linear and log amplifiers. For the measurement of fluorescence in cells generally logarithmic amplification is preferred because they produce "strong" or specific fluorescence signals by compressing the scale and also expands the scale for weak signals resulting in better amplification. After amplification of electrical pulses, an analog-digital converter (ADC) converts these electrical signals into graphical form which can be displayed on computer interface as different plots corresponding to the measurement of various events and parameters.

Table 5.3 Evaluation methods for bioadhesive multiparticulate delivery systems

Method	Comment
Direct assay techniques	
Tensiometry	Measurement of force required to dislodge two surfaces, one coated with mucus and other with bioadhesive dosage form
Flow through	Measurement of flow rate required to dislodge the two surfaces; useful for microparticulate delivery systems
Adhesion number	Measurement of ratio of number of particles attached to substrate to the total number of applied particles
In-vivo techniques	Endoscopy, gamma-scintigraphy
Molecular mucin based assays	
Viscometry and rheology	Measurement of intrinsic viscosity (related to the complex size of mucin and bioadhesive material)
Dynamic light scattering	Measurement of diffusion coefficient (related to the complex size of mucin and bioadhesive material)
Analytical ultracentrifugation	Measurement of change in molecular weight and sedimentation coefficient ratio of mucin-bioadhesive complex to mucin

5.2.1.2 Laser scanning cytometry

Laser scanning cytometry (LSC) works on the principle similar to flow cytometry but it overcomes the limitation which restricts flow cytometry to analyze the samples in liquid state only. With the provision of sample preservation with precise position of each sample this method permits automated evaluation of samples in solid phase e.g. tissue sections, adherent cultured cells, imprint of cancer tissues and cytology smears. The preservation of samples allows repeated visual inspection and cross-examination of specific cells with respect to their biochemical, morphological or genetic properties. It also allows the remeasurement of same samples after repeated treatments with drugs or other chemical reagents as per requirements of specific study.

LSC is a powerful analytical tool which allows:

- Freedom for the visualization of specimens either with simple microscopic technique or by powerful laser scanning techniques for imaging.
- Generation of stoichiometric data and analysis of heterogeneous cell populations.
- Unlimited view of individual events in population data under consideration.
- Reanalysis of same cell specimens under varying conditions i.e. chemical or drug treatment.
- Cross-examination of localized cellular constituents.
- Identification of molecular constituents in contiguous environment and correlate them with cellular processes.
- Automated analysis of tissues either in sections or in microarrays.
- Simultaneous evaluation of cultured cells at individual and colony levels.

5.2.1.3 High content screening assays

It is a very sensitive cell-based assay for imaging and analysis of multiplexed targets of interest. High content screening (HCS) assays images compound-treated cells/target of interest and processed for further analysis to an automated computer interface. It provide data based on multiple parameters i.e. intensity of fluorescence in target cells, density of cells, localization of compound, cell size and morphology. Generally, 96 or 384 wells microplates are used for HCS an assay which allows screening of more compounds against one or multiple targets. In this manner a single experiment is sufficient to evaluate multiple cellular targets against a compound for direct effects with easy correlation. This method also minimizes the wastage of reagents and other resources. For cytotoxicity evaluation, HCS assays already proved their effectiveness as they allow multiplexing targets of interest for cytotoxicity evaluation e.g. permeability, nuclear morphology, membrane potential, mitochondrial transmembrane potential, pH, apoptosis and changes in cellular concentration of Ca^{2+} and other ions or oxidative stress. To increase the effectiveness of these assays an appropriate combination of fluorescent reagents is required. With 96 well microplates, a single HCS assay can provide relevant data in about 3 hours after exposure of cells to nanoparticles. As all the steps of HCS assays, from sample preparation to graphical output are automated; this minimizes the chances of errors and provide accurate and precise results. The time of exposure is actually depends on nature of cellular targets selected for experimentation. Thus, these cell based assays are efficiently utilized as a rapid and valuable method for toxicological studies in animal experimentations.

5.2.1.4 Confocal laser scanning microscopy

With the use of confocal laser scanning microscopy (CLSM or LSCM) one can obtain optical images of high resolution. The process of optical sectioning makes this technique capable to produce in-focus images of thick specimens. A series of point-by-point acquired images is reconstructed on a computer interface which allows 3-dimensional reconstruction of topologically complex cellular objects. For CLSM analysis a laser beam is delivered through a light source orifice which is focused on a fluorescent specimen by an objective lens. The objective lens focused the laser beam within a small focal volume and specimen becomes illuminated. Then objective lens recollects the emitted fluorescent light and reflected laser light from the illuminated spot. This mixture of light is separated by a beam splitter which only passes the laser light through it while fluorescent light is reflected towards the detector unit via a pin hole. The detector unit consists of photo-detection arrangement e.g. PMTs or an avalanche photodiode which transforms the light signals into electrical signals for recording by computerized system.

The detector pin hole is arranged in such a manner that it rejects the light that is not originated from the focal point and suppresses the out-of-focus light. The pin hole blocks most part of returning light to provide sharper images in comparison to simple fluorescence microscopy. This technique also permits the imaging of various z-axis planes; known as z stacks of specimen. This detected light represents one pixel of the complete image and its brightness corresponds to relative intensity of detected fluorescent light. When total area of interest is scanned by the laser; it rises as a complete pixel-by-pixel and line-by-line image. One or more oscillating mirrors (servo-controlled) assists scanning of specimen across the horizontal plane by laser beam. The speed of scanning can be varied due to the low reaction latency of such scanning method. Slower scanning process results in better signal-to-noise ratio which produces images with better contrast and higher resolution. By adjusting the microscope stage i.e. upward or downward, one can collect the information from different focal planes. These 2-dimensional images of successive focal planes are assembled to generate a complete 3-dimensional image of the specimen under examination.

5.2.1.5 Fluorescence confocal microscopy

Fluorescence confocal microscopy (FCM) is a modified form of confocal microscopy. In this technique the specimen under examination is doped with a high-quantum yield fluorescent dye which sharply absorbs at wavelength of exciting laser beam. The dye molecules which absorbs laser beam show fluorescence at comparatively longer wavelength. This difference between the absorption wavelength and fluorescence is known as 'Stokes shift'. In case of greater Stokes shift, signals of excitation and fluorescence can be separated successfully; in such a manner that only signal of fluorescence reaches the detector unit. In case of heterogeneous specimen, the fluorescent probe concentration depends on coordinates and results high contrast images. It is possible to visualize the features of living cells and tissues with the help of FCM.

5.2.1.6 Laser capture micro-dissection

Laser capture micro-dissection (LCM) is an advanced technique for the isolation of pure cells of interest from specific microscopic regions of tissue specimens. A transferable transparent film is applied over the surface of specimen tissue section. A very thin section of tissue is mounted on a glass slide and viewed under the microscope in order to select microscopic clusters of cells to be isolated. To mark up the desired cell clusters, operator focus the region and pushes the button which activates the inbuilt near infrared laser diode. This pulsed laser beam mark up a precise spot on transferable transparent film and fused the underlying cell clusters of interest with the film. Then this transparent film is lifted in order to separate the desired cell clusters from unwanted cells.

The overall process is so precise that the morphology and chemistry of laser marked cells and surrounding cells does not altered or damaged. This attribute makes this technique quite effective to isolate the sample cells for RNA, DNA and/or protein analysis. A vast range of samples can be analyzed by LCM including cytological preparations, solid tissue aliquots, blood smears and cell cultures. Archived frozen and paraffin-embedded tissues of older studies may also be viewed.

5.2.1.7 Pharmacoscintigraphy

For pharmacoscintigraphic evaluation, the formulations are labeled with a radioactive isotope which is traced by the different visualization techniques e.g. gamma scintigraphy, positron emission tomography (PET) etc. With the aid of this technique one can easily visualize and quantify many vital parameters in animal models and humans i.e. site of adhesion, rate of drug release, mode of drug absorption and extent of absorption. Pharmacoscintigraphy is emerged as a promising approach for the evaluation of multiparticulate drug delivery systems with the benefits of non-invasiveness and repetitive measurements. Radiopharmaceuticals used for these studies are radioactive agents which generally does not elicit any harmful physiological response from animals or humans when employed for diagnostic or therapeutic purpose. In pharmacoscintigraphy, the external imaging of radiopharmaceutical is essentially independent of density of tissues in comparison to radiographic techniques which are almost or entirely depends on differences in tissue densities.

The common steps of pharmacoscintigraphic evaluation involve efficient labeling of test formulations with radioisotopes, proficient imaging, accurate determination of parameters of interest and interpretation of obtained data. Effectiveness of pharmacoscintigraphic methods relies on the efficient labeling of test formulations with radioisotopes. The commonly used radioisotopes for pharmacoscintigraphic evaluations are technetium-99m (^{99m}Tc), iodine-125 (^{125}I), iodine-131 (^{131}I), gallium-67 (^{67}Ga) and indium-111 (^{111}In). From these radioisotopes, ^{99m}Tc is generally preferred for radiolabeling of test formulations; approximately 80% of radiopharmaceuticals for nuclear medicine purpose are ^{99m}Tc labeled compounds. ^{99m}Tc is a metastable nuclear isomer of technetium-99 which emits readily detectable 140 keV gamma rays. Its half life for gamma emission is 6.0058 hours i.e. within 24 hours 93.7 % of ^{99m}Tc decays to ^{99}Tc. These characteristics make this isotope perfect for diagnostic evaluations but on the other hand limit its therapeutic use.

5.3 FACTORS AFFECTING EVALUATION OF BIOADHESIVE PROPERTIES

5.3.1 Surface Cleanliness

The impurities over the biological surface hinder the effective surface area available for bioadhesive interactions and thus affect the strength of bioadhesion. Bioadhesive behavior of biological surfaces may significantly alter in the presence of adsorbates or oxide layers. When evaluating bioadhesive properties, the biological surface under investigation must be chemically clean i.e. it should be free from any contaminants and impurities with well characterized and reproducible surface structure. To establish a controlled chemical environment, these evaluations are done within an ultra high vacuum apparatus having a base pressure of $< 6 \times 10^{-11}$ mbar. **Fgure 5.6** shows the comparison between bioadhesive force measurement of contaminated and clean biological surface. The graph represents force distance curves for single measurement with silica microsphere on Cu (100) over cleaned and contaminated surface. The adhesion force rises from about 120 nN in case of contaminated surface while it is 250 nN for clean surface; a significant difference is clearly evident in terms of pull-off force. It is concluded that the presence of even marginal extent of contamination over biological surfaces may cause considerable reduction in adhesion force which is extremely sensitive to surface condition.

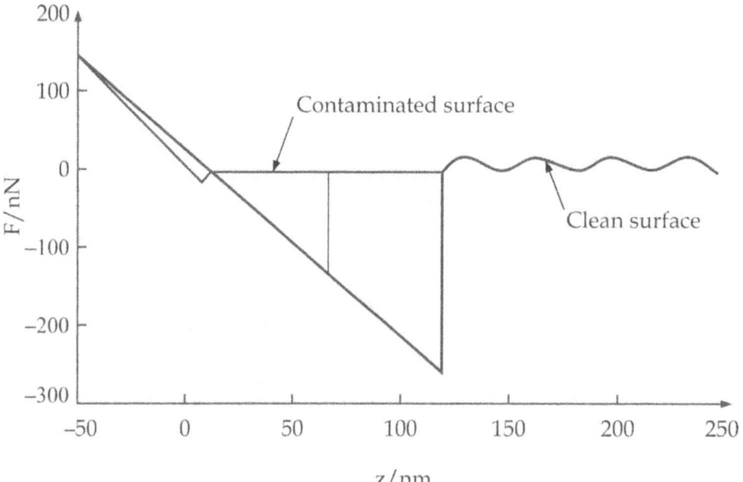

Figure 5.6 Typical force distance curves obtained for single measurements with a spherical silica tip on the contaminated (thin grey line) and the clean (solid black line) Cu (100) surface, respectively

5.3.2 Externally Applied Load

In order to perform accurate measurements of adhesion forces with AFM technique, a purely elastic contact between the tip and surface is required. On failing to maintain this condition, the relationship between adhesion force, surface energy and sphere radius become irrelevant. Externally applied loads may cause irreversible changes e.g. plastic deformations or transfer of material between tip and the surface. In order to nullify the loading effects, measurement of adhesion forces is done as a function of externally applied load. As a demonstration, adhesion forces of silica particles were measured over a single crystal surface of Ag (100) and results were plotted as a graph **(Figure 5.7)**. Silica spheres are optimal system as a model for the verification of elastic contact due to their rigidity and smooth surface with usually an elastic response output. The results of the study demonstrate that up to the external loads of 200 nN there is no significant change in adhesion force of about 90 nN. But a further increase in external load up to 350 nN results in increased adhesion force. The same experiment was performed with other metal single crystals and it was concluded that adhesion force does not depend significantly on external load as long as the load is less than adhesion force. Accordingly, the measurement of adhesion forces is performed in low external load conditions to limit or neglect the influence of externally applied load and plastic deformations.

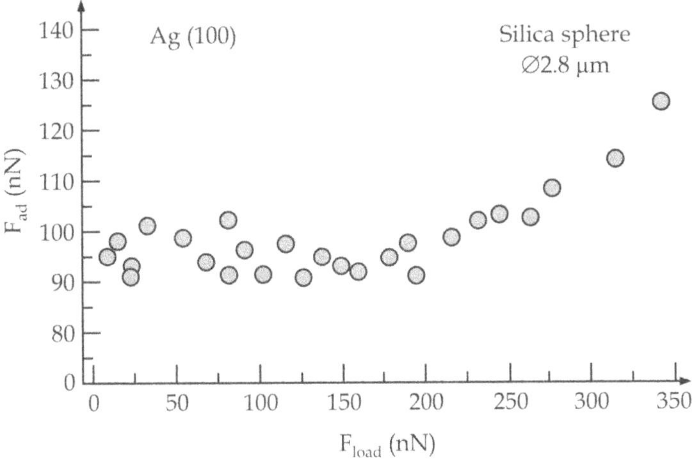

Figure 5.7 Adhesion forces vs. applied external load measured between a silica sphere (Ø 2.8 µm) and the clean Ag (100) surface

5.3.3 Probe Size

The surface area of the probe utilized for bioadhesive evaluation also plays a significant role in bioadhesive bonding of drug delivery systems. In order to investigate the effect of adhesion force on particle radius, cantilevers with silica spheres of different size were utilized for a comparative study over a clean Ag (100) surface. With these silica spheres, adhesion forces were measured in terms of force-distance measurements. With the increase in sphere radius, adhesion forces also increases **(Figure 5.8)**. Qualitatively this relationship is supported by other models of contact mechanics. On the basis of this experiment with only 3 points data, it is difficult to verify the linear relationship between size of particles and measured adhesion forces.

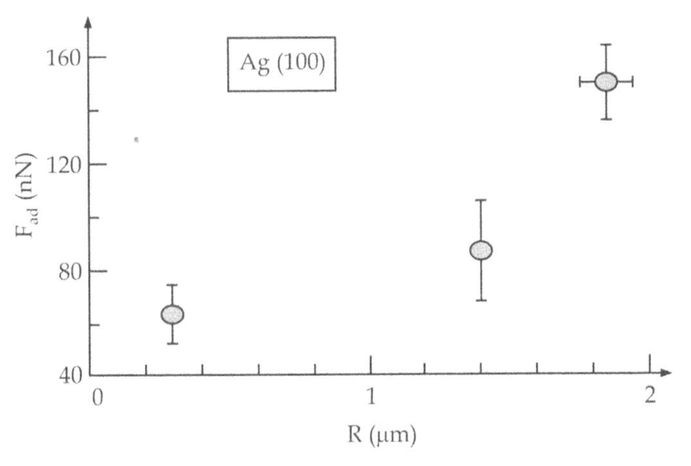

Figure 5.8 Adhesion forces between Ag (100) and silica microspheres of different size

5.3.4 Topography

With the advancements in computerized testing systems, topographic studies proved their importance in evaluation of bioadhesive forces. Generally all biological surfaces exhibit some degree of roughness which may cause a decrease in actual area of contact. In the light of this fact, the measured force of adhesion may be lower than expected values. This fact should be significant in case of *in-vitro* evaluation models where generally a probe with smooth surface is utilized for the evaluation of bioadhesive drug delivery systems.

5.3.5 Contact Time

The time allowed for the contact during evaluation has a marked effect on bioadhesive properties. The maximum detachment force as well as total work of adhesion is increased with increasing contact time.

5.3.6 pH

The pH of the medium selected for the evaluation of bioadhesive properties is important as the bioadhesive properties of hydroxy propyl methyl cellulose, carbopol, sodium carboxy methyl cellulose, guar gum and poly vinyl pyrrolidone were found to be optimal between pH 5 and 6, illustrating the effects of pH on bioadhesion.

Bioadhesive Nanoparticles

Nanosystems by means of diverse compositions and biological possessions have been expansively scrutinized for drug delivery applications. Bioadhesive nanoparticles can be used in targeted drug delivery at the site of disease to improve the uptake of poorly soluble drugs, the targeting of drugs to a specific site and drug bioavailability. Several anti-cancer drugs including paclitaxel, doxorubicin, 5-fluorouracil and dexamethasone have been successfully formulated using nanomaterials. The effectiveness of drug delivery systems can be attributed to their small size, reduced drug toxicity, controlled time release of the drug and modification of drug pharmacokinetics and biological distribution.

Nanotechnology offers the ability to observe measure, manipulate and manufacture things at the nanometer scale **(Table 6.1)**. A nanometer (nm) is a SI unit (System International Unit) of length (10^{-9} m) or a distance of one-billionth of a meter. At this scale, one can think about the size of atoms and molecules.

Table 6.1 Dimensions of some common objects in nanometers

Objects	Dimensions (approx.)
Width of an atom	1 nm
Width across a DNA molecule	2 nm
Width of a dust particle	800 nm
Length of some bacteria	1000 nm
Width of red blood cell	10000 nm
Width of hair	75000-100000 nm

The main problems with the existing drug delivery methods are the low drug loading capacity, low targeting efficiency and poor ability to control the size distribution. Utilization of nanotechnological approaches could allow manufacturing of nano/micro particles with high loading efficiency and highly homogeneous particle size. For the development of drug delivery systems, nanotechnology will become more advantageous if it is appreciated that the real potential of nanotechnology in drug delivery is based on utilization of nano/micro fabrication and manufacturing, rather than on dealing with delivery systems in the nano/micro scale. To understand the true significance of nanotechnology in drug delivery, it may be beneficial to categorize drug delivery systems on the basis of their size distribution **(Table 6.2)**. The following are the notable technological advantages of nano-carriers for drug delivery: superior stability (i.e. long shelf life); high loading capacity (i.e. more drug molecules can be assimilated in the particle matrix); incorporation of both hydrophilic and hydrophobic drugs; and feasibility of variable routes of administration, including oral administration and inhalation. These nano-carriers can also be fabricated to support controlled/sustained drug release from the polymer matrix.

Table 6.2 Nanotechnology based drug delivery systems

Systems	Nano-carriers	Size distribution (nm)
Polymeric systems	Dendrimers	1-10
	Polymer micelles	10-100
	Niosomes	10-150
	Nanoparticles	**50-500**
	Nanocapsules	100-300
	Nanogels	200-800
	Polymeric nano-conjugates	1-15
Lipid systems	Solid lipid nanoparticles	50-400
	Lipid nano-structured systems	200-800
	Cubosomes	50-700
	Liposomes	10-1000
	Polymerosomes	100-300
	Immunoliposomes	100-150
Protein/peptide nanotubes	Peptide nanotubes	1-100
	Fusion proteins and immunotoxins	3-15
Metal nano-structs	Metal colloids	1-50
	Carbon nanotubes	1-10 (diameter)
	Fullerene	1-1000 (length)
	Gold nanoparticles	1-10
	Gold nanoshells	100-200
	Silicone nanoparticles	10-130
	Magnetic colloids	100-600

6.1 NANOPARTICLES

Nanoparticles are solid colloidal particles with diameters ranging from 1-1000 nm. They comprise of macromolecular constituents and can be used as an adjuvant in vaccines or drug carriers, in which the active ingredient is dissolved, entrapped, encapsulated, adsorbed or chemically attached. Polymers originated from natural or synthetic sources both are successfully utilized for nanoparticles preparation. Depending on the preparation process nanoparticles are categorized as: nanospheres and nanocapsules. Nanospheres have a monolithic-type structure (compact matrix) in which drugs are dispersed or adsorbed on the surface **(Figure 6.1 (a))**. Nanocapsules having hollow space due to a membranous structure and drugs are entrapped in the core or adsorbed exteriorly **(Figure 6.1 (b))**.The term "nanoparticles" is adopted commonly to represent both of them.

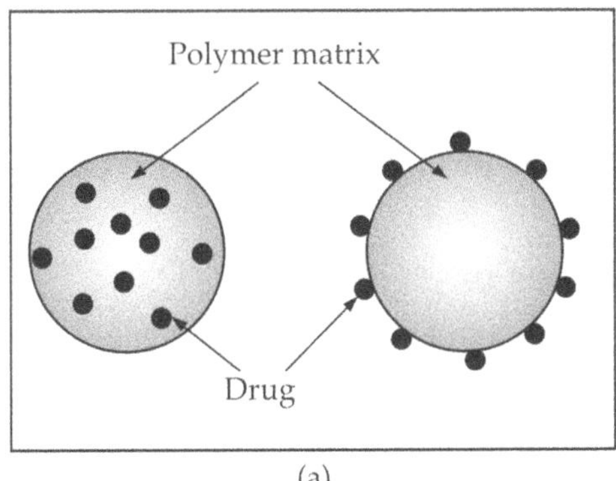

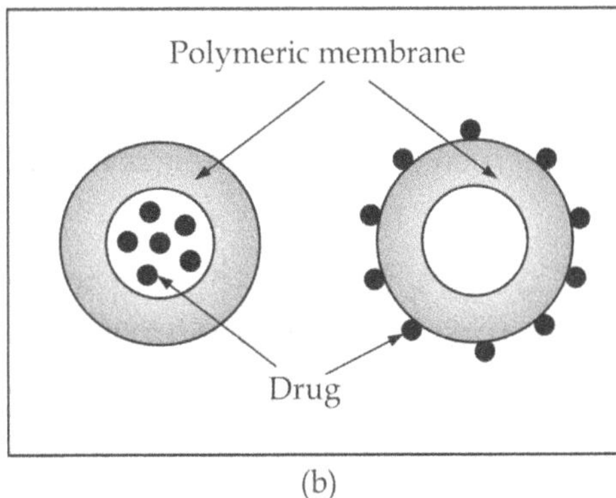

Figure 6.1 (a) Nanospheres (b) Nanocapsules

The evolution of bioadhesive materials for drug delivery purpose revolutionized the scope of nanoparticles as drug carriers. Bioadhesive nanoparticles have a tendency to adhere to the epithelial surfaces resulting in prolonged residence time at the site of absorption. This will commands the elimination at a much slower rate in comparison to conventional formulations, thus the bioavailability of drug be likely to augment. As a consequence, nanoparticles have been developed for targeted drug delivery of various therapeutic agents such as anti-inflammatory, anti-allergic and beta-blocker drugs. The uses of bioadhesive nanoparticles are immense and there are sufficient evidences that these nanoparticles display distinct characteristics from the microcrystalline structures. There is no drug delivery system where the nanoparticles are not being investigated and explored to find the advantages of their incorporation to improve the desired characteristics.

6.1.1 Advantages of Bioadhesive Nanoparticles

- Particle size and surface characteristics of nanoparticles can be easily manipulated to achieve both passive and active drug targeting.

- Controlled/sustained release of drug throughout the transportation and at the site of localization which alters organ distribution of the drug and subsequent drug clearance so as to achieve increased therapeutic efficacy with reduction in side effects.

- Controlled release and particle degradation characteristics can substantially regulated by the choice of polymers.

- Relatively high loading capacity and drug can be incorporated into the system without any chemical reaction; this is an important factor for preserving the drug activity.

- Capable of site specific targeting by surface modification i.e. attachment of targeting ligands or magnetic assistance.

- Administered via various routes including oral, nasal, parenteral and intraocular etc.

6.1.2 Factors Influencing Characteristics of Bioadhesive Nanoparticles

The various properties of different materials incorporated in the formulation i.e. nature of bioadhesive polymer (ionic, nonionic or neutral), composition of the bioadhesive polymer, solubility of the bioadhesive polymer etc., are the important factors which influence the characteristics of bioadhesive nanoparticles.

6.1.1.1 Composition of bioadhesive polymer

In addition to the properties of drug the physicochemical properties of the bioadhesive polymer also influence the preparation and characteristics of bioadhesive nanoparticles. The source of origin of bioadhesive polymer directs its composition and significantly influences the preparation and properties of nanoparticles. Commonly, polymers are composed of fractions of different molecular weight and number of these fractions is not uniform for every batch. This batch-to-batch variation also affects the characteristics of nanoparticles. For example, free thiol groups in HSA undergo oxidation in order to form dimers. Langer et al. studied the influence of dimers and higher aggregates of HSA on the preparation of albumin nanoparticles. They concluded that the batches with higher molecular weight fractions give rise to nanoparticles with larger particle size and higher polydispersity.

6.1.1.2 Polymer solubility

The method of preparation and characteristics of nanoparticles are markedly influenced by the solubility of polymer in aqueous or organic solvents. Nanoparticles are prepared by utilizing the differential solubility of the polymers in aqueous and non-aqueous solvents, as polymers can fold or unfold depending on the polarity of the solvent. Polymers exhibit pH-dependent water solubility based on their isoelectric point (pI). The pH value of the aqueous solution was found to have a significant influence on the size of the albumin nanoparticles. Particle size decreased with increasing pH above the pI of albumin (pI = 5.05). At a pH away from the pI, the hydrophobic interactions in the polymer are reduced, resulting in lesser aggregation.

6.1.1.3 Surface properties

One of the major advantages of polymers is the existence of various functional groups on the surface which can be utilized for the nanoparticle surface modification to alter their biodistribution or biocompatibility or drug loading and/or to improve enzymatic stability **(Figure 6.2)**. Particle size and surface properties of polymer nanoparticles depend on the number of bonding sites, number of functional groups, degree of unfolding, electrostatic repulsion among polymer molecules, pH and ionic strength. The conformational changes in a polymer (i.e., unfolding of polymer structure) reveal its active interaction sites/functional groups such as amine, carboxyl, and thiol groups. These active groups present on the surface can be cross-linked using cross-linking agents such as glutaraldehyde. Cross-linking assists the control of drug release from nanoparticles and also provides stabilization against proteolytic breakdown. An increase in the concentration of cross-linking agent generally decreases the particle size of nanoparticles due to the formation of denser particles. Protonation or deprotonation of the surface groups can influence the degree of cross-linking.

The surface functional groups can also be used for the drug loading by electrostatic interaction. Surface modified nanoparticles can be functionalized to respond to various stimuli such as pH, temperature etc. Thermo-responsive albumin nanoparticles were prepared by conjugating poly (N-isopropylacrylamide-co-acrylamide)-block-polyallylamine (PAN) on the surface carboxyl groups in albumin. Similarly, ligands have been attached to the surface of nanoparticles for drug targeting to specific tissues in the body. The surface functional groups of polymer can also directly interact with the biological membrane. Bioadhesiveness of Gliadin nanoparticles in the intestinal region have been reported, where hydrogen bonding and hydrophobic interactions between surface amino acids and intestinal membrane were involved.

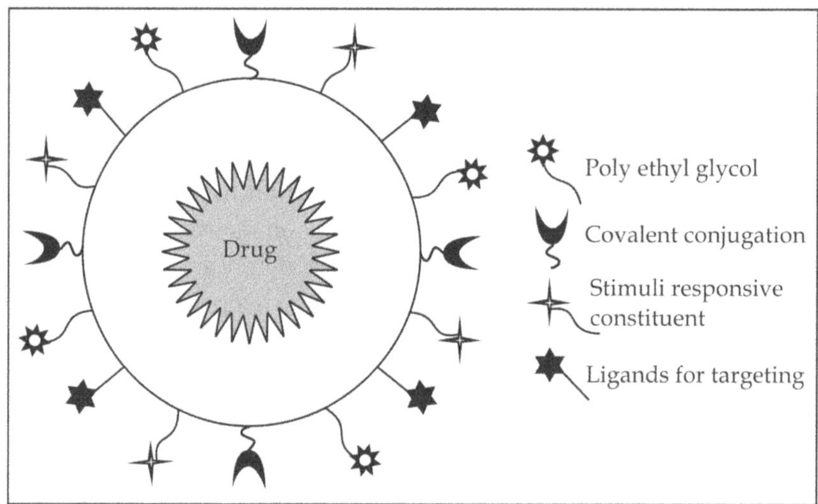

Figure 6.2 Schematic representation of surface modification of nanoparticles

6.1.1.4 Drug properties

Loading capacity of nanoparticles is markedly influenced by the physicochemical properties of the drug, such as solubility, log P and molecular weight. The loading of drugs in nanoparticles can be achieved by encapsulation or by the interaction of drug with polymer through covalent or non-covalent interactions. Extremely hydrophobic drugs have been found to interact with cysteine residues present in protein polymers by means of hydrophobic interactions. Numbers of hydrophobic drugs are known to bind to serum albumin and hence albumin appears to be a promising carrier. For example, paclitaxel a highly hydrophobic drug is loaded in albumin nanoparticles by mixing albumin and paclitaxel in a high pressure homogenizer. Gelatin offers higher encapsulation efficiency for hydrophilic drugs in comparison to hydrophobic drugs. Doxorubicin was adsorbed onto gelatin coated iron oxide nanoparticles for targeting using magnetic field. It was found that the adsorption of cationic doxorubicin onto gelatin nanoparticles increased with increasing pH owing to the negative charge of gelatin at higher pH. Some researchers studied the release of drugs of varying polarity from gliadin nanoparticles and found that hydrophobic drugs are released slowly because of their higher affinity to hydrophobic gliadin. On the other hand, hydrophilic drugs showed a burst release followed by slower drug diffusion from the nanoparticle matrix. The release of hydrophilic drugs from nanoparticles followed zero order kinetics, whereas hydrophobic drugs were released by pseudo zero-order kinetics.

6.2 METHODS OF PREPARATION

Different techniques for the preparation of nanoparticles with desired size range and good entrapment efficiency are available depending on the physicochemical properties of drugs and polymers. The drug-loaded nanospheres or nanocapsules can be prepared by simple, safe and reproducible techniques. The selection of method for the preparation of nanoparticles is based on three aspects:

- Need for less toxic reagent

- Simplification of the procedure to allow economic scale-up and

- Optimization to improve yield and entrapment efficiency

Nanoparticles preparation is based on attractive and repulsive forces balancing in the polymer. Generally increase in polymer unfolding and decrease in intramolecular hydrophobic interactions believed critical factors for nanoparticles formation. The polymer undergoes conformational changes during nanoparticles formation which depends up on composition, concentration, formulation parameters, and method of crosslinking. Nanoparticles of water insoluble polymers require surfactants to stabilize the formulation. There are numerous techniques for the preparation of nanoparticles which are given **(Table 6.3)**.

Owing to the several restrictions including post operative steps like purification, preservation, discontinuous or incomplete film, poor stability of substances face numerous challenges to select best fit single process or technique applicable for all drugs. In spite of these challenges has proven great potential for preparation of bioadhesive systems.

Table 6.3 Methods for the preparation of nanoparticles

Polymerization based methods
• Emulsion polymerization • Mini-emulsion polymerization • Micro-emulsion polymerization • Interfacial polymerization • Controlled/living radical polymerization (C/LRP)
Dispersion based methods
• Solvent evaporation • Nanoprecipitation • Emulsification/ Solvent diffusion • Salting out • Dialysis • Supercritical fluid technology (SCF)
Coacervation or ionic gelation of hydrophilic polymers

6.2.1 Polymerization based Methods for the Preparation of Nanoparticles

The formulation of polymer nanoparticles with pre-requisite characteristics can be achieved suitably when the monomers combine together to produce the polymers. Various methodologies that are used in the fabrication of nanoparticles are as follows:

6.2.1.1 Emulsion polymerization

It is one of the primitive methods, utilizing protective colloids or surfactants to prevent aggregation. Emulsion polymerization is simple and readily accessible method for the formulation of nanoparticles and can be classified as aqueous or organic depending upon the nature and type of the continuous phase/medium. When organic phase is used as the continuous media, then the monomer is dispersed as emulsion or inverse microemulsion, or any non solvent for the monomer (e.g. polyamide nanospheres). This procedure is now rarely used due to the involvement of toxic organic solvents, non-biodegradable monomers, surface active agents and initiators which needs to be removed from the final product. Newer polymers as poly (methamethacrylate) (PMMA), poly (ethylcyanoacrylate) (PECA) were used along with organic solvents as n-pentane, cyclohexane, toluene (ICH, Class 2, 3, and 2 respectively) to formulate nanoparticles.

The second method that utilizes aqueous media as the continuous phase eliminates the use of emulsifiers or surfactants and the monomer in such case is dissolved in it. Different mechanisms are used to initiate polymerization which may involve collision of monomer molecule with the initiator (generally an ion or a free radical) or transformation of monomer molecule may be done using high energy radiation (gamma, UV or strong visible light). This leads to chain growth as mentioned in anionic polymerization technique. The termination of the polymerization reaction may be preceeded or followed by the processes of phase separation and solid particle formation.

6.2.1.2 Mini-emulsion polymerization

This method has been found to be used quite frequently as per the reported literatures. Typically, it consists of monomer mixture along with surfactant, initiator and a suitable co-stabilizer with water. The basic difference between mini emulsion and polymerization method is the use of low molecular mass substance as co stabilizer and high shear device like ultra sound, as the mini emulsions exhibit stability related problems, hence to achieve a steady state high shear is required.

6.2.1.3 Microemulsion polymerization

It is a relatively new and effective way to prepare polymer nanoparticles and is advantageous over the other two techniques of emulsion and microemulsion polymerization, but differ kinetically. In this method, a water soluble polymer as initiator is added to the aqueous phase which consists of thermodynamically stable microemulsion of swollen micelle, from where the polymerization starts spontaneously and is dependent on the high quantities of the surfactant used. The surfactant, leads to an interfacial tension close to zero at the oil/water interface and completely covers the particles. Hence, the particle size and the average number of chains per particle are smaller. Polymer chains initiate in the some droplets and later the osmotic and elastic influence of chains, causes destabilization of the empty micelles, and leading to secondary nucleation. Latexes of size 5-50 nm coexists with the empty micelles in the final product. Thus, the formed product critically depends on the concentration of surfactant, monomer and initiator along with the reaction temperature.

6.2.1.4 Interfacial polymerization

Amongst the well established methods, the interfacial polymerization technique involve the polymerization of two species of reactive monomers dissolved in two phases as dispersed and continuous phase and the reaction takes place at the interface of the liquids. Interfacial cross-linking reactions like poly addition and poly condensation or radical polymerization were utilized to synthesize nanosized hollow polymer particles. Nanocapsules containing oil can be produced by monomers polymerization at the oil/water interface of a very o/w microemulsion. A totally water miscible organic solvent served as a monomer vehicle and monomer interfacial polymerization was supposed to occur at the surface of the oil droplets that produced during emulsification. The use of aprotic solvents like acetone and acetonitrile was suggested to encourage nanocapsule development while use of protic solvents like ethanol, n-butanol and isopropanol suggests nanosphere development. On the other hand nanocapsules containing water can be produced by the monomers polymerization at the w/o interface in w/o microemulsions and gets precipitated to form nanocapsule shell.

6.2.1.5 Controlled/living radical polymerization (C/LRP)

Radical polymerization use is limited due to lack of control over the molecular weight, molecular weight distribution, end functional groups and the macromolecular structural design. These limitations may be due to inevitable fast radical-radical termination reactions. The current innovation of controlled or living radical polymerization method has enlightened a new prospect. Factors that are associated with this method are incremented environmental concern and fast growth of pharmaceutical as well as medical applications for hydrophilic polymers. Owing to "green chemistry" which demands for environment friendly and chemically safe solvents like water and supercritical carbon dioxide. As a result, execution of C/LRP leads to development of polymeric nanoparticles with specific particle size as well as size distribution control in the industrially important aqueous dispersed systems. Various methods employed to study successfully C/LRP are as follows:

- Nitroxide-mediated polymerization (NMP)
- Atom transfer radical polymerization (ATRP)
- Reversible addition and fragmentation transfer chain polymerization (RAFT)

6.2.2 Dispersion based Methods for the Preparation of Nanoparticles

Drug dispersion in predeveloped polymers is a widespread procedure to develop biodegradable bioadhesive nanoparticles. It is done usually with application of poly (lactic acid), poly (D, L-glycolide), poly (D, L-lactide-co-glycolide) and poly (cyanoacrylate) polymers. Nanoparticles preparation by this method can be achieved in following ways:

6.2.2.1 Solvent evaporation

In this method volatile solvents is utilized to prepare polymer solutions and emulsion can be formulated. Earlier chloroform and dichloromethane were used as solvents to prepare polymer solution but now they are replaced with ethyl acetate solvent having superior toxicity profile. Prepared emulsion can be transformed into a nanoparticles suspension after evaporation of the solvent from polymer. Conventionally two major techniques are available to produce emulsions as formation of single emulsions or double emulsions. These techniques employ high speed homogenization or ultrasonication then evaporation of solvent takes place either by continuous magnetic stirring at room temperature or under reduced pressure. Then solid nanoparticles can be collected by ultracentrifugation followed by washing with distilled water to eliminate excipients like surfactants. Lastly obtained product is lyophilized **(Figure 6.3)**.

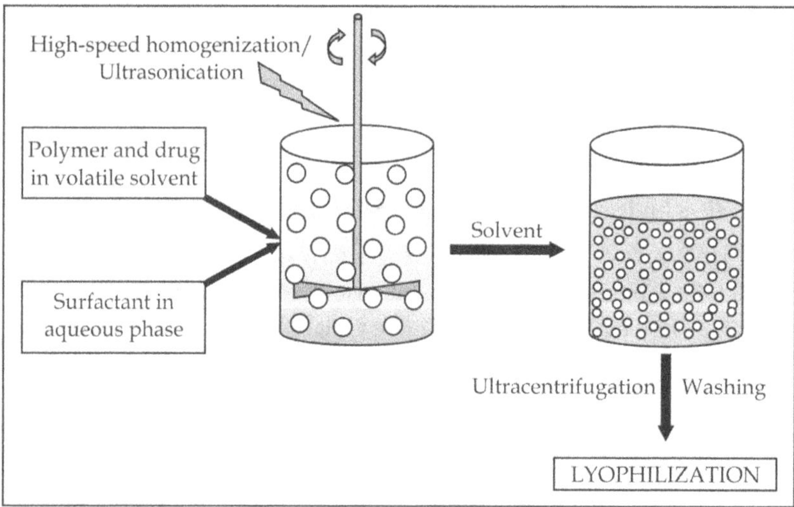

Figure 6.3 Schematic representation of solvent evaporation technique for nanoparticles preparation

6.2.2.2 Nanoprecipitation

In this method predeveloped polymer gets precipitated from an organic solution and organic solvent diffusion in the aqueous media in the presence or absence of surfactant takes place. This method is also recognized as solvent displacement method. Usually a water miscible solvent of intermediate polarity is taken to dissolve polymer which may lead to the precipitation of nanospheres. Polymer phase is injected into a stirred aqueous solution with stabilizer. Polymer gets deposited on the interface formed between water and organic solvent due to fast diffusion of the solvent and may cause formation of a colloidal suspension **(Figure 6.4)**. Phase separation is carried out with a completely miscible solvent which is a non-solvent of the polymer to facilitate the colloidal polymer particles formation during the initial stage of the procedure. When a small amount of non-toxic oil is included in the organic phase the solvent displacement method allows the formation of nanocapsules. Nanocapsule with oily central cavity greater loading capacity is reported for lipophilic drugs. The utility of this technique is limited to water miscible solvents in which the diffusion rate is sufficient to cause instant emulsification.

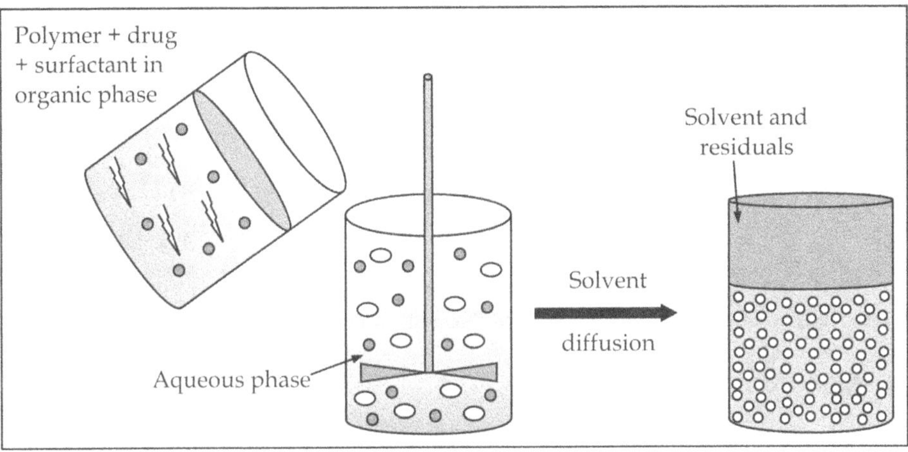

Figure 6.4 Schematic representation of nanoprecipitation technique for nanoparticles preparation

6.2.2.3 Emulsification/solvent diffusion (ESD)

ESD is a modified form of solvent evaporation process in which partially water soluble solvent like propylene carbonate is used to dissolve encapsulating polymer. This is further saturated with water to make sure the early thermodynamic equilibrium of both liquids. It is essential to encourage the diffusion of the dispersed phase solvent with an excess of aqueous phase when the organic phase is partially miscible with aqueous phase or with another organic phase in contrary to cause polymer precipitation and consequent nanoparticles development. Lastly according to the boiling point solvent is eliminated either by evaporation or filtration **(Figure 6.5)**. Advantages possess by this technique includes greater entrapment efficiency (usually > 70%), no requirement for homogenization, simple, ease of preparation, batch-to-batch reproducibility with narrow size distribution. In spite of such advantages certain limitations associated with this process are high volume of water that is to be eliminated from the suspension and water soluble drug leakage into the saturated aqueous external phase during emulsification. Various drug incorporated nanoparticles has been reported by ESD technique includes mesotetra-(hydroxyphenyl)-porphyrin, doxorubicin, plasmid DNA, coumarin, indocyanine, cyclosporine, sodium glycolate.

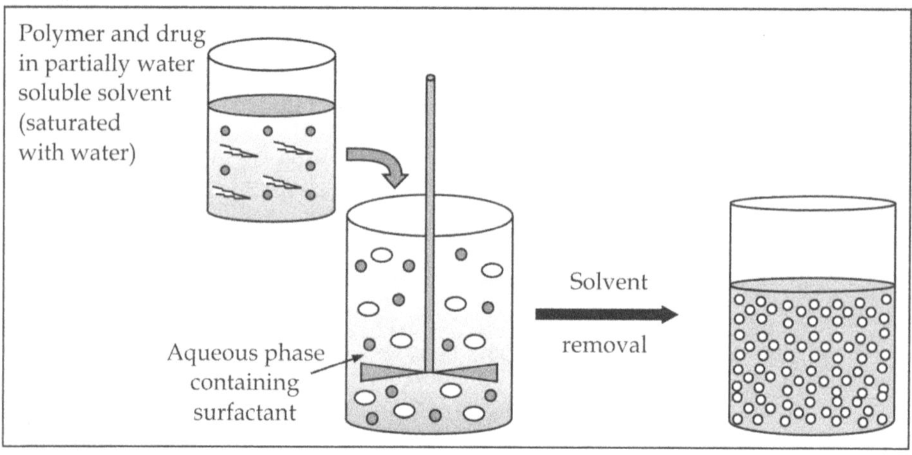

Figure 6.5 Schematic representation of ESD technique for nanoparticles preparation

6.2.2.4 Salting out

This method is based on the separation of water miscible solvent form aqueous solution. It is considered to be modification of emulsification/solvent diffusion method. Method involves dissolution of drug and polymer in a solvent like acetone followed by emulsification into an aqueous gel incorporating salting out agents (may be electrolytes like magnesium chloride, calcium chloride, magnesium acetate or non-electrolytes like sucrose) and stabilizer like polyvinyl pyrrolidone or hydroxyl ethyl cellulose and lead to the formation of oil/water type emulsion. This emulsion is further diluted with appropriate volume of aqueous solution to increase the diffusion of organic solvent into the aqueous phase and cause formation of nanospheres **(Figure 6.6)**. Salting out substances selection is important because encapsulation efficiency of the drug may be affected by it. It has been used to prepare nanospheres of PLA, poly-methacrylic acid with improved efficacy and easy scale up. The benefit of this method is less stress to encapsulation of protein materials and suitable for heat sensitive materials as it does not need an increase in temperature. The limitation of this technique is limited to lipophilic drugs only and requires extensive washing steps during nanoparticles preparation.

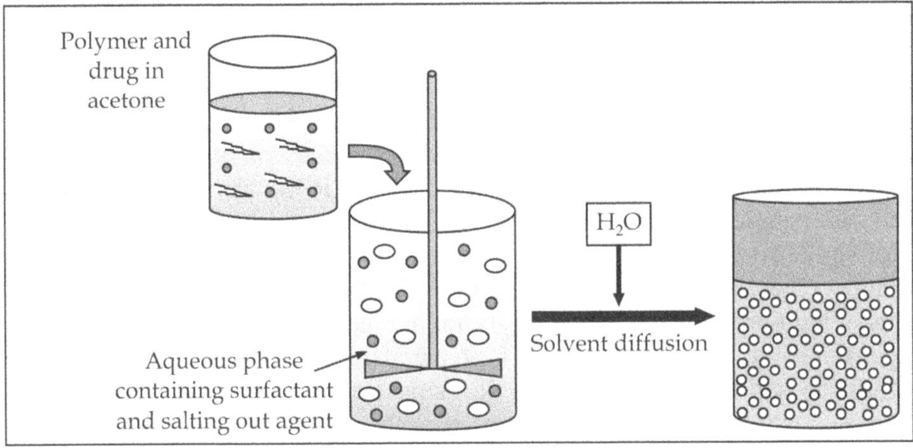

Figure 6.6 Schematic representation of salting out technique for nanoparticles preparation

6.2.2.5 Dialysis

This is very simple and efficient method for the development of small uniformly distributed nanoparticles. Dialysis tube with appropriate molecular weight cut off is taken and polymer solution prepared in organic solvent is placed in it. Then dialysis is done against a non-solvent miscible with previous one. Formation of homogeneous nanoparticles suspension takes place due to displacement of the solvent inside the membrane that is followed by polymer aggregation. The mechanism of dialysis method for nanoparticles formation is not very much clear rather believed to similar of nanoprecipitation. This technique was applied to get various polymer and copolymer nanoparticles. Various natural and synthetic polymer based nanoparticles were reported by novel osmosis based method that is based on the use of a physical barrier, usually dialysis membrane or common semi- permeable membranes. This membrane contains the polymer solution and allow the passive transport of solvents to slow down the mixing of the polymer solution with a non-solvent.

6.2.2.6 Supercritical fluid technology (SCF)

An urgent need of environment friendly method leads to the development of supercritical fluid technology method for the development of polymeric nanoparticulate system. This method possesses the potential to develop nanoparticles with highest purity and without organic solvent traces. SCF offers an innovative and interesting technique for nanoparticles production along with avoidance of conventional techniques drawbacks. SCF involves two concepts basically developed for the nanoparticles production which are as follows:

(a)   Rapid expansion of supercritical solution (RESS)

(b)   Rapid expansion of supercritical solution into liquid solvent (RESOLV)

(a) ***Rapid expansion of supercritical solution (RESS):*** RESS involves formation of solution after dissolution of solute in a supercritical fluid than rapid extension of the solution across an orifice or a capillary nozzle in to ambient air **(Figure 6.7)**. A high degree of super-saturation with rapid pressure reduction in the expansion cause homogenous nucleation and results the development of well-dispersed particles. Studies carried out using various model solutes for RESS showed that micrometer as well as nanometer sized particles were present in the expansion jet. Poly (perfluoropolyetherdiamide) droplets were reported using rapid expansion of CO_2 solution. The experimental apparatus used for RESS comprised of following three units: a high-pressure stainless steel mixing cell, a syringe pump, and a pre-expansion unit. Polymer solution is prepared in CO_2 at ambient temperature and before the solution leaves the nozzle using syringe pump, it is pumped to pre-expansion unit. This is heated isobarically to the pre-expansion temperature and now supercritical solution is allowed to expand through the nozzle at ambient pressure. Particle size and morphology of the particles produced by RESS is affected by concentration and degree of saturation of the polymer.

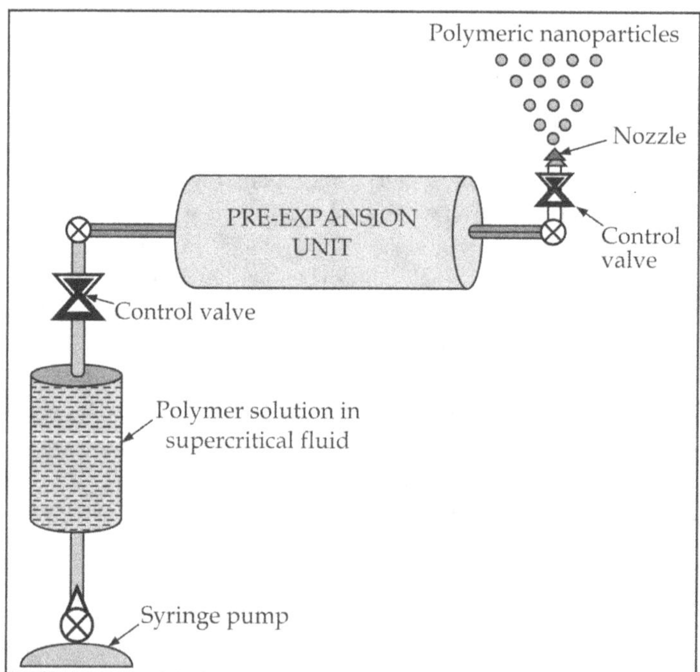

Figure 6.7 Schematic representation of RESS technique for nanoparticles preparation

(b) ***Rapid expansion of supercritical solution into liquid solvent (RESOLV):*** This method simply involves alteration to RESS with extension of the supercritical solution into a liquid solvent rather than ambient air known as RESOLV

(Figure 6.8). Development of Polyhepta decafluorodecyl acrylate nanoparticles has been reported with an average size of < 50 nm. The main drawback associated with RESS is the development of micro sized product rather than nanosized products which can be overcome with the new technique of SCF known as RESOLV. RESOLV causes suppression of particle growth in the expansion jet by liquid solvent and make possible to get nanosized particles.

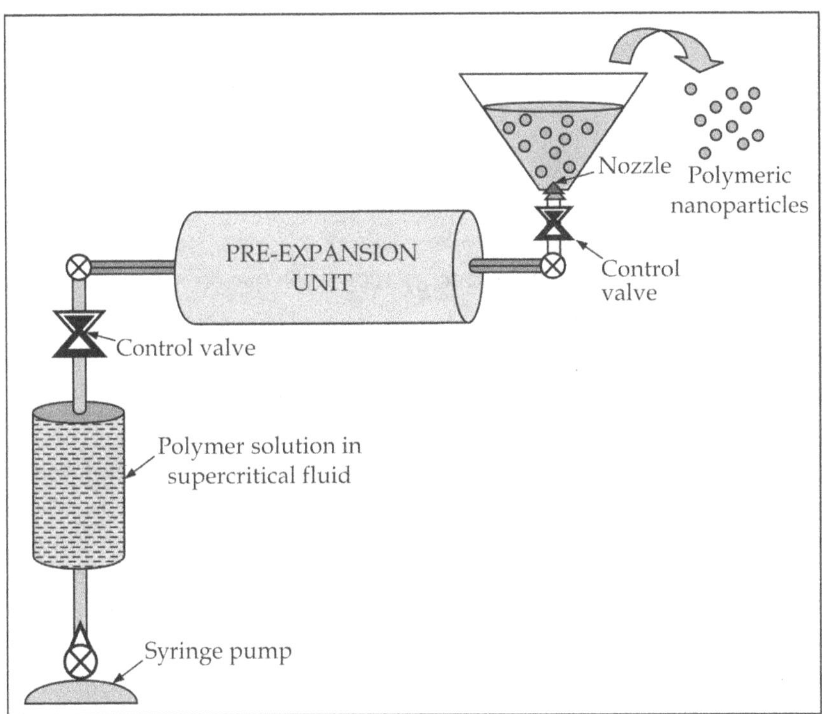

Figure 6.8 Schematic representation of RESOLV technique for nanoparticles preparation

6.2.3 Ionic Gelation or Coacervation of Hydrophilic Polymers

Biodegradable hydrophilic polymers like chitosan, gelatin and sodium alginate are used to prepare bioadhesive nanoparticles. Ionic gelation method was used to formulate Dexamethasone sodium phosphate containing chitosan nanoparticles **(Figure 6.9)**. This method utilizes mixture of two aqueous phases including chitosan polymer, a di-block copolymer ethylene oxide or propylene oxide (PEO-PPO) and poly anion sodium tripolyphosphate. This method results formation of nanosized coacervate after interaction of amino group of chitosan (+ charge) and tripolyphosphate (− charge). Ionic gelation results transition from liquid to gel because of ionic interaction at room temperature.

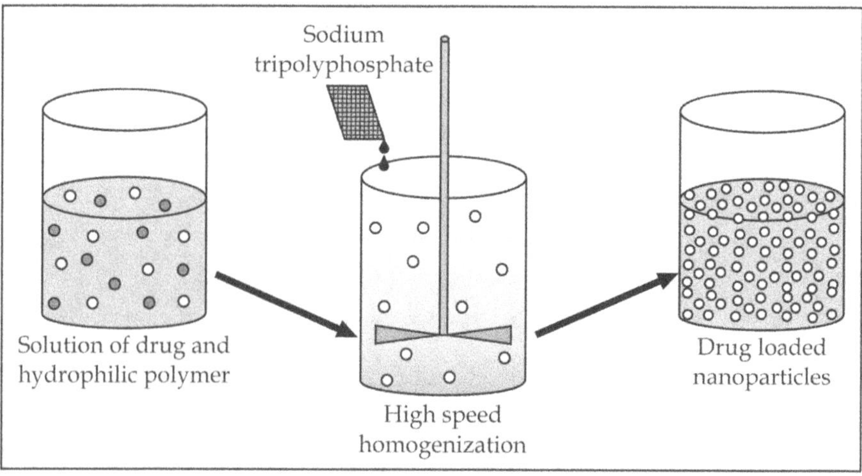

Figure 6.9 Schematic representation of ionic gelation technique for nanoparticles preparation

6.3 PROTEIN STABILIZED NANOPARTICLES

Several researchers have utilized protein as stabilizer because of its complete compatibility with even the injectable formulations. This process of protein stabilization is illustrated in **Figure 6.10** for producing protein stabilized drug loaded nanoparticles. The choice of organic solvent and the extent of homogenization can be used to further tailor the nanoparticle size. A variation of the process is also developed, in which the aqueous phase was presaturated with the organic solvent and a small amount of ethanol was added to the organic phase. In this variation, smaller nanoparticles of 140-160 nm are obtained. The advantage with nanoparticles smaller than 200 nm is that they can be easily sterilized by filtering with standard 0.22 mm filter. Thus, the whole process can be carried out in a sterile environment and the sterilization can be done just before the lyophilization step. To form a solid and stable layer of albumin onto drug nanoparticles, the protein needs to be cross-linked (or denatured) onto the particle surface. Typically, protein crosslinking can be achieved by heat, use of cross-linker such as glutaraldehyde or high shear. Fortunately, in the emulsification, solvent evaporation process high shear is already in use, hence it can also be used for cross-linking protein stabilizers. High-shear cross-linking works for the protein-bearing sulfhydryl or disulfide groups (e.g. albumin). The high-shear conditions produce cavitation in the liquid, which causes tremendous local heating and results in the formation of hydroxyl radicals that are capable of cross-linking the polymer, for example, by oxidizing the sulfhydryl residues (and/or disrupting the existing disulfide bonds) to form new, cross-linking disulfide bonds.

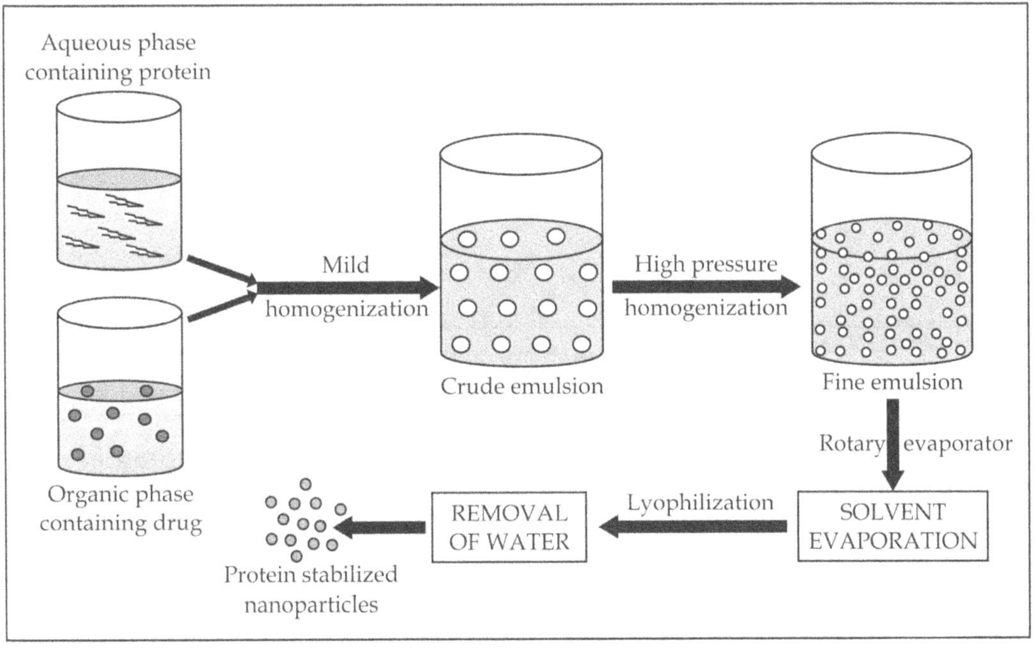

Figure 6.10 Schematic representation of protein stabilized nanoparticles preparation

6.3.1 Biological Characteristics of Protein Nanoparticles

6.3.1.1 Biocompatibility

Nanoparticles performance biologically determined through opsonization and particles clearance by mononuclear phagocytic system (MPS) or the reticuloendothelial system (RES). Process utilized in the opsonization and particles clearance from the blood is presented in **Figure 6.11**. In the opsonization process foreign particle or organism is sheltered with the protein called opsonin.

Generally albumin, fibrinogen are found to be dominating on the surface of the particle but afterward displaced by greater affinity proteins like immunoglobulins (IgG & IgM), fibronectin, laminin, C-reactive protein and type-I collagen. Particles uptake by immune system cells and their interaction with blood components determined by these bound proteins.

Opsonization may complete within few seconds to many days. Binding of opsonins to nanoparticles involves the use of Vander walls, electrostatic and hydrophobic/hydrophilic forces. Nanoparticles surface properties like charge, composition, hydrophobicity, preparation method affects the opsonin adsorption to their design and development of protein based response and T-cells activated response.

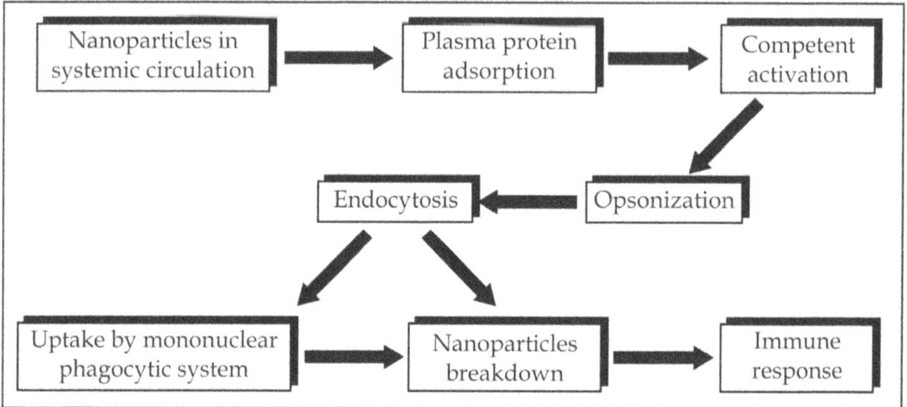

Figure 6.11 Opsonization and clearance of nanoparticles from systemic circulation

Immune response can be induced by biologically important substances that can act as antigens like proteins, sugars, lipids and nucleic acids. Humoral type of response to above substances may be T-cell dependent or independent. Generally proteins that are processed and presented by antigen presenting cells (APCs) to T cells through major histocompatibility complex (MHC) are T-cell dependent antigens. Then antibodies are formed against these antigens from antigen specific B cells that are helped by antigen activated T-cells. Immune stimulation or suppression characteristics of protein nanoparticles are affected by variety of factors.

6.3.1.2 Biodegradation

Biodegradability of protein polymers is one of the important advantages and it is affected by protein physicochemical properties. Hence it is necessary to analyze the impact of proteolytic enzymes on release characteristics from nanoparticles of protein. The degradation of human serum albumin (HSA) in presence of different enzymes was studied by researchers. In presence of various enzymes extent of cross-linking affected the stability of HSA. An increase in cross-linking may lead to decline in the enzymatic degradation of nanoparticles since enzymes face difficulty to penetrate into cross-linked particles. PEG chains attachment on gelatin nanoparticles surface provides slow release with greater proteolytic stability. PEG coating or PEGylation cause steric repulsion from proteolytic degradation for protein matrix.

6.3.2 Biodistribution and Applications

Protein nanoparticles of various therapeutic agents are developed with different size ranges **(Table 6.4)**. The smaller particles (< 500 nm) are generally accepted for systemic applications as they can avoid RES uptake and cause long circulation. For solid tumors smaller nanoparticles may easily extravasate through the leaky vasculature. It is generally found that tumor vascular pore size varies from 200 to 600 nm and explored for nanoparticles passive targeting to tumors. Moreover larger molecules are retained because of the poor lymphatic drainage when they reach the tumor interstitium. A further level of targeting can be achieved by attaching targeting ligands to the nanoparticles.

Table 6.4 Examples of protein polymers used for nanoparticulate delivery systems

Protein polymer	Drug	Particle size (nm)
Human serum albumin	Ganciclovir	200-300
	Paclitaxel	130
	Loperamide, encapsulated targeting ligands: apolipoprotein A-1, B-1000 and E-3	218-240
Bovine serum albumin	Bone morphogenetic protein (BMP-2)	200-400
Gelatin	Doxorubicin	135-301
Casein	Curcumin	<200
Gliadin	Lectin conjugates	587±35
	Vitamin E	900
	Acetohydroxasamic acid	412±35
	Benzalkonium chloride, linalool, linalyl acetate	900-950
Zein	Essential oils	100

Long circulatory gelatin nanoparticles has been prepared after surface manipulation with PEG and also known as PEGylated nanoparticles. These PEGylated gelatin nanoparticles attained two times higher blood levels when compared to non-PEGylated nanoparticles. Enhanced tumor accumulation of gelatin nanoparticles was also achieved after PEGylation. When tumor half-life was compared it was six times higher in case of PEGylated than non-PEGylated nanoparticles.

Oral drug delivery can be improved by the use of Gliadin nanoparticles a bioadhesive system. In gliadin neutral amino acids are present that possibly through hydrogen bonding interact with the intestinal mucosa while through hydrophobic interactions lipophilic amino acids present in gliadin interact with mucus. Greater binding affinity to colonic mucosa is achieved through attachment of lectin to gliadin nanoparticles. Colon targeted system can be prepared by exploring such properties. Recently a new nanoparticulate-in-microsphere oral system (NiMOS) was developed by researchers for gene delivery to GIT. In this system gelatin nanoparticles was used encapsulating plasmid DNA followed by encapsulation in microspheres of polycaprolactone (PCL) **(Figure 6.12)**. This PCL layer protects nanoparticles in stomach from acidic and enzymatic degradation while release its contents in intestine by the action of lipases presents in it.

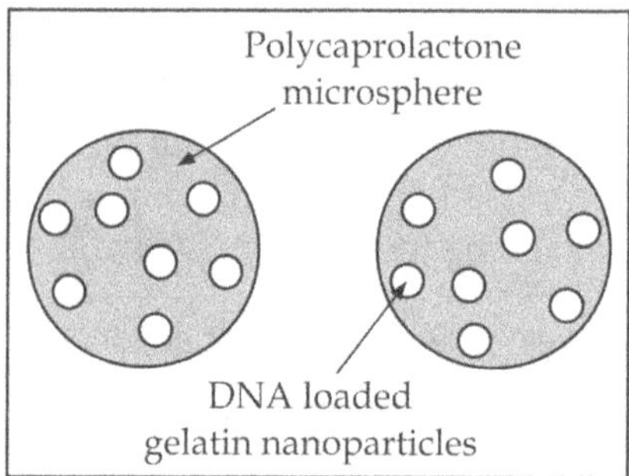

Figure 6.12 Schematic representation of nanoparticle-in-microsphere oral system (NiMOS)

6.4 DRUG LOADING

To be a successful nanoparticulate system it must have the ability of high drug loading. The drug loading can be imparted by two ways:

1. At the time of nanoparticles production (During procedure)
2. Incubation with preformed nanoparticles (Absorption/adsorption of drug)

Drug loading and entrapment efficiency is based on drug solubility in polymer or matrix material that is related with molecular weight of polymer, polymer composition, polymer drug interaction and existence of end functional groups. Generally PEG moiety has less or no effect on drug loading. When proteins or macromolecules are loaded at or near their isoelectric point they show highest loading capacity. Based on studies ionic interaction between matrix material and drug for small molecules could be very effective mode to improve the drug loading.

6.5 DRUG RELEASE

Drug release and biodegradation of polymer are considered as prominent factors for development of successful nanoparticulate system. Generally release rate of drug is affected by drug solubility, diffusion of drug through nanoparticle matrix, matrix erosion/degradation, desorption of surface bound or adsorbed drug, combination of erosion and diffusion process. Hence diffusion, solubility and biodegradation of matrix govern the release process.

Drug release in case of nanospheres occurs by diffusion or erosion of the matrix under sink conditions. When the drug diffusion is quicker than erosion of matrix then release is largely governed by a diffusion process. Instant release or burst release is mainly ascribed to weakly bound or adsorbed drug to the nanoparticles surface. It is striking that the method of incorporation has an impact on release profile. If loading of the drug is done by incorporation method then system has a relatively lesser burst effect and greater sustained release properties. When the nanoparticles are coated by polymer then release is governed by drug diffusion from the core across the polymeric membrane. This membrane coating acts as a barrier for release, therefore the solubility and diffusivity of drug in polymer membrane becomes decisive factor in drug release. Additionally the ionic interaction between the drug and auxiliary ingredients can also affect the release rate.

In-vitro drug release can be studied by various methods which are as follows:

1. side-by-side diffusion cells with artificial or biological membranes;
2. dialysis bag diffusion technique;
3. reverse dialysis bag technique;
4. agitation followed by ultracentrifugation/centrifugation;
5. Ultra-filtration or centrifugal ultra-filtration techniques.

6.6 CHARACTERIZATION OF BIOADHESIVE NANOPARTICLES

The bioadhesive nanoparticles are generally characterized for size, surface morphology, specific surface area, surface charge, surface hydrophobicity, entrapment efficiency, density, electrophoretic mobility and angle of contact.

6.6.1 Size and Surface Morphology

The size of the nanoparticles is most important parameter as it decides the compatibility with delivery routes and their therapeutic efficiency. The particle size of nanosized particulates of sub-optical range depends on the surface associated properties and the variability due to the method of preparation which may even change during sizing procedure. The size distribution of the nanoparticles can be determined by two main techniques which involves the principles of electron microscopy and photon correlation spectroscopy. The electron microscopy method includes transmission electron microscopy (TEM), scanning electron microscopy (SEM) and freeze fracture methods. For quantitative purposes photon correlation spectroscopy and freeze fracture microscopy are preferred due to the better results.

In freeze fracture microscopy the sample dispersion of nanoparticles is confronted with poly (methyl methacrylate) and interrupted by in process particle aggregation which results into only a few discrete particles for size distribution analysis. With this method morphological characterization of internal structure is also possible. The electron microscopy methods are the alternative methods in which size measurement of individual particles give better information about the size distribution with less time consumption. For the differentiation between nanocapsules, nanospheres and emulsion droplets TEM is effectively used. SEM is much less time consuming comparatively but as the nanoparticles are composed of organic materials which are non-conductive, gold coating is required. This gold coating varies from 30-50 nm in thickness. Therefore the size of the nanoparticles by this method includes the additional thickness of gold coating.

Another advanced microscopic method, Atomic force microscopy (AFM) is effectively utilized for the characterization of solid lipid nanoparticles (SLN) and PLA nanospheres. As the aqueous medium is employed in AFM for the analysis, this method is effective for the analysis of nanoparticulate behavior in biological fluids.

6.6.2 Surface Charge and Electrophoretic Mobility

The interaction of nanoparticles with biological components is greatly depends on the nature and intensity of surface charge. The surface charge of nanoparticles can be determined by the measurement of particle velocity in an electric field. The techniques based on laser light scattering like Laser Doppler Anemometry or Velocimetry are effective methods which allows fast and high-resolution measurement of velocities of nanoparticles.

The surface charge of nanoparticulates could also be determined in terms of electrophoretic mobility. For the measurement of electrophoretic mobility the removal of residual surfactant and free drug adherent or solubilized in aqueous phase is required before the measurement. This can be done by repeated washing with centrifugation however it may lead to aggregation. Nevertheless, the aggregation of nanoparticles favored the measurement of electrophoretic mobility as aggregation contributes to well visible bands. The aggregated bands of nanoparticulates are visualized distinctively.

Commonly, phosphate saline buffer (pH 7.4) is used for the measurement of electrophoretic mobility of nanoparticulates which relatively reduces the absolute charge due to ionic interaction between buffer components and charged surface of nanoparticles. Zeta potential is also determined from electrophoretic mobility with the help of Helmholtz-Smoluchowski equation. In a steady Poiseuille flow through a capillary channel, a relation between the ratio of streaming potential difference (ΔE) to pressure gradient (ΔP) and the zeta potential (ς) is described by the equation:

$$\frac{\Delta E}{\Delta P} = \frac{\varepsilon \varsigma}{\mu \lambda_0 + \lambda_s / R}$$

where, λ_0 is the electrolyte conductivity,

λ_s is the specific surface conductivity,

ε is the dielectric constant,

μ is the viscosity of electrolyte solution, and

R is the capillary radius.

6.6.3 Specific Surface Area

Generally, Sorptometer is utilized for the measurement of specific surface area of freeze dried nanoparticles. The specific surface area can also be calculated by the following formula:

$$A = \frac{6}{\partial.d}$$

where, A = specific surface area,

∂ = density and

d = diameter

In most cases, calculated and measured specific surface areas are approximately same but sometimes there is a deviation in measured values due to the presence of residual surfactants. It appears that the specific surface area is reduced owing to surfactant coating.

6.6.4 Surface Hydrophobicity

This property has great impact on the interaction of nanoparticles with the biological environment (e.g. cell adhesion and protein adsorption). The bio-fate of nanoparticles and their contents can be determined collectively by hydrophobicity and hydrophilicity. The extent and the type of hydrophobic interaction of nanoparticles with blood components are mainly regulated by hydrophobicity. Surface hydrophobicity can be evaluated by several methods including hydrophobic interaction chromatography, two-phase partition, adsorption of hydrophobic fluorescent or radiolabelled probes and contact angle measurements. The measurement of angle of contact suggests about the hydrophobicity or hydrophilicity of the nanoparticles. The water contact angle is measured only on plain surface hence nanoparticles are compressed as tablet/pellet. Effect of blood components on resultant *in-vivo* hydrophilicity or hydrophobicity can be studied by incubation of the particles with blood serum followed by centrifugation and lyophilization. Collected dried nanoparticles are compressed then angle of contact with water can be determined. The serum component decreased the contact angle by 20^0. This suggests that the drug components are adsorbed strongly and affect subsequent wettability characteristics of the nanoparticulates. Currently various methods for analysis of surface chemistry have been used like X-ray photoelectron spectroscopy (XPS) allows the identification of specific chemical group presents on the surface of nanoparticles.

6.6.5 Density

In addition to SEM, TEM following freeze fracture microscopy could successfully be used in morphological investigation of nanoparticulates. The interiors are continuous or some structural imperfections exists that gives an idea related to density distribution across the matrix. Some polymeric nanoparticles especially polycynoacrylate and poly (methyl methacrylate) seem to have porous interior and they also exhibit more irregular and rough surface. The density of nanoparticulates is determined with helium or air using gas pycnometer. The value may differ from each other as obtained with air and with helium. The difference is much more pronounced due to specific surface area and the porosity of the structure.

6.6.6 Entrapment Efficiency and Nanoparticle Recovery

The nanoparticle recovery, which is also referred to as nanoparticle yield in the literatures, can be calculated using following equation:

$$\text{Nanopaticle Recovery (\%)} = \frac{\text{Mass of nanoparticles recorvered}}{\text{Mass of nanoparticles, drug and added excipients}} \times 100$$

Drug entrapment efficiency has been expressed as drug content, which is also referred as drug loading in literatures and drug incorporation efficiency, represented by following equation:

$$\text{Entapment efficiency (\%)} = \frac{\text{Conc. of drug in nanoparticles}}{\text{Conc. of drug added}} \times 100$$

6.6.7 *In-vitro* Release

This can be estimated using standard dialysis, diffusion cell or recently introduced modified ultrafiltration technique. Nanoparticles *in-vitro* drug release can be determined in phosphate buffer utilizing double chamber diffusion cells on a shaker stand. A Millipore hydrophilic low-protein binding membrane is situated between the donor chamber and receptor chambers. The donor and receptor chambers are filled with nanoparticles suspension and plain buffer respectively. Drug release from the receptor compartment is analyzed at different time intervals using standard methods.

In-vitro release behavior of the nanoparticles by modified ultrafiltration technique is reported by Magenheim and coworkers. In ultrafiltration cell containing buffer direct addition of nanoparticles suspension is done and aliquots of dissolution medium at different time intervals are filtered to the ultrafiltration membrane using less than two bar positive nitrogen pressure and analyzed for the drug release using standard methods.

6.7 APPLICATIONS

Liposomes probably the first nanoparticulate system when discovered gave the several breakthrough discoveries employing nanoparticles as drug delivery system. Several applications have been reported by researchers using nanoparticulate drug delivery system. Some major or important applications are discussed below:

6.7.1 Cancer Therapy

Drugs that do not cross the blood brain barrier (BBB) causes insufficient drug delivery across it and lead to ineffective brain chemotherapy. Poly (butyl cyanoacrylate) nanoparticles coated with polysorbate-80 has been explored for effective brain targeting with potential of BBB crossing. Albumin nanoparticles covalently bonded with apolipoprotein A-I and apolipoprotein B-100 has been also utilized for brain delivery. For cancer therapy injectable drug delivery nano-vectors are also used when multiple drug therapy is used. To evade the body defense these vectors must be large enough but they should be sufficiently small also to avoid blockages in the capillaries. Size plays major role in capillary blockage. The blockages can be efficiently prevented as these vectors are smaller than the capillary diameters.

Nano vectors can be used for anticancer drugs and they can also be functionalized in order to bind with specific sites and cells after extravasation through ligand-receptor interactions. Sometimes surface markers are overexpressed on target cells to maximize the specificity.

6.7.2 Antibody Targeting

Nanoparticles mediated antibody delivery for targeting has been reported by many researchers, especially in case of cancer treatment. This type of antibody targeting may improve the therapeutic efficacy of the active moiety as well as distribution and concentration of the moiety at targeted site. Novel approaches have been applied to develop immune-nanoparticles with better therapeutic efficacy against colorectal tumor cells. Similarly for treatment of cancer dendrimer magnetic nanoparticles showed efficient gene targeting.

6.7.3 Vaccine Delivery

To improve the output of therapeutics nanocarriers containing therapeutics with potential of molecular targeting as well as diagnostic imaging capacity are emerging as the upcoming generation of functional nanomedicines. Nanoparticles a novel carrier based on poly-glutamic acid were prepared and applied for the cancer treatment as carriers for vaccines. In vaccine research compounds that shows enhanced immune responses to recombinant or synthetic epitopes are considered very important.

6.7.4 Drug Delivery

Lipid nanoparticulate systems have been explored from many years and still proving its potential for deliverance of drugs and similarly nanostructured lipid carriers are also used for drug delivery. Lipid nanoparticles for topical delivery of psoralen were reported by one research group in which they compare lipid nanoparticles with nanostructured lipid carriers consist of precirol and squalene. They observed the particle size nearly 200-300 nm for both carriers and used for the treatment of psoriasis. In their study it was also reported that nanoparticulate systems containing 8-methoxy psoralen can minimize the permeation differentiation between normal and hyper proliferative skin in comparison with free drug in aqueous control.

6.7.5 Improvement in the Gastrointestinal Tract Absorption

A novel type of nanoparticulate system has been reported to overwhelm intestinal degradation and drug transport-limited absorption of P-glycoprotein substrate drugs. One interesting report was found on mucoadhesive, self-nano-emulsified drug delivery system (SNEDDS) of cyclosporine A, quality by design for understanding the product variability. This is most probably very first report on this type of research on quality by design in the field of pharmaceutical nanotechnology. They utilized near infrared, chemometric analysis and several other well established processes for specification of emulsions during processing. The impact of nano-droplets size on the SNEDDS variability was also investigated.

6.7.6 Diagnostic Medicine

Role of Nanoparticles has been reported for diagnostic medicine also by various researchers. In one study antibody-conjugated, hydrophilic, magnetic nanocrystals were used as smart nano-probes for the ultrasensitive detection of breast cancer via magnetic resonance imaging (MRI). MRI contrast agents (Manganese ferrite nanocrystals) were synthesized by thermal decomposition for MRI. Amphiphilic triblock copolymers were applied to modify the surfaces. They were found to be advantageous as a contrast medium for detection of breast cancer tumors. In another study different methods were exercised for detection of streptavidin by attachment of a molecule to dielectric particles composed of a rare earth oxide core and a polysiloxane shell containing fluoreschein for biodetection. New type of magnetic nanoparticles, gadolinium hydroxide and dysprosium oxide, can be characterized by different techniques by use of X-ray diffraction, magnetometry, and NMR relaxometry at multiple fields. They have been reported for diagnostic purposes and showed very good applications. Very first time new technique was employed by the use of Nanotube and antibody for detection of cancer.

Bioadhesive Microspheres

Microspheres represent a worthy subdivision of particulate drug delivery systems by virtue of their small size and efficient drug carrier capacity. Microspheres can be designed for controlled delivery of therapeutics to overcome the problem of limited bioavailability associated with some marketed conventional dosage forms. In order to capitalize maximum therapeutic effectiveness, the delivery system should release the optimum concentration of active drug at particular biological site within a specific duration and also kept no or minimal extent of toxic adverse effects. Bioadhesive microspheres are successfully employed to achieve these objectives for drug delivery through different routes of administration.

As a dosage form, microspheres appear as free flowing powders and generally composed of biodegradable polymers or proteins. The polymers may be from natural or synthetic origin and the size of microspheres is ideally less than 200 μm. The bioadhesive formulations for oral administrations are generally designed for prolonged stay at desired site throughout the gastrointestinal tract which results in better bioavailability profile of incorporated therapeutic agent especially in case of drugs with low solubility in intestinal fluids. As a drug carrier bioadhesive microspheres of biodegradable polymers usually follow sustained release kinetics. More precise control over the drug release rate from bioadhesive microspheres can be achieved by the incorporation of novel bioadhesive polymers. Depending upon the polymer utilized for the preparation of bioadhesive microspheres, they are utilized for the drug delivery and other biomedical applications.

The therapeutic success of simple microspheres is restricted due to short residence time at absorption site despite of their high drug loading capacity. This shortcoming associated with simple polymeric microspheres can be resolved by the utilization of bioadhesive polymers to provide an intimate contact with absorptive surface. The addition of bioadhesive assets to microspheres results in several advantages such as efficient absorption and enhanced bioavailability owing to high surface to volume ratio, a much more intimate contact with mucosal surface and target specificity. The biological hurdles i.e., short gastric emptying time can also be effectively managed in order to improve drug localization for controlled or sustained release. Microspheres of biodegradable and non-biodegradable polymers have been investigated for sustained release. An important requirement of polymers is that degradation products should be nontoxic because such products eventually enter systemic circulation or result in tissue deposition.

7.1 ADVANTAGES OF BIOADHESIVE MICROSPHERES

- Reliable means to deliver the drug to the target site with specificity, if modified, and to maintain the desired concentration at the site of interest without untoward effects.

- Solid biodegradable microspheres have the potential throughout the particle matrix for the controlled release of drug.

- Microspheres received much attention not only for prolonged release, but also for targeting of anticancer drugs to the tumor.

- The size, surface charge and surface hydrophilicity of microspheres have been found to be important in determining the fate of particles *in-vivo*.

- Studies on the macrophage uptake of microspheres have demonstrated their potential in targeting drugs to pathogens residing intra-cellularly.

- Blood flow determination: Relatively large microspheres (10-15 μm in diameter) are useful for regional blood flow studies in tissues and organs. In most cases the microspheres are injected at desired locations in the circulatory system and eventually lodge in the capillaries. The microspheres and fluorescent dyes they contain are first extracted from the tissue sample, and then fluorescence is quantities on a spectrofluorometer or fluorescence microplate reader. Traditionally, this type of study has been carried out using radiolabled microspheres; however fluorescent microspheres have been shown to be superior in chronic blood flow measurements.

7.2 MECHANISM OF DRUG RELEASE

Theoretically the release of drug from biodegradable microspheres classified but in actual practice the mechanism is more complex and combination of different mechanisms may operate

- (a) Degradation controlled monolithic systems
- (b) Diffusion controlled monolithic systems
- (c) Diffusion controlled reservoir systems
- (d) Erodible poly agent system

Release pattern of incorporated active drug from bioadhesive microspheres is critical to confirm its effectiveness at the site of absorption. The release kinetics of active constituent is markedly influenced by the physicochemical properties of active drug and nature of polymer utilized for the preparation of bioadhesive microspheres. The structure and micro-morphology of polymeric network of both biodegradable as well as non-biodegradable polymers plays an important role in drug release from intact microsphere.

The drug release from bioadhesive microspheres possibly follow one of the three suggested mechanisms i.e. pore-diffusion mechanism, osmotically driven burst mechanism and polymer erosion/degradation mechanism. In case of pore-diffusion, the surrounding aqueous media diffuse towards the core containing active drug and dissolves it. The concentration gradient acts as driving force for the release of drug by diffusion process through polymeric network. The osmotically driven burst mechanism utilizes the self originated osmotic pressure to rupture polymeric coating in order to release incorporated drug. The required osmotic pressure is created due to the diffusion of aqueous media into the core through polymeric coating. This burst effect is mainly controlled by factors related to drug and polymer properties such as drug-polymer ratio, particle size of incorporated drug and size of the bioadhesive microspheres. In case of polymer erosion/degradation mechanism, drug is dispersed within the polymer which is eroded by the surrounding fluids leading to release of drug. This mechanism is accompanied by accumulation of monomer in release medium. The erosion process cause changes in polymeric microstructure of bioadhesive microspheres leading to plasticization of polymer matrix.

The drug release from bioadhesive microspheres composed of non-biodegradable polymers depends upon the type of polymeric network i.e. matrix or reservoir type. In reservoir type systems, drug-core is coated with polymer while in matrix type systems drug is dispersed throughout the polymeric network. Diffusion or erosion or combination of both mechanisms governs the drug release.

7.3 POLYMERS FOR BIOADHESIVE MICROSPHERES

As discussed earlier, biodegradable and non-biodegradable polymeric materials have been utilized for the preparation of bioadhesive microspheres. On the basis of their origin, these polymeric materials are divided into two groups:

- Synthetic Polymers
- Natural polymers

However, the derivatives of both synthetic and natural polymeric materials are also employed as carriers for the preparation of bioadhesive microspheres. The commonly used bioadhesive polymeric materials as carriers include chitosan, albumin, collagen, agarose, gelatin, starch, carrageenan, ethylene vinyl acetate copolymer, poly anhydrides, lactide, methyl acrylate, acrolein, glycolides and their copolymers etc.

7.3.1 Synthetic Polymers

The polymers of synthetic origin are subdivided into two categories:

7.3.1.1 Non-biodegradable polymers

Acrolein

Epoxy polymers

Glycidyl methacrylate

Poly methyl methacrylate (PMMA)

7.3.1.2 Biodegradable polymers

Poly anhydrides

Lactides

Poly alkyl cyano acrylates (PACA)

Glycolides and their copolymers

Poly alkyl cyano acrylates are synthetic polymeric material with a great potential as a drug carrier for bioadhesive formulations meant for parenteral as well as oral and ophthalmic administration. For sustained release of narcotic antagonist, anti-cancer agents like cyclophosphamide, doxorubicin, cisplatin etc, poly lactic acid is a suitable polymer as a drug carrier. Copolymers of poly glycolic acid and poly lactic acid are also utilized for the development of sustained release formulations for the delivery of anti-malarial agents and other similar therapeutic agents.

Bioadhesive microspheres composed of poly anhydride polymers were evaluated to overcome the problem of short precorneal residence time associated with the ocular administration of therapeutic agents. Timolol maleate loaded microspheres were prepared using poly adipic anhydride as a bioadhesive material for ophthalmic deliverance. A novel concept of functionalized microspheres is also reported which utilizes poly acrolein as a polymeric base. These functionalized microspheres avoid the activation process due to the presence of free CHO groups over poly acrolein surface which form Schiff's base on exposure to NH_2 groups of proteins.

Synthetic polymers are now also choice for the controlled release as well as targeted microparticulate carriers.

7.3.2 Natural Polymers

These polymers are obtained from different sources like proteins, carbohydrates and chemically modified carbohydrates.

7.3.2.1 Proteins

Albumin

Gelatin

Collagen

7.3.2.2 Carbohydrates

Agarose

Carrageenan

Chitosan

Starch

7.3.2.3 Chemically modified carbohydrates

Poly-dextran

Poly-starch

Biological protein, albumin is widely accepted as a potential carrier for the development of bioadhesive systems to deliver drugs as well as therapeutic proteins. Albumin is successfully employed for either local or targeted deliverance of therapeutic agents to discrete anatomical sites. Its applications for the delivery of antitumor agents are widely accepted as a targeting approach to the tumor cells. Another natural polymer, gelatin is also utilized for the preparation of microspheres to efficiently deliver therapeutic agents or biological response modifier i.e. interferon to phagocytes.

As a carbohydrate, starch consists of gluco-pyranose unit and its hydrolysis yields D-glucose. This poly saccharide offers a large number of OH groups which are advantageous for the incorporation of active therapeutic agents within the microspheres or may interact with functional groups of different therapeutic agents to bind them on the surface of microspheres.

Chitosan is produced by deacylation of chitin. The surface charge of chitosan plays an important role for the development of different drug delivery systems. At alkaline or neutral pH conditions, chitosan remains insoluble but it forms salts with organic and inorganic salts. In solutions, its NH_2 groups become protonated and provide a net positive charge on the surface of the polymeric chain.

Non-biodegradable polymeric materials are associated with the problem of carrier toxicity due to the accumulation of polymeric material in body after complete release of incorporated drug. The carrier toxicity is of great concern in case of chronic therapy and parenteral administration. Whereas biodegradable carriers do not possess such accumulation of carrier polymeric material as they degrade into non-toxic degradation products after complete release of loaded drug. Therefore biodegradable polymers are generally preferred for drug delivery systems especially in case of parenteral administration.

7.4 PREPARATION OF BIOADHESIVE MICROSPHERES

With the technological advancement in pharmaceutical manufacturing processes, a number of techniques are available for the preparation of microspheres. The technique for preparation of microspheres is adopted on the basis of nature of selected polymer. The selection of polymer depends on intended use, duration of therapy and type of release i.e. sustained or delayed. Moreover, the choice of technique for microsphere preparation is mainly guided equally by some formulation as well as technique related factors.

For the selection of suitable technique following points should be considered:

- Capable to incorporate reasonably high drug concentration.
- Post synthesis stability in terms of clinically acceptable shelf life.
- Control over particle size and dispersability, especially in case of parenterals.
- Control over drug release as per the requirement of therapy.
- Economic in terms of production yield.
- Ease of product recovery.
- Reproducibility.
- Complete removal of toxic solvents from final product.

Methods: Different types of methods are employed for the preparation of microsphere. These include:

- Single emulsion technique
- Double emulsion technique
- Polymerization technique
  - (a) Normal polymerization
  - (b) Interfacial polymerization
- Phase separation coacervation technique
- Spray drying and spray congealing
- Solvent extraction

7.4.1 Single Emulsion Technique

This technique is generally adopted for the preparation of particulate carriers of micron range. Bioadhesive microspheres of natural polymers i.e. carbohydrates and proteins are prepared by single emulsion technique. For the preparation of microspheres, bioadhesive polymer is dissolved or dispersed in aqueous medium. This aqueous dispersion is then dispersed in a non-aqueous or oily medium followed by cross linking of dispersed polymeric globules. Polymer cross linking can be accomplished by heating or chemical cross linking agents i.e. formaldehyde, glutaraldehyde etc. Chemical cross linking agents are utilized for thermolabile substances because heating method may cause denaturation of such materials. However, use of chemical cross linking agents result in excessive exposure of active drug to chemicals followed by centrifugation, separation and washing for complete removal of un-reacted chemicals which may increase the manufacturing cost.

7.4.2 Double Emulsion Technique

The preparation of bioadhesive microspheres by double emulsion technique involves formation of double/multiple emulsion i.e. w/o/w or o/w/o. The w/o/w type double emulsions are best suited for peptides, vaccines, proteins and hydrophilic drugs. This method is compatible with both synthetic as well as natural bioadhesive polymers. In this technique, an aqueous protein solution is dispersed in a lipophilic organic continuous phase. Active drug(s) may be added in the aqueous protein solution. The organic continuous phase generally contains bioadhesive polymer which eventually encapsulates the protein and active constituents present in dispersed aqueous phase. This primary emulsion is then sonicated and homogenized before its dispersion into aqueous poly vinyl alcohol (PVA) solution leading to the formation of multiple/double emulsion. Finally, this double emulsion is processed for removal of solvents either by solvent extraction or by solvent evaporation method for the recovery of bioadhesive microspheres. This technique is reported for the incorporation of vaccines, peptides, proteins and a number of conventional hydrophilic drug molecules into microspheres.

7.4.3 Polymerization Techniques

On the basis of polymerization process, polymerization techniques for the preparation of bioadhesive microspheres are generally classified as:

- Normal polymerization

- Interfacial polymerization.

7.4.3.1 Normal polymerization

In normal polymerization, different processes of polymerization i.e. precipitation, bulk, emulsion, micellar and suspension polymerization are employed. For bulk polymerization, a monomer or a mixture of monomers is heated in the presence of catalyst which initiates the process of polymerization. Drug may also be loaded during the process of polymerization. Suspension polymerization process is also known as pearl or bead polymerization. This process also utilizes heating of monomer or mixture of monomers. Here monomer or mixture of monomers is dispersed in a continuous aqueous phase and heating is applied for polymerization. The droplets of monomers may also accompanied with an initiator and other additives.

Another polymerization process i.e. emulsion polymerization, slightly differs from suspension polymerization process. In emulsion polymerization initiator is added to the aqueous phase instead of monomer droplets which later on diffuses to the surface of micelles. Among all of the polymerization processes, purest form of polymers is obtained by bulk polymerization.

7.4.3.2 Interfacial polymerization

Interfacial polymerization process involves reaction between the different monomers at interface of two immiscible liquid phases which results into the formation of bioadhesive polymeric film. This formed polymeric film essentially envelops the dispersed phase which may contain active drug.

7.4.4 Phase Separation Coacervation Technique

This technique is based on the concept of polymer solubility decrement in organic phase which leads to formation of a polymer rich phase termed as coacervates. Methodologically, the active drug candidate is dispersed in a polymer solution followed by addition of a non-solvent which separate out the polymer from the organic phase with the engulfment of drug particles within the formed bioadhesive microspheres **(Figure 7.1)**. This addition of non-solvent results in rapid solidification of polymer. Several successful attempts have been reported for the preparation of poly lactic acid (PLA) microspheres by this method using butadiene as an incompatible polymer. The formed microspheres tend to stick with each other leading to agglomeration. This agglomeration of formed microspheres must be avoided by stirring of contents at a suitable speed. Process variables i.e. stirring speed and stirring time etc, plays a critical role to control the kinetics of microspheres formation as there is no definite conditions for the attainment of equilibrium. These process variables are also affects the formation of coacervates which determines the distribution of polymeric film, particle size and agglomeration.

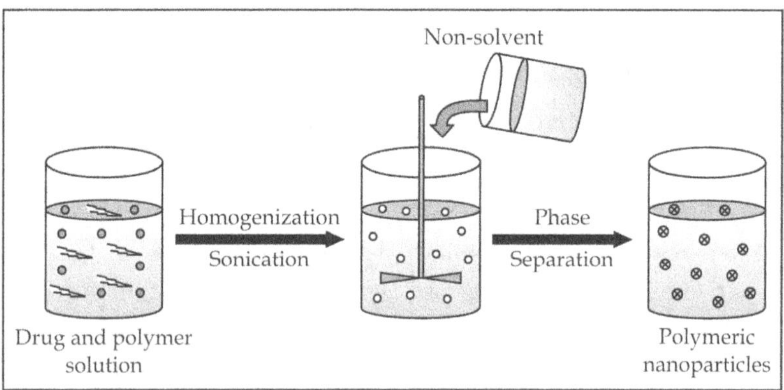

Figure 7.1 Schematic representation of phase separation coacervation technique

7.4.5 Spray Drying and Spray Congealing

Principally these techniques depend on drying rate of fine spray of drug and polymer solution. The drying may be achieved by solvent removal or cooling. When solvent removal is adopted for drying, the technique is known as spray drying whereas cooling process is adopted for spray congealing technique. A suitable volatile organic solvent such as acetone, dichloromethane etc., is selected to dissolve the polymer. The active therapeutic agent is dispersed in polymeric solution by homogenization at high speed in order to obtain a homogenous dispersion. Then atomization of this homogenized polymeric dispersion in a hot air stream leads to the formation of small droplets or fine mist which is instantly exposed for solvent removal or cooling process. Generally, these techniques yields bioadhesive microspheres in the size range of 1-100 μm.

Finally, prepared microspheres are withdrawn from the stream of hot air with the assistance of cyclone separator and subjected to vacuum drying in order to completely remove the traces of solvent. However, very high rates of solvent removal results in the formation of porous microparticles. Feasibility of complete operation under aseptic conditions is counted as a major advantage of these techniques. Some of the penicillins were formulated as microspheres by spray drying process. Spray congealing method is utilized for the encapsulation of thiamine mono-nitrate and sulphaethylthiadizole in a mixture of mono and di-glycerides of stearic acid and palmitic acid.

7.4.6 Solvent Extraction Technique

This technique utilizes the basic principle of extraction for the removal of organic solvent to yield bioadhesive microspheres. Generally, water miscible organic solvents such as isopropanol are utilized to dissolve the polymer. The organic phase is removed with the aid of extraction with water. This technique usually decreases the overall hardening time for microspheres. Occasionally, drug or protein is directly added to the organic phase containing polymer. The rate of solvent removal is affected by the ratio of organic polymeric solution to water, solubility profile of polymer and the temperature of water.

7.5 DRUG LOADING

Generally two processes are adopted for the efficient loading of the drug over bioadhesive microspheres i.e. drug may be added during the preparation of microspheres or the prepared microspheres may be incubated with drug solution. The drug can be loaded by the course of chemical linkage, physical entrapment, surface adsorption or combination of these incidents. The overall loading efficiency of microspheres markedly depends on nature of drug/polymer and the technique of preparation.

Of the two methods, drug incorporation during the preparation of microspheres yields maximum drug loading but associated with several drawbacks i.e. the drug may be affected by process variables like heat of polymerization, vigorous agitation etc., and presence of other additives e.g. surfactants, cross linking agent, stabilizers etc. On the other hand, incubation of preformed microspheres with drug solution yields relatively low loading efficiency but avoid the effects of process variables of preparation techniques. In incubation method, preformed microspheres are incubated with a highly concentrated drug solution in a suitable solvent. The drug is loaded to preformed microspheres by penetration or diffusion process through pores present within the polymeric network. Drug loading by surface adsorption is also possible which depends on the nature of polymer utilized. Drug loaded microspheres are then removed by filtration, centrifugation or solvent removal followed by drying.

7.6 EVALUATION OF BIOADHESIVE MICROSPHERES

In order to develop efficient microspheres for the delivery of proteins, antigens or other therapeutic molecules, strict evaluation of microspheres is essential. The microstructure of prepared microspheres varies to a great extent which ascertains the drug release behaviour and stability of the microspheres. A number of evaluation parameters are utilized to assess the efficiency of microspheres.

7.6.1 Particle Size and Shape

Particle size and distribution of microspheres are determined by light microscopy (LM), scanning electron microscopy (SEM), electron microscopy (EM) etc. Commonly SEM and LM are used for the visualization and analysis of size, shape and surface morphology of microspheres. From several decades, these techniques provide reliable and reproducible results for microparticulate systems.

Examination with light microscopy provides important information in case of double walled microspheres which is helpful to control coating parameters at the time of preparation. The surface morphology of intact or cross sectioned microspheres can be revealed by SEM investigation. The high resolution of SEM in comparison to LM allows detailed analysis of microsphere surface. In case of double walled microspheres, visualization of microspheres before and after coating helps to assess and measure significant changes in surface morphology.

Confocal lasers scanning microscopy is applied as a nondestructive visualization technique for microparticles and characterization of structures not only on the surface, but also inside the particles. Confocal fluorescence microscopy is generally employed for the characterization of multiple walled microspheres. Some other methods e.g. laser light scattering and multi size coulter counter can also be used for the characterization of size, shape and morphology of microspheres.

7.6.2 Electron Spectroscopy for Chemical Analysis

Electron spectroscopy for chemical analysis (ESCA) is preferably used to analyze surface chemistry of microspheres and to reveal the type of interactions involved. By the means of ESCA, atomic composition of the surface can be determined which eases the prediction of degradation pattern of polymeric network. The ECSA spectra can be used to determine surfacial degradation of biodegradable microspheres.

7.6.3 Attenuated Total Reflectance Fourier Transform-Infrared Spectroscopy

The assessment of polymeric matrix degradation of microspheres can be done by the utilization of FT-IR. For this purpose, the surface of microspheres is subjected to alternated total reflectance (ATR) measurement. When infrared beam passed through the ATR cell containing microspheres, it reflected several times and give rise to IR-spectra. The IR-spectra obtained by ATR FT-IR analysis mainly corresponds to the surface material of microspheres and reveals the information about its composition. The surface composition of microspheres depends on the adopted manufacturing technique and conditions.

7.6.4 Density Determination

A pychnometer with multi volume function is generally used for the density measurement of microspheres. To measure the density of microspheres, accurately weighed sample is placed in multi volume pychnometer chamber and helium is introduced at a constant pressure. The expansion of helium causes a pressure decrement within the pychnometer chamber which is measured. Two consecutive readings of pressure decrement at different initial pressure are noted and the volume of microspheres is calculated. The density of microspheres is represented as g/ml.

7.6.5 Isoelectric Point

Isoelectric point of microspheres can be determined by measuring their electrophoretic mobility. The commonly used apparatus for the measurement of electrophoretic mobility of microspheres is micro electrophoresis. This apparatus measures the time of particle movement over a distance of 1 mm at different pH values over a wide range, generally 3-10 and the mean velocity of particles is calculated. These values are used for the determination of electrophoretic mobility which corresponds to ionization behaviour, net surface charge and ion absorption nature of microspheres under examination.

7.6.6 Surface Carboxylic Acid Residue

Radioactive glycine conjugates are used for the determination of surface carboxylic acid residues. These radioactive glycine conjugates are prepared by reaction between C_{14}-glycine ethyl ester hydrochloride and microspheres to be evaluated. The glycine residue links with microspheres by condensation of water soluble 1-ethyl-3 (3-dimethyl amino propyl) carbidiimide (EDAC). Then the radioactive emission of these conjugates is measured by liquid scintillation counter. This radioactivity measurement is correlated to carboxylic acid residues. The free carboxylic acid residues play an important role for hydrophilic or hydrophobic or any other type of derivatized microspheres.

7.6.7 Surface Amino Acid Residue

For the determination of amino acid residues associated to microsphere surface, radioactive conjugates of C_{14}-acetic acid. The method is similar to the determination of free carboxylic acid residues and based on indirect estimation. Here radioactivity of C_{14}-acetic acid conjugates is measured instead of C_{14}-glycine conjugates. EDAC is for condensation of amino groups and C_{14}-acetic acid residues. The radioactivity of carboxylic acid residues is measured by liquid scintillation counter and free amino acid residues are calculated. However, the accuracy of this method relies on time allowed for the conjugation of microspheres with radioactive moiety and the reactivity of free functional group available on the surface of polymeric carrier.

7.6.8 Entrapment Efficiency

To exert the therapeutic effect of incorporated drug, sufficient amount of drug should be entrapped within the polymeric carrier. The drug entrapment efficiency of microspheres is determined by lysing accurately weighed sample of microspheres in a suitable solvent. Then amount of drug in the solvent is analyzed spectrophotometrically or as per the corresponding monograph. The percent entrapment of drug is calculated by following formula:

$$\% \text{ entrapment} = \frac{\text{Actual content}}{\text{Theoretical content}} \times 100$$

7.6.9 Angle of Contact

The angle of contact is an important parameter which governs the wetting property of polymeric microspheres. The hydrophilic or hydrophobic nature of microspheres is markedly influenced by angle of contact. The presence of components adsorbed on the surface of bioadhesive microspheres influences the angle of contact which is a thermodynamic property and specific to solid polymeric carriers. The measurement of angle of contact is made at solid/air/water interface. A droplet of microsphere suspension is taken in a circular cell and examined for the measurement of advancing and receding angle of contact within a minute of deposition at 20 °C.

7.6.10 Release Studies

The experimental methods for the assessment of *in-vitro/in-vivo* release kinetics of bioadhesive microspheres are adopted as per the objectives of developed delivery system i.e. oral, topical or rectal administration. There is still a need of experimental methods which allows efficient assessment of release characteristics and permeability of drug released from bioadhesive polymeric particulate carriers. For the drug release studies of bioadhesive microspheres several *in-vitro* and *in-vivo* techniques have been reported.

7.6.10.1 *In-vitro* methods

At the stage of product development and large scale production, *in-vitro* drug release data assist quality control measures to ensure the proper drug release from bioadhesive microspheres. *In-vitro* maintenance of defined hydrodynamic and biological conditions is necessary for sensitive and reproducible assessment of release characteristics. Simulation of similar *in-vivo* conditions for *in-vitro* methods is somewhat difficult due to which a very few *in-vitro* methods are available for drug release studies of microspheres. These methods are modified or tailored as per the requirement of study protocols. However, no standard *in-vitro* method has been developed till date. Different research groups adopted different apparatus of varying designs according to their study protocols.

Beaker method

In this method, bioadhesive microspheres are taken in a beaker containing suitable media and stirred continuously at a constant speed using overhead stirrer. Due to bioadhesive properties microspheres sticks to the bottom of beaker. Suitable aliquots are withdrawn at predetermined intervals and analyzed spectrophotometrically or as per the corresponding monograph. The equivalent volume of fresh media is added on each sample withdrawn in order to maintain sink condition. The total volume of media taken in the beaker is varied from 50-500 ml and the speed of stirring ranges between 60-300 rpm. In case of non-bioadhesive systems, some modification in this method are also reported i.e. use of cellophane or dialysis membrane to kept the microspheres in beaker.

Interface diffusion system

Interface diffusion technique was proposed by Dearden and Tomlinson for the evaluation of bioadhesive microspheres developed for buccal delivery. However, this technique is also adopted for bioadhesive microspheres meant for administration through other routes. The apparatus used by Dearden and Tomlinson, consists four compartments which represents four different sections of biological system. First compartment containing buffer solution represents oral cavity and appropriate amount of bioadhesive formulation to be evaluated is added to this compartment. The second compartment containing octanol represents buccal membrane and the third compartment represents biological fluids. The fourth compartment also contains octanol and represents protein binding of the incorporated drug. A syringe is generally used for the withdrawal of samples from first compartment at different time intervals and the samples are analyzed for the amount of drug by suitable techniques.

Modified keshary chien cell

This apparatus is especially designed for the evaluation of trans-membrane drug delivery systems in a laboratory setup. It is a modified form of Keshary Chien cell and equipped with thermal regulatory system to maintain the temperature of filled media at body temperature i.e. 37 °C. Generally, water is used as release media and the volume of filled media is around 50 ml. The system to be evaluated is added to a tubular section of the apparatus which has fitted with a 10# sieve towards bottom. This arrangement reciprocates the medium at a speed of 30 strokes/min.

Dissolution apparatus

Traditional dissolution apparatus described in IP or USP i.e. basket and paddle type apparatus are also utilized for the evaluation of bioadhesive systems for *in-vitro* drug release. The volume of dissolution media is varied in the range of 100-500 ml according to the requirements of bioadhesive system to be evaluated. The rotation speed of basket or paddle is generally kept between 50-100 rpm to maintain the homogeneity of the medium throughout the evaluation. The samples are withdrawn at suitable time intervals and analyzed for the drug amount. The equivalent sample volume is replaced on each sample withdrawal with fresh media to maintain sink condition.

Other methods

Several of methods are also designed by different research groups for the precise evaluation of drug release from bioadhesive systems. These methods includes agar gel method, dissolution apparatus USP-III, blocks of plexi glass arranged in a flask, Valia-Chein cell etc and reported in different research literatures. Despite of a wide range of evaluation methods, an ideal method is still to be designed which maintains the sink conditions perfectly to represent almost similar biological conditions of human body.

7.6.10.2 *In-vivo* methods

In-vivo methods for drug release studies of bioadhesive systems, principally depends on the permeability of the mucosal surface to be exposed for the absorption. The permeability of penetrants across the biological membranes depends on their interaction with mucin, membrane components and microorganisms present over the surface. In earlier times, several researchers measure systemic pharmacological effects due to the absorption of drugs after application to the biological/mucosal surface. In recent times, animal models have gained the interest for more accurate measurement of drug release or permeability of the drug in biological environment.

Animal models

Animal models e.g. rats, hamsters, sheep, rabbits, cats, dogs and pigs are dominantly utilized for the assessment of drug release or permeability from bioadhesive systems. These animal models are also utilized for screening of compounds, exploration of absorption mechanisms and to evaluate the effectiveness of permeation enhancers. All the protocols for the evaluation of bioadhesive dosage forms in animal models are designed in the view of ethical guidelines prescribed for experimentation on animals. Sometimes, such evaluation requires surgical process e.g. ligation of oesophagus to restrict the dosage form within the oral cavity for the assessment of buccal absorption. Generally, such evaluations are carried out on the animals in anesthetized condition to minimize the degree of discomfort to animal and ease of animal handling. Methodologically, the dosage form is administered via desired route i.e. buccal, oral, rectal, ocular, vaginal or topical and blood samples are withdrawn by suitable technique at predetermined intervals. Blood samples are analyzed for drug amount by highly efficient techniques like HPLC.

Buccal absorption test

In 1967, Beckett and Triggs develop an evaluation method for bioadhesive formulations meant for buccal delivery which is known as buccal absorption test. This simple method is quite effective for the evaluation of either single or multi-drug dosage forms. By this method one can easily and reliably measure the loss of drug from oral cavity after administration of dosage form. This test is also effectively employed for the investigation of contact time, relative importance of molecular structure of drug, biological pH and initial drug concentration.

7.6.11 In-vitro-In-vivo Correlations

In-vitro assessment of drug release from a dosage form provides an idea for its *in-vivo* performance in biological conditions. However, these *in-vitro* predictions does not reflects the actual performance completely but sometimes correlated closely with the results in animal models or human studies. Such correlations between *in-vitro* assessment (dissolution) and *in-vivo* outputs (bioavailability determined by blood-plasma concentration and/or urinary excretion data) are acknowledged as '*in-vitro-in-vivo* correlations'. These correlations are very important for the development of products with better and specific bioavailability requirements. Several methods are utilized for the prediction of *in-vitro-in-vivo* correlations.

7.6.11.1 Percent of drug dissolved *in-vitro* v/s peak plasma concentration

In order to check the extent of *in-vitro-in-vivo* correlations one can compare *in-vitro* percent drug release from different dosage forms with peak plasma concentrations obtained from *in-vivo* experimentations. The formulation factors i.e. additives, process variables; markedly affect the performance of dosage forms. A poorly formulated dosage form provides low concentration of drug in comparison to a well formulated dosage forms and hence the amount of drug available for absorption is low. In such cases it is difficult to correlate *in-vitro* predictions with *in-vivo* experimentations.

7.6.11.2 Percent of drug dissolved v/s percent of drug absorbed

When dissolution rate acts as a limiting factor for the absorption of drug and after dissolution the drug is absorbed completely, the comparison of percent drug dissolved with percent drug absorbed may give rise to a linear correlation. On the other hand, when rate of absorption acts as a limiting factor for the bioavailability of drug, variation in dissolution rate may not be reflected in terms of change in rate and extent of drug absorption during *in-vivo* predictions.

7.6.11.3 Dissolution rate v/s absorption rate

The determination of absorption rate is somewhat more difficult in comparison to the determination of absorption time. The inverse relationship between absorption rate and absorption time may be utilized to correlate the dissolution data of *in-vitro* studies to the absorption data of *in-vivo* predictions. In such *in-vitro-in-vivo* correlation analysis one can easily distinguish the rapid drug absorption from slower drug absorption on the basis of observed absorption time for the dosage form under evaluation. Lesser absorption time represents rapid absorption of certain amount of drug available in the dosage form. The time required for the absorption of similar amount of drug from a dosage form is correlated.

7.6.11.4 Percent of drug dissolved v/s serum drug concentration

Dissolution rate limited absorption of the drugs from gastrointestinal tract may give rise to a linear correlation between percent drug dissolved at specified time intervals and drug concentrations in serum at corresponding time intervals.

7.6.11.5 Percent of drug dissolved v/s percent of the dose excreted in urine

If there is a linear correlation between percent drug dissolved and the percent drug absorbed then one can easily correlate the drug amount in body to the drug amount excreted via urine. Furthermore, a linear relationship may be established between percent drug dissolved and percent dose excreted in the urine. Such correlations play an important role for the prediction of dose related toxicity profile of a given dosage form.

7.6.12 Evaluation of Bioadhesive Properties

The efficiency of bioadhesive systems resides in their bioadhesive properties therefore precise and accurate assessment of these properties is necessary. Different *in-vitro, in-vivo* and *ex-vivo* methods are adopted for the evaluation of bioadhesive properties of a polymeric matrix. These methods are generally based on the measurement of tensile strength and/or shear strength. Recently, several chip based systems and imaging techniques are gaining the interest for the assessment of bioadhesive properties in an *in-vitro* setup.

In case of bioadhesive microspheres, the *in-vitro* tensile strength is measured by dipping a filter paper in 8% mucin solution and this mucin coated filter paper is then placed in the contact of hydrated sample of bioadhesive microspheres for a definite time period to allow bioadhesive interaction between mucin and microspheres. Then maximum force required for the detachment of filter paper from polymeric surface of microspheres is determined. Similar process is used for *ex-vivo* tensile strength measurement with a modification that mucin coated filter paper is replaced by mucosal/biological surface obtained from a suitable animal model. For bioadhesive microspheres, wash off technique may also be employed for the evaluation of bioadhesive properties. In this technique, an excised mucosal/biological surface is first rinsed with buffer solution over which precounted bioadhesive microspheres are sprinkled and kept for a specified time to allow bioadhesive interactions. Then buffer solution is allowed to run again over the mucosal/biological surface in order to wash off the microspheres which do not adhere to the surface efficiently. The percentage retention of microspheres is calculated and acknowledged as percent bioadhesion. Bioadhesive properties of other bioadhesive systems can also be evaluated by incubating them with a viscoelastic solution of mucin e.g. 30% w/w solution of mucin followed by maximum detachment force determination required for the separation of polymeric system from mucin surface. An integrated chip (IC) based system; BIOCORE is also reported for the computerized measurement of bioadhesive properties. In this system the polymeric system to be evaluated is immobilized on the surface of an IC and mucin solution is allowed to pass over it. This process causes development of bioadhesive interactions between polymer and mucin which are measured by an optical phenomenon. This optical phenomenon is called as surface plasmon resonance which measures the change in refractive index due to the binding of mucin to the polymeric surface.

7.7 APPLICATIONS

7.7.1 In Vaccine Delivery

Vaccines are preferred to gain the protection against microbial infections. An ideal vaccine must be efficacious, safe and convenient to apply with lowest possible cost.

Bioadhesive microspheres are widely investigated for their potential for vaccination against several infectious diseases. This biodegradable system is suitable for mucosal delivery of vaccines and overcomes the problem of short retention associated with conventional vaccine delivery systems. In vaccination process, the safety and minimization of adverse reactions is a complex issue and depends on the degree of antibody production. Bioadhesive microspheres offer several advantages over conventional systems for vaccination in terms of:

- Improvisation of antigenicity.
- Modulated antigen release.
- Stabilization of antigen.

7.7.2 Targeting using Bioadhesive Microspheres as Carriers

The development of novel systems for drug delivery is generally focused on the targeted delivery of therapeutics in order to achieve site specific drug delivery. In recent times, this well established dogma of targeted drug delivery has attracted the scientific community to develop drug delivery systems against some deadly diseases e.g. cancer, inflammatory bowel diseases etc. The role of carrier system for targeting purpose is to carry the drug to the desired site and maintain its concentration as long as possible at the site of action/absorption. Bioadhesive microspheres may adhere to the region of interest due to their bioadhesive properties and hence fulfill the requirements for targeted drug delivery.

7.7.3 Monoclonal Antibodies Mediated Microspheres Targeting

As we know that monoclonal antibodies (Mabs) are extremely specific molecules. Attachment of Mabs on the surface of bioadhesive microspheres increases their targeting efficiency towards the specific sites. The direct attachment of Mabs to bioadhesive microspheres can be achieved by covalent coupling which involves the interaction of free aldehyde groups, hydroxyl groups or amino groups present on the surface of microspheres with Mabs. Such microspheres comprising Mabs are known as immuno-microspheres. Several methods are reported for the attachment of Mabs to microspheres, some of them include;

- Non-specific adsorption.
- Specific adsorption.
- Direct coupling.
- Reagents mediated coupling.

7.7.4 Chemoembolization

The use of bioadhesive microspheres in chemoembolization is recently reported in literature. It is an endovascular therapy in which selective arterial embolization of a tumor is achieved in addition to simultaneous or subsequent delivery of chemotherapeutic agent. Chemoembolization is an advanced form of traditional embolization techniques which brings sustained therapeutic levels of chemotherapeutic agent in tumor region in addition to vascular occlusion action.

7.7.5 Imaging

By the labeling of bioadhesive microspheres with radioisotopes one can employ them for imaging purpose. The imaging of various cells, cell lines, tissues and organs is successfully done by the utilization of such radiolabled bioadhesive microspheres. Radiolabled microspheres are generally used for diagnostic purposes e.g. scintigraphic imaging of tumor masses in lung with the help of radiolabled human serum albumin microspheres. According to the size range of microspheres, these can be used for the imaging of several other specific sites.

7.7.6 Topical Porous Microspheres

The microspheres having numerous interconnected voids are acknowledged as micro-sponges. These microsponges are capable of entrapping a wide range of active ingredients in the size range of 5-300 μm including essential oils, emollients, fragrances etc. Therefore, these micro-sponges are successfully employed as topical carriers in the form of creams, powders and lotions. The porous and non-collapsible structure of micro-sponges released the entrapped active ingredients in a controlled manner.

7.7.7 Surface Modified Microspheres

Bioadhesive microspheres can be tailored by changing the surface properties of polymer which results in protection against phagocytic clearance and also alters their biodistribution. Such surface modifications of microspheres provide the ability to target discrete organs and to avoid their rapid clearance from the body. The surface modification of polystyrene, polyester or poly methyl methacrylate microspheres with the aid of poloxamer results in enhanced hydrophilicity which decreases their uptake by macrophages. Another example of surface modified microspheres is covalently modified protein microspheres by the utilization of PEG derivatives which shows a decrease in clearance and immunogenicity. The surface modifiers which are frequently used for surface modification of microspheres include:

- Proteins.
- Synthetic soluble polymers.

- Carbohydrates (mono, oligo and polysaccharides) and their derivatives.
- Antibodies and their fragments.
- Chelating compounds e.g. DTPA, EDTA or Desferroxamine.

The future of therapeutics delivery will be based on advanced and novel systems, bioadhesive microspheres are one of them. The ongoing researches in the field of bioadhesive microspheres give a glimpse of shining future of these polymeric systems, particularly for safe, targeted and effective *in-vivo* delivery of genes and other genetic materials. Their role in the diagnostics and sorting of diseased cell is also under the review.

Bioadhesive Nanogels

Introduction

For the last few decades, pharmaceutical field has witnessed quantum jump in the fields of drug discoveries, product developments, analytical methods, and packaging technologies. Not only had this, but the dedicated efforts of pharmaceutical researchers given an up thrust and lead to the augmentation of technologies from conventional drug delivery to pharmaceutical nanotechnology. This technological face-lift improves patient safety, compliance and provide more promising drug delivery route.

Pharmaceutical nanotechnology (PN) deals with the study of carriers (Drug delivery, diagnostic tools, biomarkers etc) that falls in the range of nanoscale (i.e. 10^{-9} m). It is basically dealing with design, fabrication, evaluation and applications of carrier or device or structures ranging in nanoscales. They have excellent capabilities to deal with the target site at molecular or supramolecular level. PN leads to the development of multifarious dosage forms like nanoparticles, nanocapsules, nanoshells, nanofibers, nanowires, Q-dots, nanotubes etc. The overall effect of these nanostructures is now further amplified by the amalgamation of gel technology. Nanogel is the best example of this amalgamation.

Nanogels (NGs) are basically a unique and effective articulation of nanostructures with hydrogels. NGs possess an extensive crosslinking matrix and excellent capacity to get imbibed in water and hence can easily modulate the drug release profile as per quest of patient. Its hydrophilic front, excellent colloidal stability, pharmacological inertness, high drug loading capacity, and targeted delivery make it as ideal drug delivery candidate. NGs are polymeric networks with three-dimensional configuration that absorb large quantities of water or biological fluids. Their water affinity is attributed to the presence of hydrophilic groups - such as ether, amine, hydroxyl, sulfate and carboxyl - in the polymer chains. NGs can be formulated as polymeric networks and confined to smaller dimensions **(Figure 8.1)**. Self-assembled NGs are promising nano-biotechnological tools with potential application in the drug delivery and diagnostics.

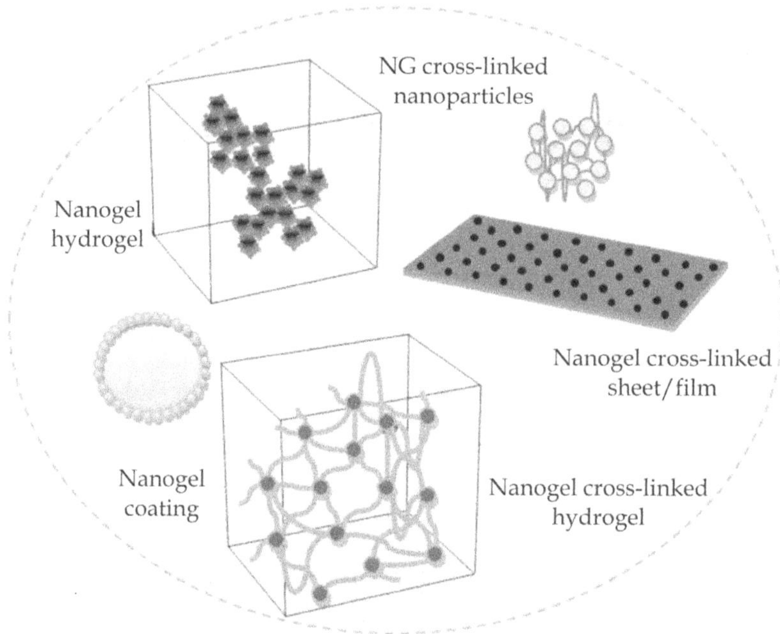

Figure 8.1 Different types of NGs for drug delivery

NGs are better drug delivery vehicles which offer following merits:

- Potential for administration through various routes, including oral, pulmonary, nasal, parenteral, intra-ocular etc;

- The particle size and surface properties can be manipulated to evade fast clearance by phagocytic cells, that allows passive and active drug targeting both;

- Targeted drug delivery with improved therapeutic efficacy and reduced side effects. Drug pay load is relatively high and may be obtained without chemical reactions; this is an important part for preserving the drug activity;

- Competent to reach the smallest capillary vessels, owing to its tiny volume and ability to penetrate the tissues either through the paracellular or the transcellular pathways.

Above mentioned merits presents NGs as promising drug delivery vehicles. In spite of this various facets like tissue toxicological profile, NGs-cell interactions and clinical safety need to be explored. Factors like selection of drug candidate, selection of suitable polymer as well as crosslinker are responsible for overall behavior of NGs.

8.1 MATERIALS FOR NGs

NGs can be prepared by multitudinous range of excipients. These excipients may be of natural, semi-synthetic or synthetic origin. They can be briefly portrayed as below (**Figure 8.2**).

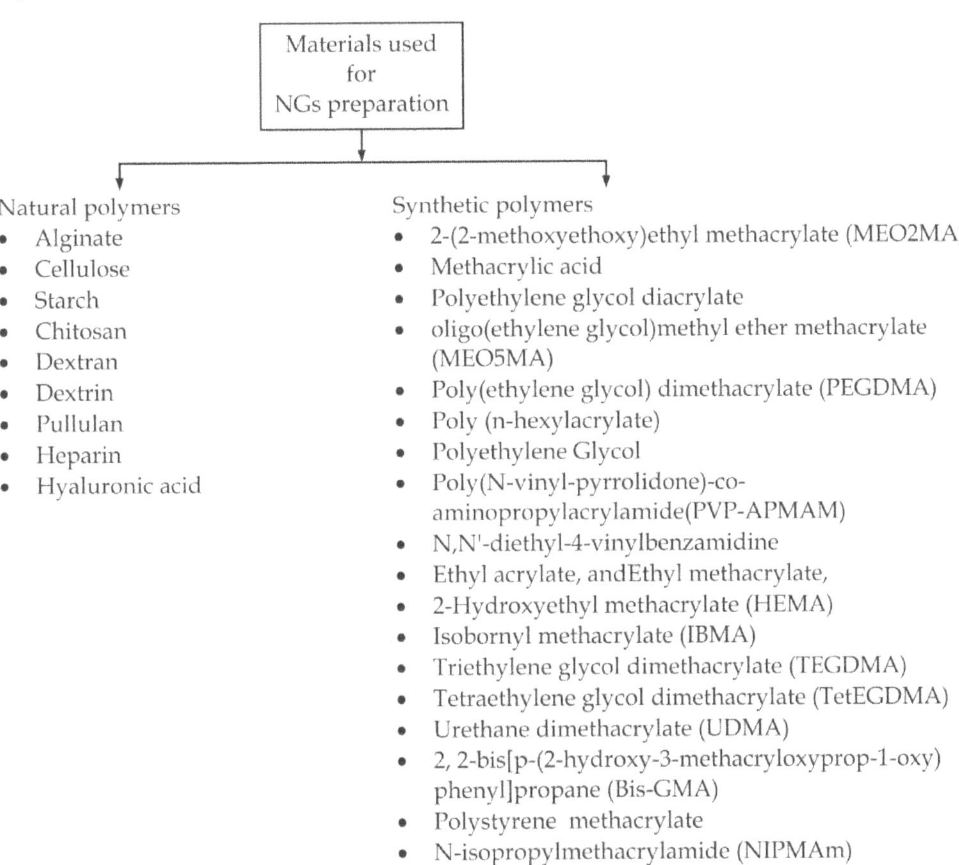

Figure 8.2 Classification on excipients used for preparation of NGs

8.2 PROPERTIES OF NGs

Human body and its complex physiochemical processes are a cumbersome task for drug delivery system in order to achieve a targeted delivery. The case became more sensitive when it is concern with NGs because the overall efficiency is dependent on various vital factors like particle size, its charge, zeta potential, swelling index, dissolution profile, toxicity consideration, polydispersity etc. The expedient properties of NGs are summarized in the **Figure 8.3**.

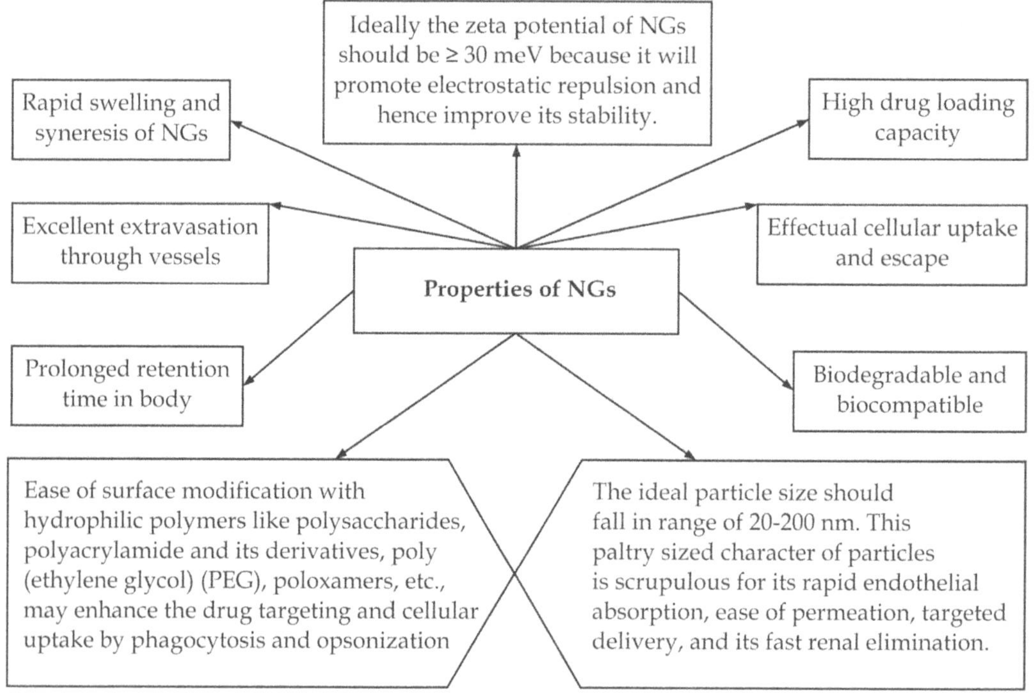

Figure 8.3 Properties of NGs

8.3 METHODS OF PREPARATION

NGs/hydrogels are generally prepared from hydrophilic polymer matrices that are cross-linked by several methods. One method is physical cross-linking. Hydrogen bonds, crystallized domains, hydrophobic interactions, stereo-complexation, temperature-induced sol-gel transition, host-guest interaction, aggregation and self-assembly have been utilized for the synthesis of ''bulk NGs''. But this method of preparations are still striving with barriers like toxicological profile generated due the employment of organic solvent and some surfactants during the preparation of NGs. Hence, there is a strong need to develop some process modifications that are able to expunge these types of techno-troubles.

8.3.1 Photolithographic Techniques

This technique is basically employed in the production of surface treatment of stamps, or to prepare replica molds for molded gels. But now it is effectively implemented for preparation of hydrogel particles (3D), microgels, and NGs ring. This process operates in cascade fashion which is consisting of five basic steps **(Figure 8.4)**.

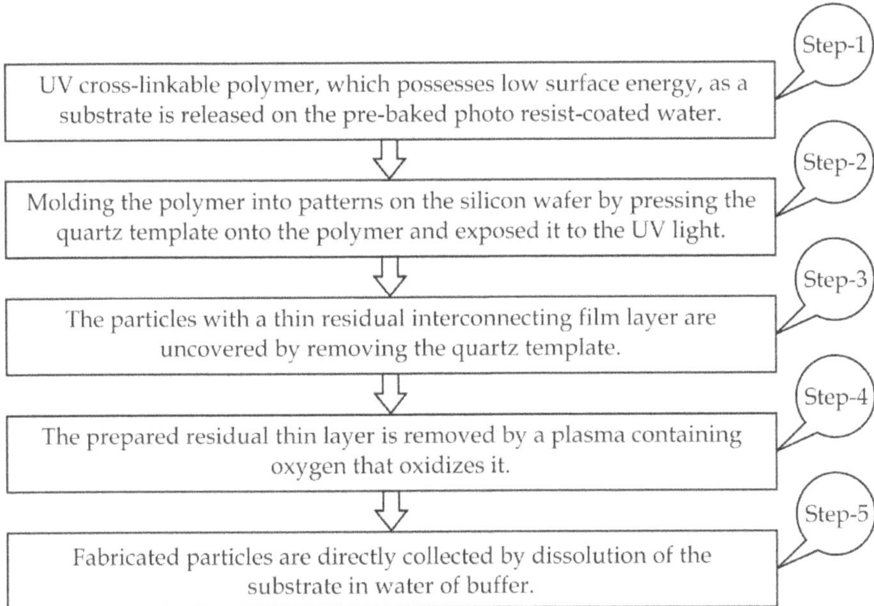

Figure 8.4 Flow chart of steps involved in photolithography technique

A top-down method called ''Particle replication in non-wetting templates (PRINT)'' was developed to fabricate NGs with control over particle size, shape and composition. A photocurableperfluoro polyether (PFPE) replica was used as the molding material. This eliminated the formation of a residual interconnecting film between molded objects, thus allowing for the preparation of isolated objects **(Figure. 8.5)**. In the approach, silicon master templates were mainly made by using electron beam lithography. Dimethacrylate-functionalized PFPE oligomers containing a photo-initiator were poured onto various patterned silicon master templates and then photo-chemically cured to form patterned elastomeric PFPE replica mold. PFPE-based materials have many advantageous properties including solvent resistance, chemical robustness and durability. They have also been used for different applications to fabricate organic solvent resistant microfluidic devices with features on the order of hundreds of microns. Using PRINT, monodisperse NGs of poly (ethylene glycol diacrylate) (PEGDA), triacrylate resin, PLA and poly pyrrole were prepared. Their sizes were ranged from 200 nm to micron-scale in diameter with various shapes such as trapezoidal, bar, conical and arrow **(Figure 8.6)**. In addition, DNA, proteins and small-molecule therapeutics were incorporated into 200 nm PEG-based NGs using a simple encapsulation technique to demonstrate the compatibility of PRINT with biomolecules.

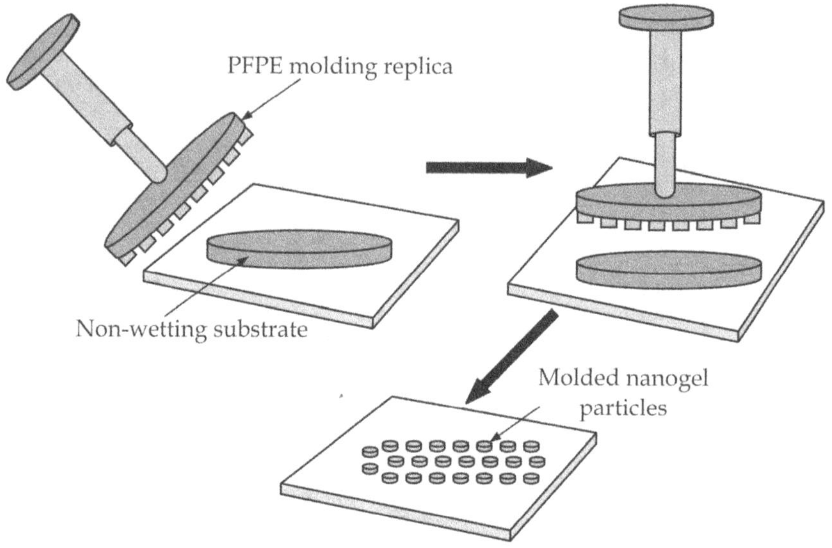

Figure 8.5 Schematic representation of PRINT technique for NG preparation

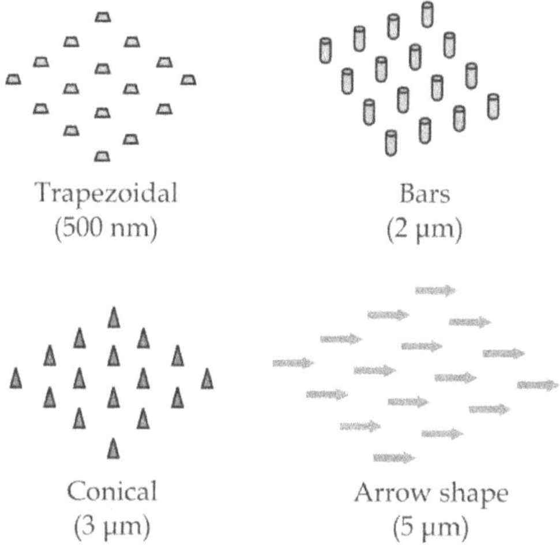

Figure 8.6 Schematic representation of different NG shapes and their size ranges

8.3.2 Micro-Molding Methods

Micro-molding of hydrogels has been examined as a potential method to fabricate NGs. The method is synonymous to photolithographic techniques. Moreover, by controlling the features on a mold stamp, they enable control over the size and shape of NGs, which are important for biomedical applications. The preparation of shape-controlled, harvestable hydrogel particles encapsulated with mammalian cells was demonstrated using micro-molding method. In the process, subjects were dispersed in a hydrogel precursor aqueous solution consisting of either methacrylated polymers or their derivatives and a photo-initiator. The resulting mixture was poured onto plasma-cleaned hydrophilic molds and finally cross-linked via exposure to high frequency UV light. The resulting NGs were removed, hydrated and then harvested. They can be obtained in multitudinous shapes like square, needle, spherical, cubic, prisms, and strings.

A similar method was reported for the preparation of cell-laden chemically and physically cross-linked hydrogel particles for tissue engineering. This approach utilized the controlled release of gelling agents from the mold to enable rapid gelling upon contact of hydrogel-forming precursors with the gelling agent in the mold. Ionically cross-linked hydrogels of alginate, a naturally occurring carbohydrate-based polymer, were prepared from cross-linking of alginates molded between PDMS and calcium-containing Agarose slab upon the release of calcium ions from the slab. The obtained micro-structured hydrogel particles had lateral dimensions between 5-2000 µm and vertical dimensions between 10-200 µm.

8.3.3 Microfluidic Preparation

Microfluidic methods have been recently explored for the preparation of monodisperse NGs. The methods require the fabrication of microfluidic devices by soft lithography using elastomeric materials, particularly PDMS or polyurethane elastomers as building blocks. The devices generally consist of inlets for monomers (or oligomers) and continuous phase and micro-channels with a tapered junction where two immiscible phases are merged **(Figure 8.7)**. Emulsification of monomers by breaking up liquid threads to droplets and *in-situ* cross-linking of the resulting droplets by photo-polymerization or poly-condensation are the two general steps involved in the continuous microfluidic preparation of NGs. Confinement of droplets, variation of flow rates of liquids and precise control of reaction time are key parameters to generate monodisperse particles with a variety of shapes and morphologies. More recently, the microfluidic preparation of complicated nanostructured particles has been reported. Nano structured gels can be prepared by various methods and use of plentiful polymers, but the aspired physiochemical properties are solely dependent on gelation methods.

Physical gelation by ionic cross-linking can be achieved in a micro-channel using two approaches; internal and external gelation. For the former, droplets consist of a gelling polymer and a crosslinking agent precursor in inactive form. Continuous phase contains an activator that can diffuse into droplets and react with cross-linking agent precursors, triggering the release of cross-linking agents. The released cross-linking agents can cause gelation. For the latter, droplets are emulsified in continuous phase that contains a cross-linking agent. Diffusion of cross-linking agents to emulsified droplets leads to gelation. As a consequence, the cross-linking agent should be soluble in aqueous droplet phase. Recently, physical gelation by ionic cross-linking using internal and external cross-linking approaches was explored for the microfluidic preparation of NGs of alginate cross-linked with calcium ions (Ca^{2+}). For internal gelation, an aqueous sodium alginate dispersion containing $CaCO_3$ as a cross-linking agent precursor was supplied from the central channel and soybean oil containing acetic acid as an activator was supplied from the side channels. Two liquid streams passed through a tapered junction to form emulsified droplets in soybean oil continuous phase. Acetic acid that diffused to the aqueous droplets reacted with $CaCO_3$. The generated Ca^{2+} ions as cross-linking agents involved in cross-linking reactions with carboxylic acid residues of sodium alginate, resulting in the formation of alginate NG particles. However, weak gelation was identified as the most important shortcoming, along with poor control over NG morphology for the method. For external gelation, aqueous sodium alginate solution was emulsified in soybean oil containing sodium acetate. Downstream of the channel, Ca^{2+} ions diffused to aqueous droplets to cross-link alginate. Contrary to internal cross-linking, this method resulted in the successful preparation of stable monodisperse spherical alginate NGs. In addition, control over the diffusion time of cross-linking agent in aqueous phase and the concentration of cross-linker in organic phase allowed for the preparation of various alginate NGs with capsular, gradient and uniform structures.

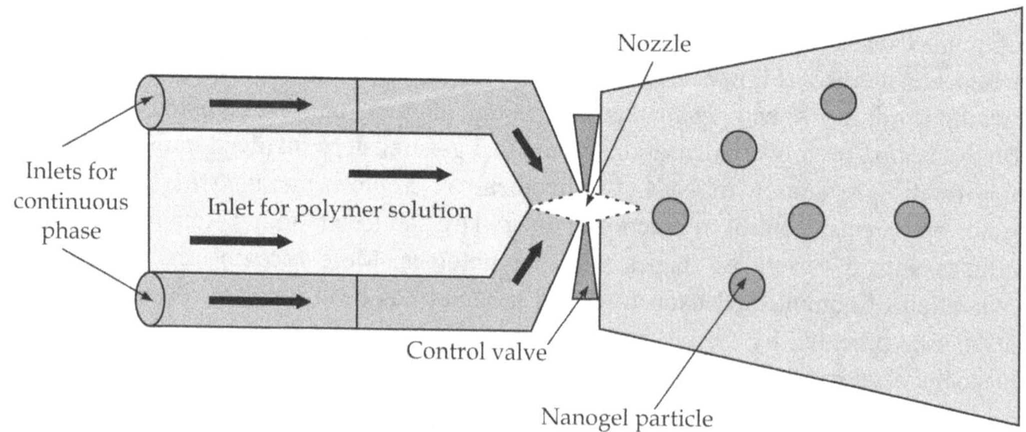

Figure 8.7 Schematic representation of microfluidic device for NG preparation

8.3.4 Preparation of NGs using Biopolymers

Chitosan, hyaluronan (HA) and dextran (Dex) are naturally occurring carbohydrate-based biopolymers. Chitosan is a polysaccharide composed of 2-amino-deoxy-D-glucan combined with glycosidic β (1-4) linkages. It is commercially obtained by hydrolysis of amino-acetyl groups of naturally occurring chitin, which is the main component of shells, crabs, shrimp and krill. Due to their unique properties like high water solubility, non-toxic, biocompatibility and biodegradability, these biopolymers have been used for various applications in biomedicine, pharmaceutics, materials science, cosmetics and food industry. Another feature of these biopolymers is a high content of functional groups, for example amino groups in chitosan. These functional groups can be utilized in cross-linking with additional functional cross-linkers, resulting in the formation of functional NGs of biopolymers. Furthermore, the residual functional groups can also be utilized for further bio-conjugation with cell targeting agents.

The successful methods that are required for the preparation of NGs utilizing the above biopolymers are discussed here below:

- Water in oil (w/o) heterogeneous emulsion method
- Aqueous homogeneous gelation method
- Spray drying method and
- Chemical cross-linking method

8.3.4.1 Water-in-oil (w/o) heterogeneous emulsion method

This process operated in a two tier fashion: firstly the emulsification of aqueous droplets of hydrophilic biopolymers upon addition of oil soluble surfactants in continuous oil medium followed by cross-linking agent addition.

(a) *Inverse (mini) emulsion method*: In this process, w/o type of emulsion is prepared using hydrophilic biopolymer aqueous droplets and continuous oil medium mixture by homogenizer or a high-speed mechanical stirrer. Then polymer solution is cross-linked by an appropriate agent. Finally the nanoscalar particles are dispersed in suitable organic solvent and subjected for further purification by either precipitation or centrifugation.

(b) *Reverse micellar method*: The process is somewhat similar to the inverse (mini) emulsion method, but fundamentally differs in that it involves the incorporation of relatively large amount of oil-soluble surfactants which not only impart thermodynamic stability to solution but also facilitate the preparation of 10-100 nm size range NGs particles **(Figure 8.8)**.

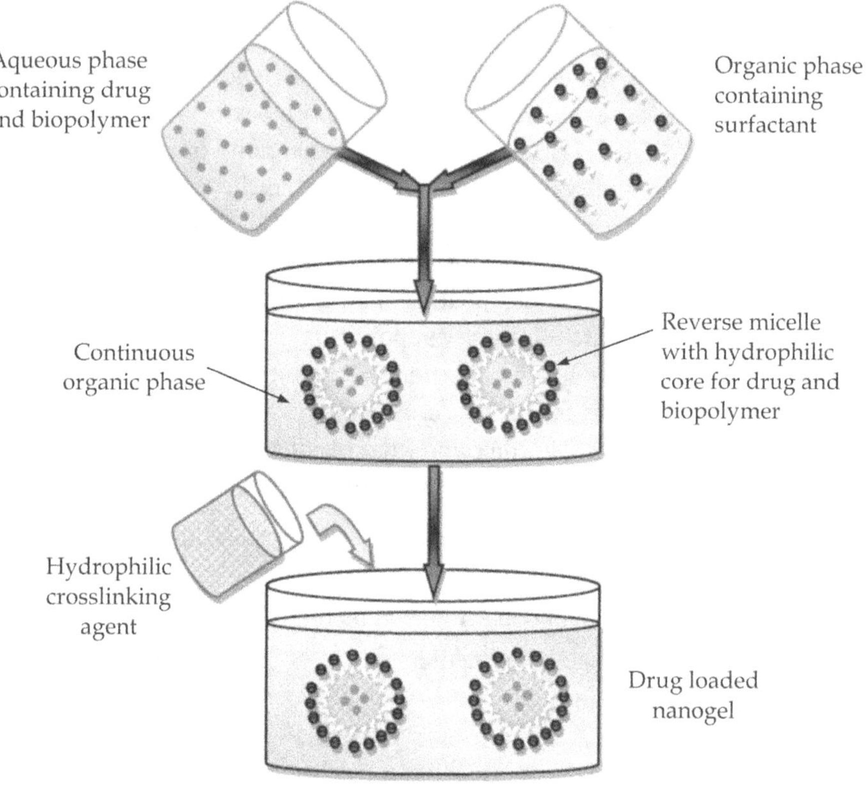

Figure 8.8 Schematic representation of reverse micellar technique for NG preparation

(c) *Membrane emulsification*: It is a comparatively novel method for the formation of spherical particles having uniform size distribution. This method utilizes a membrane, initially Shirasu porous glass (SPG) membrane with uniform pore size ranging from 0.1 to 18 μm that allows liquid to permeate under adequate pressure. It may lead to emergence of uniform sized droplets which dispersed in the continuous phase, causing development of simple w/o and o/w emulsions, multiple emulsions such as o/w/o and solid/o/w dispersions and the corresponding particles with various shapes including microspheres, hollow spheres, core-shell microcapsules and organic–inorganic hybrid materials **(Figure 8.9)**.

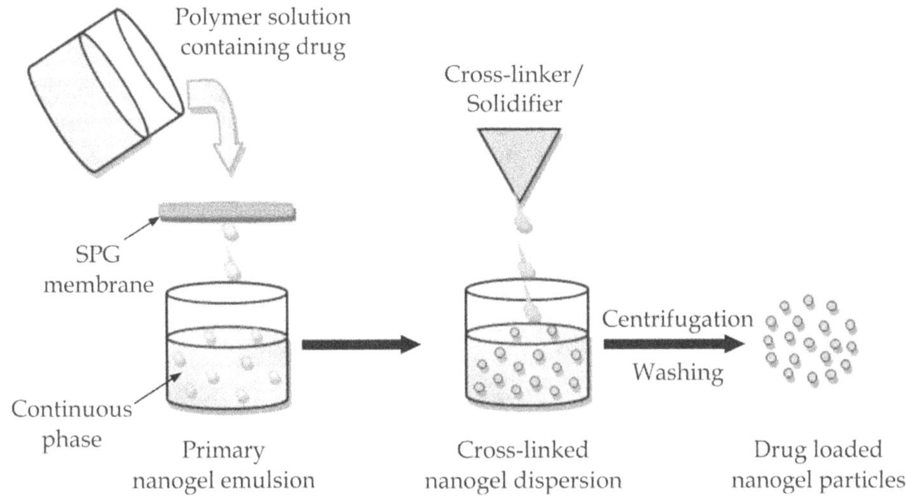

Figure 8.9 Schematic representation of membrane emulsification technique for NG preparation

This technique combined with a step-wise crosslinking method was recently developed to prepare NG particles with an uniform size distribution. Chitosan nanospheres containing insulin were prepared by this process. First, a stable w/o emulsion with a uniform droplet size was formed by passing an aqueous chitosan/acetic acid solution containing insulin through the uniform pores of a porous glass membrane into paraffin/petroleum ether mixture containing hexaglycerinpentaester (PO-500) emulsifier. Next, the uniform droplets of chitosan were hardened by both ionic cross-linking with tripolyphosphate (TPP) and chemical crosslinking with glutaraldehyde. The solidification condition was optimized based on nanospheres morphology, encapsulation efficiency, drug activity and *in-vitro* release profile. A similar method was applied to prepare chitosan based NGs incorporated with BSA and more recently, agarose beads with different particle size ranges.

8.3.4.2 Aqueous homogeneous gelation method

Covalent chemical crosslinking was utilized for the preparation of biopolymer-based nanoparticles in water. An example includes the utilization of a facile carbodiimide coupling reaction of chitosan with a PEG dicarboxylic acid as a water-soluble cross-linker, resulting in the formation of chitosan based NGs with a diameter of 4-24 nm by transmission electron microscopy (TEM) and 50-120 nm by dynamic light scattering (DLS). In another example, ethylene diamine tetra acetic dianhydride (EDTAA) was used to react with chitosan for the preparation of pH-sensitive NGs with a diameter of 70-80 nm. They enabled reversible switch of their surface upon pH change to be positive at pH<4.8 and negative at pH>5.2 and were stable in the entire pH range. These characteristics suggest that they are an effective candidate for encapsulation of pH-sensitive anticancer agents such as highly water-insoluble camptothecin (CPT).

Reversible physical crosslinking has also been explored to prepare fine nanoparticles. In particular, ionic gelation involves electrostatic interaction of cationic chitosan with polyanion, polyethyleneimine (PEI) and typically TPP in water. The method is advantageous in that it avoids the possible toxicity of cross-linkers and reagents that are involved in chemical cross-linking method. For the development of drug delivery carriers to target tumors, chitosan was recently modified with glycidyltrimethyl ammonium chloride to form N-[(2-hydroxy-3-trimethylammonium) propyl] chitosan chloride, which was in turn cross-linked with TPP in the presence of methotrexate, an anticancer drug. The resulting NGs underwent a change in volume upon decreasing pH, varying the diameter from 180 nm at pH 7.4 to 450 nm at pH 5. This volume transition is effective for targeted drug delivery of cancer therapeutics in that methotrexates are physically entrapped in chitosan-based NGs at physiological pH 7.4, while they are released from the NGs in tumor cells under acidic conditions. In addition, these NGs were conjugated with transferrin, a cell-targeting protein, in aqueous media, which facilitates receptor-medicated endocytosis. The resulting methotrexate-loaded NG bio-conjugates could be used for targeted pH-mediated intracellular release of cancer therapeutics.

8.3.4.3 Spray drying method

It is widely employed method that utilize spray dryer, consist of atomizer and drying chamber. To get nanospheres or NGs, material in form of solutions or suspensions is atomized to fine droplets and hot air stream may lead to immediate drying of solvent from the droplets in drying chamber. The dried particles are settled in to a bottom collector which may be further dried by vacuum. The particle size can be varied by nozzle size, atomization speed, spray discharge rate and extent of cross-linking.

8.3.4.4 Chemical cross-linking method

The NGs can also prepared by chemical cross-linking which principally operates on basic organic chemistry named reaction principles like free radical polymerization and Michael addition. Out of which Michael addition gained a wide attention by researchers.

(a) ***Michael addition reaction***: Michael addition-type reaction has been explored to prepare hydrogels with thiol-acrylate networks. This method requires the modification of hydroxy groups of Dex with either thiols or acrylates. Thiol-functionalized Dex (Dex-SH) was prepared by a two-step reaction: activation of hydroxy groups of Dex with 4-nitrophenylchloroformate and then reaction of the resultant nitrophenyl-substituted Dex (Dex-NP) with cysteamine. The thiol-Dex was then added into a PEG tetra-acrylate, resulting in the formation of Dex-based hydrogels. In another case, vinylsulfone functionalized Dex (Dex-VS) was prepared by reaction of Dex with vinyl sulfonealkanionic acid, which was prepared by the reaction of a mercaptoalkanoic acid with divinylsulfone. They were cross-linked with linear and four-arm star mercaptopoly (ethylene glycol), which was prepared by multi-step organic synthesis, to form Dex-hydrogels.

(b) *Free radical polymerization*: Dextran based hydrogels as well as NGs can be prepared using free radical polymerization of methacrylate functionalized dextran. By the use of hydroxyl groups of dextran and various methacrylate precursors different methacrylated dextran scan be synthesized. They may contain methacrylated dextran derivatives of hydroxy-terminated HEMA-lactate (Dex-LA-HEMA), glycidyl methacrylate (Dex-GMA) and 2-hydroxyethyl methacrylate (Dex-HEMA).

8.3.5 Heterogeneous Free Radical Polymerization

This method involves the reaction of hydrophilic or water soluble monomers in the presence of cross linkers (difunctional or multifunctional) to prepare NGs. They include number of methods which are as follows: Dispersion, precipitation, inverse (mini) emulsion and inverse microemulsion polymerization.

8.3.5.1 Dispersion polymerization

This is a technique that authorized for the development of nano-sized particles with narrow size distribution. In this process most of the ingredients like monomers, polymeric stabilizers and initiators are found to be soluble as a continuous phase. Initially polymerization occurs in a homogeneous reaction mixture and later on formed polymers may become insoluble in the continuous medium. Finally it may lead to the preparation of stable dispersion of polymeric particles with aid of colloidal stabilizers. The method has been mainly utilized to develop uniform microspheres of hydrophobic polymers including polystyrene (PS) and poly methyl methacrylate (PMMA).

8.3.5.2 Precipitation polymerization (PP)

PP initiate with the preparation of non swellable homogeneous polymer mixture. Then a system compatible cross-linker is added to polymer solution. Finally the polymerization of monomers and cross-linkers in aqueous solution is initiated by free radical polymerization at a temperature over lower critical solution temperature (LCST). It ultimately results in development of irregular shaped nano-structured particles with narrow size distribution range **(Figure 8.10)**. Preparation of hydrogels and NGs by precipitation polymerization in water has been extensively explored for biomedical applications. NGs for oral delivery of protein was prepared and reported by Peppas et al. During experiment the researches has fabricated nanostructure of poly (methacrylic acid-g-ethylene glycol).

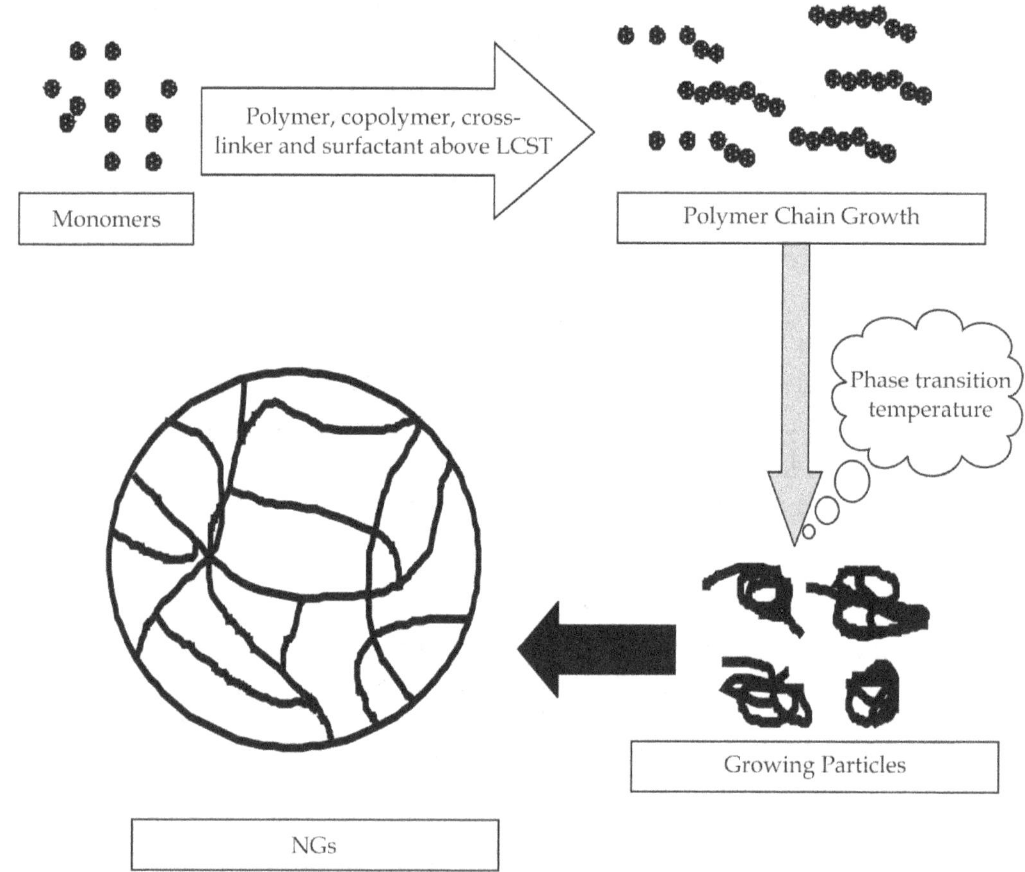

Figure 8.10 NGs preparation by precipitation polymerization

8.3.5.3 Inverse (Mini) emulsion polymerization

It is a w/o type emulsion polymerization which consists of aqueous droplets (water soluble monomers) stabilized with addition of oil soluble surfactants in a continuous organic phase. Mechanical stirring cause formation of stable dispersions for inverse emulsion while sonication cause inverse mini emulsion polymerization **(Figure 8.11)**.

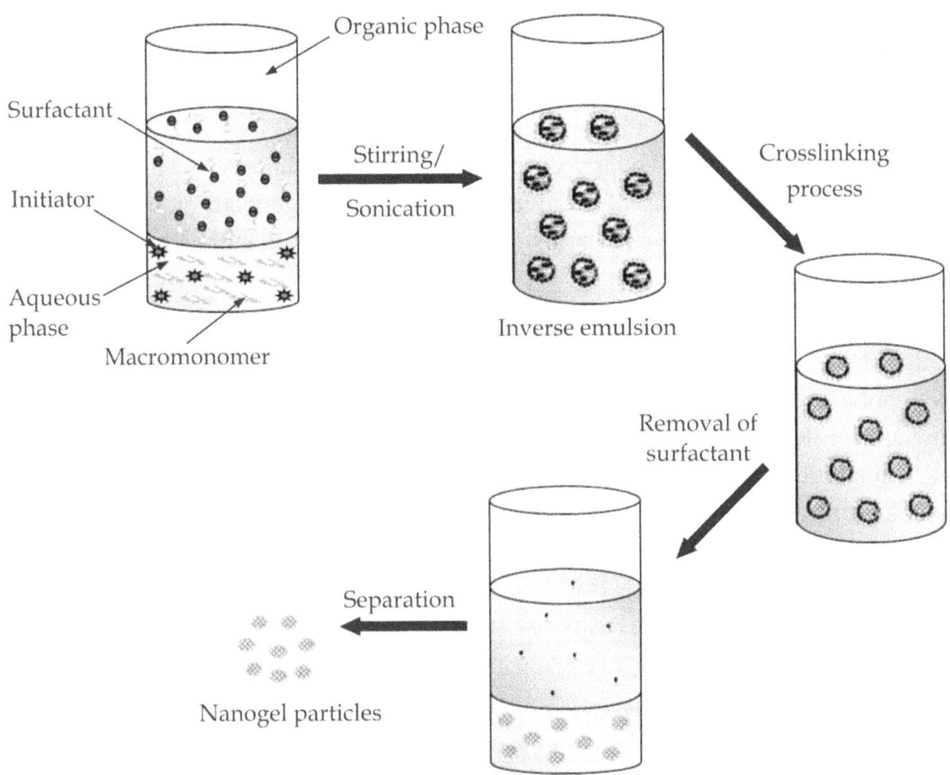

Figure 8.11 Schematic representation of inverse emulsion polymerization technique for NG preparation

8.3.5.4 Inverse microemulsion polymerization

Inverse microemulsion polymerization forms thermodynamically stable emulsion above critical micellar concentration (CMC) upon further addition of emulsifier while inverse mini emulsion produces stable macro-emulsion at below or around the CMC. This method also utilizes aqueous droplets, dispersed with the aid of bulk amount of oil soluble surfactants in a continuous media. This technique was exploited for the synthesis of well established NGs. NGs containing Dex as water soluble macromolecule was prepared with poly vinyl pyrrolidone. Modified NGs (cationic preparation) was prepared using poly (HEA-co-AETMAC) with oligoethylene glycol dimethacrylate (OEGDMA) as cross linking agent.

8.3.6 Heterogeneous Controlled Radical Polymerization (HCRP)

HCRP is a means of co-polymers preparation with optimized molecular weight, narrow molecular weight distribution, useful end functional groups and designed structures. It has been employed as an important technique for preparation of optimized polymer-protein bioconjugates. This can be done by several methods including stable free radical polymerization (SFRP), reversible addition fragmentation chain transfer (RAFT) polymerization and atom transfer radical polymerization (ARTP). ARTP initiators were found to be modified peptide sequences, biotin and streptavidin. Many HCRP reactions of hydrophobic monomers have been investigated in heterogeneous aqueous dispersion including microemulsion, miniemulsion, dispersion, conventional emulsion and suspension media.

This method has also been applied for the synthesis of stable nanoparticles of well-controlled hydrophilic block copolymers. Interestingly, the resulting doubly hydrophilic block copolymers self-assembled to form well defined micelles with a diameter of 10–20 nm in water. CRP techniques have been explored for the synthesis of gels and cross-linked nanoparticles of well controlled polymers in the presence of cross-linkers. ATRP in inverse miniemulsion for the synthesis and functionalization of stable biodegradable cross-linked NGs of well controlled water soluble polymers in the presence of a disulfide-functionalized dimethacrylate (DMA) was reported. This approach allowed for the preparation of biomaterials with many useful features.

Several other ways are available for the preparation of novel functional NGs using the method involving ATRP in inverse miniemulsion. They include the use of functional ATRP initiators and the facile copolymerization with functional monomers. The latter approach was successfully demonstrated with the preparation of OH-functionalized NGs by copolymerizing with 2-hydroxyethyl acrylate (HEA).

Well-defined functional NGs prepared by this newly developed method hold great potential as drug delivery carriers to target-specific cells for biomedical applications. Future NGs will contain targeting residues such as peptides, proteins and antibodies for delivery to specific regions and cells.

8.4 DRUG LOADING IN NGs

NGs have proven excellent potential as a drug delivery system. Properties like biodegradability, biocompatibility, high drug loading capacity, better cell and tissue permeation capabilities gave it a leading edge over existing conventional gel technologies. Its high water retention capacity makes it as ideal candidature capable of inclusion of bulky drugs and macromolecules like proteins, peptides, oligonucleotides etc. It offer dualistic drug delivery front and provide time dependent release profile with active targeting of drugs. Drug loading in NGs can be achieved by following methods:

8.4.1 Covalent Conjugation

In this method the desired moiety is covalently conjugated either to the pre-formed NGs or the conjugation is achieved during the formulation. Matsumoto et.al. reported NGs preparation by reversible addition fragmentation chain transfer (RAFT) random copolymerization. They used poly (ethylene glycol) methyl ether methacrylate (PEGMA) and pyridyl disulfide methacrylate (PDSMA) as polymers and together they were copolymerized. PDSMA acted as cross-linker and also facilitated the surface amelioration with bovine serum albumin as therapeutic moiety (BSA).

8.4.2 Self-Assembly

It is highly suitable for drug with poor aqueous solubility profile. It was prepared by the assistance of dextran modified polymer (hydrophobic in nature). Here an aqueous dispersion of modified polymer is prepared in water, or buffered saline solution, with continuous stirring, until a clear solution is obtained. If it is required a suitable hydrophilic cross-linker can be added to obtain desired size range of NGs. Gonçalves et.al. reported curcumin loaded NGs using Dex-16 as modified polymer and drug loading was done by self- assembly mechanism.

8.4.3 Physical Entrapment

Proteins was incorporated in cholesterol transformed pullulan NGs using physical entrapment method. Additionally hydrophobic molecules can be incorporated into non-polar domains produced by hydrophobic chains existing in selected NGs.

8.5 DRUG RELEASE

Drug release from the prepared NGs ultimately affects the overall therapeutic efficacy of products. Various factors like its biodegradable nature, size, etc., affects the overall release profile of drug from NGs. In biodegradable NGs the drug is released with the degradation of polymer in biofluids. It facilitate not only the targeted drug release but also effective in removing the dump mass from body in order to avoid any toxicological issue. Influence of particle size on drug release also astonish to a considerable extent. Smaller the size of particle, it is readily available at the surface for diffusion, while larger particle allow greater encapsulation with hasten drug release profile. The drug release profile also dependent on polymer, copolymer and cross-linker that are used for preparation of NGs.

Release mechanism is perplexing phenomenon that cannot be clearly explained by using one phenomenon. But the basic mechanisms that are able to explain the release pattern are discussed here below:

8.5.1 Diffusion Controlled Release Systems

It is the fundamental mechanism which controls the release of drug from NGs based system. The active moiety is dispersed in NG architecture and release may occur due to the diffusion of moiety through pores or macromolecular mesh. The active substances containing NGs can be further encapsulated in a reservoir system for controlled delivery.

8.5.2 Chemically Controlled Systems

These systems principally works on two mechanisms i.e. Erodible and pendent system which can be explained as follows:

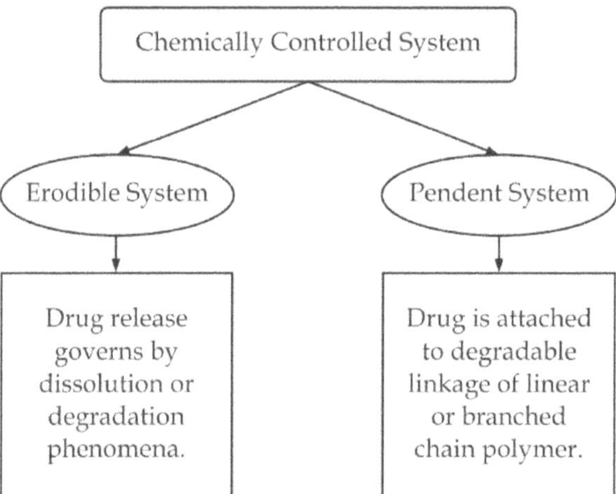

8.5.3 Swelling Controlled Release System

This system entirely depends upon swelling behavior of polymer used in preparation of NGs. When NGS, targeted to a tissue and NGs get exposed to biological fluids. A series of biophysical phenomena occurs. Fluid enters in polymeric mesh of gels and finally lowers the glass transition temperature which ultimately extricates the drug via diffusion.

8.5.4 Environmentally Responsive Systems

The drug release by NGs can also be modulated via some external stimuli response. But the adorable and imperative character of rapid swelling and shrinking is required for it. The system modulates their swelling ratio as per the intensity of stimulus projected like pH, temperature, light, electromagnetic field etc. These characters make it the most suitable candidate to delivery of macromolecules like amino acids, proteins, peptide, DNA, RNA, SiRNA in gene delivery or gene therapy.

8.6 CHARACTERIZATION OF NGs

NGs are characterized in terms of size distribution, surface charge, surface morphology, hydrophobicity, optical activity, mechanical strength and swellability. Different techniques are utilized for the determination of these properties.

8.6.1 Dynamic Light Scattering (DLS)

It is synonymously known as Photon Correlation Spectroscopy (PCS) or quasi-elastic light scattering (QELS). This technique is used to carry out the size distribution profiling of nanostructured particles in NGs. The variation in the intensity of scattered light on the microsecond time scale is recorded by this technique. This may also use to measure the influence of cross-linking agent and charged monomer concentration as well as effective hydrodynamic radius of the particles. DLS analysis also showed swelling behavior of NGs in different mediums as NGs swell nearly four times of their parent dimensions. To carry out the measurements Brookhaven BI goniometer and BI 900 digital correlate like instruments can be used. Average time scattered light intensities are measured at scattering angle of 20 to 150°at different NG concentrations.

8.6.2 Surface Charge Studies

The surface charge of the NG is analyzed by measuring the electrophoretic mobility and expressed as zeta potential. The surface charge on the NGs may be because of polymer type used and manipulation by distinct functional groups. For example: poly (acrylic acid) nanoparticles have negative zeta potential on their surfaces owing to the presence of anionic carboxylate ions. For zeta potential measurement NGs are generally dispersed in 1 mM suspension of 10^{-3} M KNO_3 and analyzed using Zeta plus meter. To keep the conductivity of the medium constant KNO_3 is used. This study may also be used for carrying out drug binding and stability study of NGs. Drug binding interaction with the NG depends on the functionality of the NG and the drug. As poly (acrylamide) NGs could extract approximately 80% of the amitriptyline when compared with non-modified nanoparticles. The binding between the polymer backbone and cationic amitriptyline is found to be less because the non-modified NG has a relatively neutral polymer backbone. For negatively charged NGs, extraction is high due to the electrostatic interaction with the positively charged drug substances.

8.6.3 Scanning Electron Microscopy (SEM)

This study is performed to determine any structural defects which may hasten the drug release profile. It gives detail of morphological characteristics of nanoparticles surface.

8.6.4 Fluorescence Analysis

The florescence emission spectrum is obtained by using fluorescence spectrometer. It can be obtain by two methods:

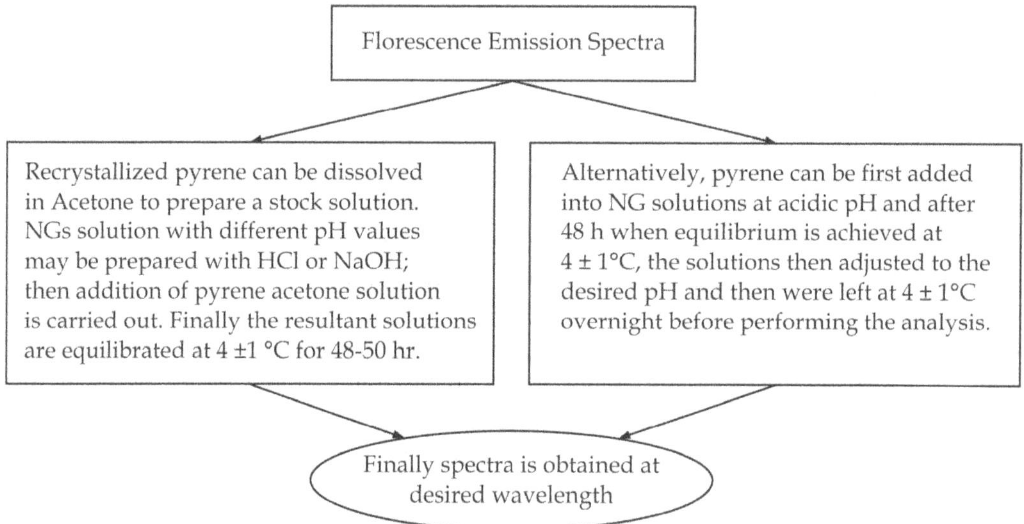

8.6.5 Atomic Force Microscopy (AFM)

This technique utilizes a probe tip with atomic scale sharpness across a sample to produce a topological map based on the forces at play between the tip and the surface. The probe can be permitted to hover just above the sample or dragged across the sample. NGs morphology can be effectively analyzed by this technique. The effect of cross-linking agent on the NGs surface and effective measurement of height and diameter of NGs can be effectively determined using this technique.

8.6.6 Nuclear Magnetic Resonance (NMR)

NMR technique can be applied to determine the size as well as the qualitative nature of nanoparticles. This technique analyzes the coupling between the polymer backbone and cross-linking agent. Physicochemical status of components within the nanocarrier can be computed by selectivity of chemical shift.

8.6.7 Circular Dichroism (CD)

CD gives an idea about optical activity of the resulting product. This is examined as a probe for chiral molecule detection embedded in NGs. It may lead to macromolecular structures with a helical twist correlates with chiral center which in turn able to induce CD signal.

8.6.8 Size Exclusion Chromatography (SEC)

NGs are considered as swellable polymer as well as highly branched structures ranging between 1-100 nm. SEC technique can be used for fractionation of materials in this range and for measurement of NG molecular distribution which is used to calculate the particle size distribution.

8.6.9 Force Spectroscopy

This is a dynamic analytical technique which can be used for the study of mechanical characteristics of polymer and de-bonding force of NGs.

8.6.10 Swelling Studies

This character is a decisive factor of all as it governs the drug targeting and its release profile. It measures the water absorbing property of system. It is determine on the basis of swelling ratio, which is ratio of weight of wet swollen gel to dry weight of gel.

$$\text{Swelling Ratio} = \frac{\text{Weight of wet gel}}{\text{Weight of dry gel}}$$

8.7 STABILITY STUDIES OF NGs

The stability of non-modified and modified NGs in different solvents is determined and is seen that all NGs form easily dispersible suspensions in water. Non-modified NGs are clear dispersions while modified NGs are cloudy due to hydrophobic or ionic interactions within the NGs forming aggregates. The stability of NG suspensions is analyzed by using a Turbiscan instrument **(Figure 8.12)**. The Turbiscan head consists of a pulsed near infrared light source ($\lambda = 850$ nm) and two synchronous detectors: a transmission detector which receives the light going across the sample (at $0°$ from the incident beam) and a back scattering detector which receives the light scattered backward by the sample (at $135°$ from incidence beam). Stability is indicated if no particle size of volume fraction occur and back scattering and transmitting peaks superimpose on each other. Instability is indicated by flocculation, coalescence, sedimentation or creaming showing differentiation in transmittance and back scattering peaks.

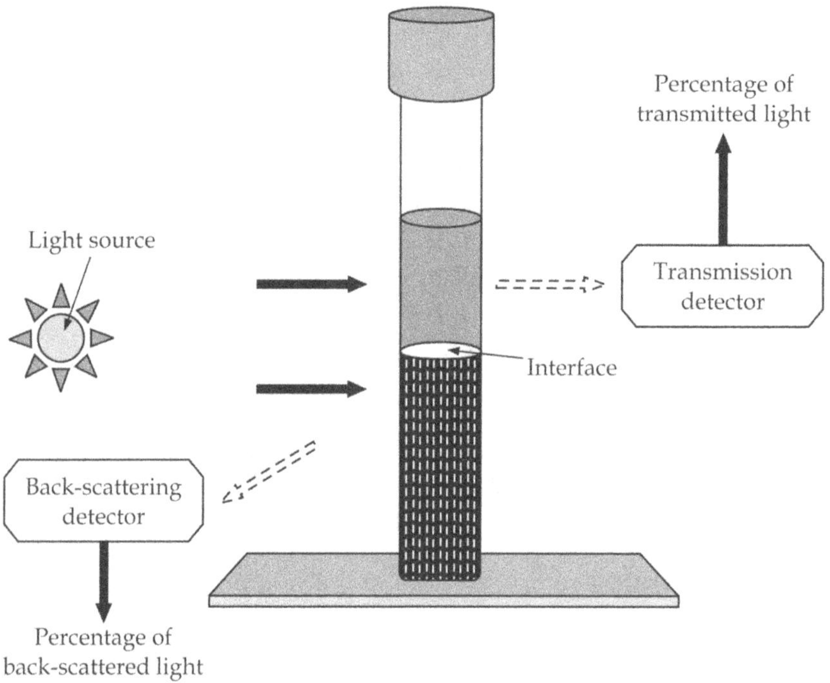

Figure 8.12 Schematic representation of Turbiscan instrument

8.8 APPLICATIONS

NGs as carriers have varied applications in the delivery of drugs, enzymes, proteins (insulin), artificial chaperones and artificial vaccines. NG based systems are also proved their effectiveness in cancer therapy, treatment of neuro-degenerative disease, bone therapy and Alzheimer's disease. NGs can be further utilized for targeted delivery with advancement in the research technology.

8.8.1 NGs as Potential Gene and Antisense Delivery Agents

The developments in the area of gene and antisense therapy imparted safe and effective drug delivery systems. It is known that many diseases like cancers are caused by mutations of single gene and genetic material insertion into the cell nucleus. For successful targeted delivery various biological barriers are to be by passed. Currently various viral and non-viral vectors have been tested for oligonucleotide delivery but owing to restrictions of viral carriers such as toxicity and immune response more impact is given to non-viral vectors. Non-viral vectors are also limited due to poor stability, heterogeneity and size considerations. Hence there is a need of an alternative like polymeric NGs size below 200 nm to form monodisperse complexes with DNA. This

DNA complex causes improved physical stability, cellular distribution and targeted delivery of oligonucleotide.

8.8.2 Toxic Scavengers

Toxicity of drugs is considered as major health care problems in human, which can be incorporated by drug miscalculation, illicit drug usage, suicide attempts. So there is a need of such systems for detoxification of overdosed patients by removal of drug as much as possible. This can be done by the application of small biodegradable carrier which can be easily extracted from human body after removal of drug. Biodegradable polymeric NGs are considered as potential candidates for overdosed drug scavenging as they fulfill these requirements. NGs are promising candidates for toxic scavenging by appropriate manipulation to absorb large quantity of desired molecules from body fluids and respond faster. As NGs can pass through tiniest blood capillaries, they have been explored for drug binding and delivery application.

8.8.3 Bone Medicine

In bone medicine recovery from bone loss is a major issue hence there is a need for efficient measures for bone gain that can be completed by peptide growth factors and non peptidyl agents. Prostaglandin E_2 is a non-peptide anabolic agent for bone but its application is limited in bone therapy due to the side-effects like diarrhea, need of frequent dosing due to short half-life. When PGE_2 in cholesterol bearing pullulan NGs were administered they induced new bone formation and also explored as a novel carrier for delivery of drugs including proteins and non-peptide molecules.

8.8.4 NGs in Alzheimer's Disease

Formation of fibrils of amyloid β-proteinis one of the major etiological causes involved in Alzheimer's disease. Hence inhibition of aggregation of amyloid β-protein is a most appealing approach for Alzheimer's disease treatment. Cholesterol bearing pullulan NGs act as artificial chaperones to inhibit the formation of amyloid fibrils, which have amyloidgenic activity. NGs incorporate amyloid β-proteins and induce a conformational change from random coil to α-helix or β-sheet structure.

8.8.5 Encapsulation of Enzyme in NGs to Enhance Bio-Catalytic Activity and Stability

Genetic approaches such as directed evolution and site mutation, chemical modification via conjugation or encapsulation provide an efficient route to enhance enzyme stability at high temperature or in the presence of organic solvent. Enzymes stability can be improved by encapsulation in silica, polymer and organo-clay particles. Low bio-catalytic activity is observed with these coating materials due to hindrance of the conformational transition of enzyme and the transport of substrate and product. It can be avoided by fabrication of a single-enzyme containing capsulate with a thin, permeable coating. Nanoparticles have obtained enhanced enzyme stability in the fabrication of enzyme at an insignificant increase in mass transfer resistance. Nevertheless, a simple, effective and versatile procedure that yields a single enzyme capsule with enhanced stability, high activity and uniformed size is being pursued to provide robust enzymes for industrial bio-catalysis.

8.8.6 Insulin Delivery by NGs

Some researchers are reinforcing to develop smart NGs for delivery of insulin. The propose system is so smart that it will detect the glucose level and then customize the insulin release. The nanoparticles are composed of an inner core of insulin, modified dextran and glucose oxidase enzymes. When it is administered to patient with high blood glucose level, it triggers the enzyme which converts glucose into gluconic acid. The acid so formed facilitates the disintegration of dextran spheres and finally results in releases of insulin. The released insulin then lowers the glucose level of the blood to the normal.

8.8.7 NGs for Treatment of Neurodegenerative Disorders

Development of therapeutic and diagnostic modality for the treatment of neurodegenerative disorders requires systemic delivery of oligonucleotide to the central nervous system (CNS). Generally when macromolecules are injected in blood they are poorly transported from the blood brain barrier (BBB). Researchers explored NGs as a novel system for oligonucleotide delivery to the brain. Oligonucleotide, negatively charged can be bind and encapsulated with Polyethyleneimine NGs which is cationic in nature and forms stable aqueous dispersion of polyelectrolyte complex.

8.8.8 Antiviral Therapy

Nucleosidase reverse transcriptase inhibitor (NRTIs), are delivered via NGs to brain and they are reported to reduce the mitochondrial toxicity by 3 folds and hence prevent neurotoxicity of system. NGs basically act on macrophages which are observed to promote latent activation of HIV in patient; hence it is most effective tool for treatment of HIV.

8.8.9 Small Molecular Weight Drug Delivery

Sustained drug delivery from polymeric formulation has opened a new avenue for the treatment of numerous diseases like cancer. Polymers that have been explored for these formulations include PLA, PLGA, PGA etc. PEG has been explored to manipulate the release profile, blood stream clearance, biodistribution and biodegradation. Typically betamethasone disodium 21-phosphate was entrapped by PLA/PLGA homopolymers and PEG engineered nanoparticles. The vascular circulation time and release profile could be modulated by variation in the composition or molecular weight of the polymer.

8.8.10 Protein, Peptide and Oligosaccharide Delivery

Oral route is considered to be as most convenient and comfortable means of drug administration however poor bioavailability due to lack of stability in GIT and low mucosal permeability may lead to degradation before absorption limits its use for protein and peptide administration. One alternative way could be to improve protein and peptide administration is the encapsulation of these agents in nanocarriers. This will protect their degradation in GIT as well as facilitate the transportation into systemic circulation.

8.8.11 Vaccine Delivery

Nanocarriers have emerged as novel carriers for antigen delivery with the advancement of technology. Primary challenge is the induction of immune response capable of safeguarding from infection or disease and ultimately to provide effective immunization after single dose of vaccine. Nanocarriers containing antigen is well recognized and uptaken from antigen presenting cells (APCs). Activated APCs migrate to regional lymph node and present antigen to T- cells which may cause induction of immune response that is the main goal of vaccination. Several studies have confirmed that APCs can internalize polymeric nanoparticles. Targeted delivery to lymph node is an effective way to avoid premature antigen presentation that can be achieved by the use of nanocarriers. Particle size is considered to be as important factor for lymphatic uptake from the interstitial space. Now a day's vaccine for cancer is considered as very promising approach for anti-cancer therapy. It may avoid the side effects associated with other therapies and provide ample opportunity for development of long lasting immunity.

8.8.12 Targeting

Targeting is an effective means of delivery of moieties to a specific site. Nanocarriers have been explored for drug targeting. One such approach is surface modification of nanoparticles with an antibody; it may interact with specific antigen site. It is reported by some authors that antibody targeting increases internalization rather than tumor localization. Internalization is thought to be very important for bioactive delivery like gene delivery, gene silencing. Other specifically designed carriers based on target site properties like pH, enzymes presence or tissue markers. Receptor mediated endocytosis is another mechanism that has been employed to confer cell or tissue specificity to nanocarriers. Cellular uptake is enhanced by interaction between specific ligand and receptor and this enhanced uptake improve the therapeutic efficacy. Targeting ligands that has been explored are galactose, lactose, mannose, lactoferrin, RGD peptide. Different targets have also been explored for cancer like diseases. Angiogenesis targeting, a major focused area causes inhibition of tumor growth. Most considered angiogenic targets are vascular endothelial growth factor receptors, matrix metalloproteinase receptors and vascular cell adhesion molecule-1.

9 Bioadhesive Patches/ Films

The flexibility and comfort offered by the bioadhesive patches/films is advantageous for drug delivery purpose especially in case of wound dressing. Moreover, bioadhesive patches/films effectively treat topical diseases by protecting the wound surface thus minimizing pain. In last two decades the research and development in the field for bioadhesive drug delivery systems revolutionized the use of these delivery systems for transdermal and buccal delivery of therapeutics to achieve local and systemic effects. Many transdermal and buccal patches/films are marketed successfully. For oral delivery bioadhesive patches/films may be preferred over bioadhesive tablets in terms of flexibility, ease of application and patient compliance. Additionally they prolong the residence time on the mucosa and not easily washed away and removed by saliva as oral gels. It may also be possible to avoid the first pass effect and presystemic elimination in the gastro intestinal tract and liver.

Bioadhesive patches that are applied directly to the affected region have the potential to supply effective drug levels at the site of action and sustain these levels over a long period of time. A bioadhesive patch for the systemic administration of a drug will, in general, be designed with much more emphasis on controlled release rates and on achieving fairly even plasma level over a predetermined period of time. In general, this type of bioadhesive patch would require relatively long adhesion times at least a few hours to achieve the desired systemic effects.

Characteristics of an ideal bioadhesive patch include elasticity, flexibility, and soft yet sufficiently strong to resist breakage due to stress from the environment at the site of adhesion. Moreover, it must also exhibit good bioadhesive strength so that it can be retained for a desired duration. As such, the mechanical, bioadhesive and swelling properties of mucoadhesive patches are critical and essential to be evaluated.

9.1 TYPES OF BIOADHESIVE PATCHES

On the basis of drug incorporation methods the bioadhesive patches can be of:

9.1.1 Matrix Type

This type of system is designed by mixing drug, adhesive and additives. Bioadhesive patches for drug delivery purposes can be bidirectional or unidirectional **(Figure 9.1 and 9.2)**. Bidirectional patches are applicable for the delivery of drug over buccal mucosa. Drug is released by these patches in both mucosa and mouth.

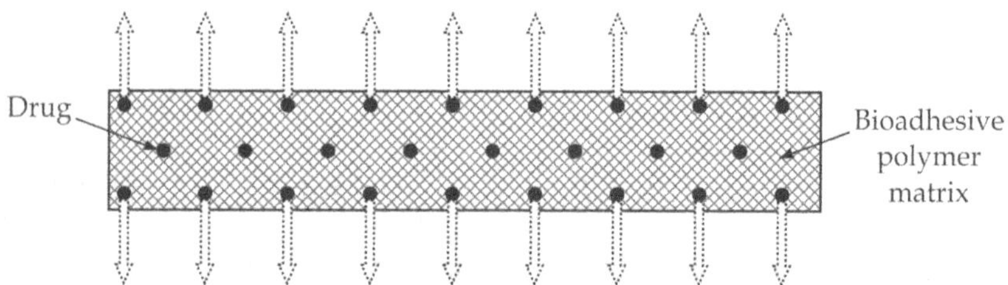

Figure 9.1 Buccal patch designed for bidirectional drug release

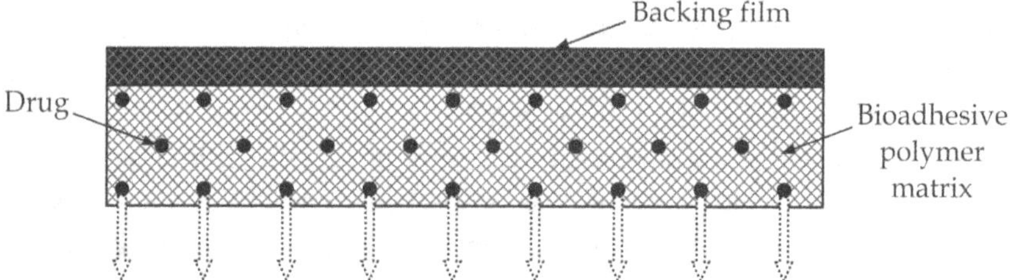

Figure 9.2 Buccal patch designed for unidirectional drug release

9.1.2 Reservoir Type

Reservoir system is designed containing a cavity for drug and additives separated from the adhesive. In order to prevent drug loss, to reduce patch deformation and disintegration, and control of drug delivery direction is done by application of impermeable backing membrane. Additionally, the patch can be constructed to undergo minimal degradation or can be designed to dissolve almost immediately.

9.2 COMPONENTS OF BIOADHESIVE PATCHES

The basic components of bioadhesive patches are:

- Drug substance
- Bioadhesive polymers

- Backing membrane
- Permeation enhancers

9.2.1 Drug Substance

Formulation and designing of bioadhesive patches as drug delivery systems should be decided on the basis of desired action as instant action/prolonged action and local/systemic action. Selection of suitable drug candidates is based on pharmacokinetic properties that are as follows:

- Drug dose should be small.
- Biological half-life between 2-8 h is considered appropriate candidates for controlled drug delivery.
- Greater fluctuations or elevated values of T_{max} shown by drug in case of oral delivery.
- Pre systemic drug elimination or hepatic first pass effect.
- Passive drug absorption.

9.2.2 Bioadhesive Polymers

Selection and characterization of bioadhesive polymer is prerequisite for the development of bioadhesive patches. Further these polymers are used in matrix devices where drug is embedded in the polymer matrix to control the duration of drug release. Bioadhesive polymers have significant benefits on patient health and treatment. Drug is released into the biological membrane (skin/mucosal) by means of rate controlling layer or core layer. For effective topical/oral drug delivery these polymers must adhere to the mucin/epithelial surface. Characteristics of an ideal polymer for bioadhesive patches include:

- Inert and environment compatible.
- Non-toxic degradable end product.
- Quick adherence and site specificity to biological surface.
- Stable during storage and shelf-life.
- The polymer should be economical and easily available.
- Easy incorporation of drug into the formulation.

Criteria followed in polymer selection

- It should form a strong non-covalent bond with the mucin/epithelial surface.
- High molecular weight and narrow distribution.
- Compatible with the biological membrane.

9.2.2.1 Semi-natural/natural bioadhesive polymers

Agarose, chitosan, gelatin, hyaluronic acid, and various gums (guar, xanthan, gellan, carrageenan, and pectin) are the example of semi-natural/natural bioadhesive polymers.

9.2.2.2 Synthetic bioadhesive polymers cellulose derivatives

Some cellulose derivatives like CMC, thiolated CMC, sodium CMC, HEC, HPC, HPMC, MC and methyl hydroxyl ethyl cellulose are categories under synthetic bioadhesive polymers.

Poly (acrylic acid)-based polymers

CP, PC, PAA, polyacrylates, poly (methylvinylether-co-methacrylic acid), poly (2-hydroxyethyl methacrylate), poly (acrylic acidco-ethylhexylacrylate), poly (methacrylate), poly (alkylcyanoacrylate), poly (isohexylcyanoacrylate), poly (isobutylcyanoacrylate), copolymer of acrylic acid and PEG are the poly (acrylic acid)-based polymer categories under synthetic bioadhesive polymer.

Others

Other example of synthetic bioadhesive polymers are Polyoxyethylene, PVA, PVP, thiolated polymers.

9.2.2.3 Water-soluble bioadhesive polymers

Some polymer such as CP, HEC, HPC (waterb38 8C), HPMC (cold water), PAA, sodium CMC, sodium alginate are example of water-soluble bioadhesive polymers.

9.2.2.4 Water-insoluble bioadhesive polymers

Some polymer such as Chitosan (soluble in dilute aqueous acids), EC and PC are example of water-insoluble bioadhesive polymer.

9.2.2.5 Cationic bioadhesive polymers

Cationic bioadhesive polymer includes Aminodextran, chitosan, (DEAE)-dextran, TMC.

9.2.2.6 Anionic bioadhesive polymers

Anionic bioadhesive polymer includes Chitosan-EDTA, CP, CMC, pectin, PAA, PC, sodium alginate, sodium CMC, xanthan gum.

9.2.2.7 Non-ionic bioadhesive polymers

Non-ionic bioadhesive polymer includes Hydroxyethyl starch, HPC, poly (ethylene oxide), PVA, PVP, and scleroglucan.

9.2.2.8 Covalently bonding bioadhesive polymers

Cyanoacrylate is the example of covalently bonding bioadhesive polymer.

9.2.2.9 Hydrogen bonding bioadhesive polymers

Some polymers are showing their bioadhesion through hydrogen bonding. Examples are Acrylates [hydroxylated methacrylate, poly (methacrylic acid)], CP, PC, PVA.

9.2.2.10 Bioadhesive polymers with electrostatic interaction

Chitosan is such a bioadhesive polymer showing its bioadhesion with electrostatic interaction.

Abbreviations

CP = Carbopol 934P, HPC = Hydroxypropyl cellulose, PVP = Poly vinyl pyrrolidone, CMC = Carboxymethyl cellulose, HPMC = Hydroxypropyl methyl cellulose, HEC = Hydroxy ethyl cellulose, PVA = Poly vinyl alcohol, PIB = Poly isobutylene, PIP = Polyisoprene.

9.2.3 Backing Membrane

Backing membrane plays a major role in bioadhesive devices by protecting the leaking of drug from the patch and also from the environmental factors during its application and storage. Excipients selected as backing membrane should be inert and drug impermeable. The usually employed materials as backing membrane include carbopol, magnesium stearate, HPMC, HPC, CMC, polycarbophil etc. This membrane prevents the drug loss and offers better patient compliance.

9.2.4 Permeation Enhancers

Permeation enhancers are the substances that facilitate the permeation through mucosal surface and their selection depends on the physicochemical properties of the drug, nature of excipients, site of administration and nature of the vehicle. Several of the permeation enhancers are enlisted in the **Table 9.1** with their respective mechanisms.

Table 9.1 Examples of permeation enhancers with mechanism

Category	Examples	Mechanism(s)
Surfactants and bile salts	Sodium glycodeoxycholate	Acting on the components at tight junctions; Increasing the fluidity of lipid bilayer membrane
	Sodium dodecyl sulphate	
	Sodium lauryl sulphate	
	Polysorbate 80	

Table 9.1 *Contd...*

Category	Examples	Mechanism(s)
Fatty acids	Oleic acid	Increasing the fluidity of lipid bilayer membrane
	Cod liver oil	
	Capric acid	
	Lauric acid	
Polymers and polymer Derivatives	Chitosan	Increasing the fluidity of lipid bilayer membrane;
	Trimethyl chitosan	
	Chitosan-4-thiobutylamide	Increased retention of drug at biological surface
Others	Ethanol	Acting on the components at tight junctions;
	Azone®	
	Octisalate	Increasing the fluidity of lipid bilayer membrane
	Padimate	
	Menthol	

9.2.4.1 Mechanisms of action of permeation enhancers

The mechanisms by which the compounds enhance permeation are still not clearly defined. It is believed that these agents cause alteration of the protective permeation barrier of the biological membrane either by interacting with the lipid domain of the epithelial cell without significant tissue damage or by damaging the mucosa tissue as well as perturbing the plasmatic cell membrane. Some possible mechanisms for permeation enhancers include:

- *Alteration in mucus rheology*: Barrier can be overcome by reducing the viscosity of the mucus and the saliva.

- *Increase in fluidity of lipid bilayer membrane*: Due to interaction with lipid or protein components intracellular lipid packing may disturbed.

- *Action on the components at tight junctions*: Owing to inhibition of various components of biological membranes (peptidases and proteases present in buccal mucosa), cause disturbance in the tight junctions or overcome the enzymatic barrier. Further changes in membrane fluidity can also alter the enzymatic activity indirectly.

- *Increase in thermodynamic activity of drugs*: Alteration in the partition coefficient may increase the solubility of the drug.

9.3   METHODS OF PREPARATIONS

Bioadhesive patches should be uniform in thickness. Following methods are utilized for the preparation of bioadhesive patches:

- Solvent-film casting
- Hot-melt extrusion

9.3.1 Solvent-Film Casting

Solvent-film casting method is the widely applied process for manufacturing of bioadhesive patches/films owing to easy manufacturing and minimum setup cost incurred at the laboratory scale. The process consists of six steps:

- Preparation of the casting solution;
- De-aeration of the solution;
- Appropriate volume of solution transfer into a mold;
- Casting solution drying;
- Cutting of final dosage form containing desired amount of drug and
- Final dosage form packaging.

In this technique the required amount of bioadhesive polymer and solvent system are treated and vortexed that cause swelling of polymer. This swelled polymer mixture is treated with required amount of plasticizer (propylene glycol or glycerin or dibutyl phthalate) followed by vortexing. Required amount of drug is dissolved in small volume of solvent system and added to polymer solution with mixing. Then this solution is keep aside to remove an entrapped air and transferred in to a previously cleaned and treated Petri plate. Prepared film/patch can be dried in oven at 40^0C and stored in desiccators till the evaluation. Some of the therapeutic agents developed as buccal patches by solvent casting technique are listed in **Table 9.2**.

Table 9.2 Some therapeutic agents processed by solvent-film casting

Drug	Bioadhesive polymer used
Felodipine	HPMC E15, Eudragit RL100
Miconazole nitrate	SCMC, Chitosan, PVA, HEC and HPMC
β-galactosidase	Noveon, Eudragit S-100
Nifedipine	Sodium alginate
Buprenorphine	CP-934, PIB and PIP
Oxytocin	CP 974P
Carvedilol	HPMC E15, HPC
Terbutaline sulfate	CP 934, CP 971, HPMC, HEC or SCMC
Chlorpheniramine maleate	HEC
Triamcinolone acetonide	CP, Poloxamer and HPMC
Chlorhexidine	Chitosan
Isosorbide dinitrate	HPC, HPMC
Ipriflavone	PLGA, Chitosan

During the manufacturing process of the bioadhesive films, emphasis is given to the rheological behavior of solution or suspension, entrapped air bubbles in solution, residual solvent in final dosage form and content uniformity. Drying rate, appearance of film and uniformity in terms of active content can be determined by rheological behavior of casted liquid. Air bubbles are accidentally introduced to the liquid and their removal is a critical step as far as homogeneity is concern. Casting of film from aerated solutions may exhibit an uneven surface and heterogeneous thickness.

Presence of organic solvents is another concern in the manufacturing of films and its use is questioned, not only because of issues related to solvent selection and residual solvents, but also due to they are hazardous for the environment and health. Content uniformity has been considered as a major challenge for formulation scientist since early development of medicated films. One of the earliest approaches to increase the drug uniformity of medicated films is proposed by some scientist, by stating that the non-uniformity of films is inherent to their monolayered nature. They proposed a multistep method for the manufacturing of multilayered films. This multistep method overcomes the heterogeneity of the monolayered form. Problem of self-aggregation may occur due to intermolecular attractive and convective forces are favored during an inherently long drying process. Addition of viscous agents such as gel formers or polyhydric alcohols is proposed to alleviate potential self-aggregation and to avoid non-uniformity. Currently, one of the major challenges addressed in film casting process is content uniformity along with casting surface. Characterization of film in terms of bioadhesiveness, mechanical strength, release and permeation characteristics has been widely investigated. Content uniformity is generally determined by weight and not by casting area.

9.3.2 Hot-Melt Extrusion

Hot-melt extrusion (HME) technique offers many advantages over other pharmaceutical processing techniques and can be used as an alternative to traditional processing methods. In this method solvents and water are not necessary, numbers of processing and time-consuming steps are also reduced. Molten polymers can function as a thermal binder during the extrusion process and may act as drug depots and/or drug release retardants upon cooling and solidification. A matrix independent of compression properties can be massed into a larger unit. Deaggregation of suspended particles is caused due to intense mixing and agitation imposed by the rotating screw in the molten polymer. It further results in a more uniform dispersion and process is continuous and efficient. Drug substance bioavailability (BA) may be improved when it gets solubilized or dispersed at the molecular level in HME dosage forms. HME can be further categorized as ram extrusion or screw extrusion. List of drug substances processed by hot melt extrusion techniques is listed in **Table 9.3**.

Table 9.3 Some therapeutic agents processed by hot melt extrusion techniques

Drug	Melting temperature (^{o}C)
Carbamazepine	192
Nifedipine	175
Chlorpheniramine maleate	135

Table 9.3 *Contd...*

Drug	Melting temperature (°C)
Piroxicam	204.9
Diclofenac sodium	284
Tolbutamide	128.4
Cetylsalicylic acid	135
Indomethacin	162.7
Ethinyl estradiol	144
Lidocaine	68.5
Hydrochlorothiazide	274
Ibuprofen	76
Hydrocortisone	220
Diltiazem hydrochloride	210
Itraconazole	166
Acetaminophen	168
Ketoconazole	150
Zidovudine	127.5
Ketoprofen	94
Lamivudine	176.8
Lacidipine	184.8

9.3.2.1 Ram extrusion

A ram (or a piston) extrusion is a method of positive displacement that generates high pressures to push materials through the die. It involves introduction of material into a heated cylinder after which ram pressurizes the soft materials through the die and transforms it into the required shape. The major drawback of ram extrusion in comparison is limited melting capacity that causes poor temperature uniformity in the extrudate and resulting in lower homogeneity.

9.3.2.2 Screw extrusion

The process of screw extrusion can be achieved by two types of extruders:

- Single screw extruder
- Twin screw extruder

(a) *Single screw extruder*

Single screw extruder is the most extensively used extrusion system in the world. This method involves rotation of single screw inside the barrel which is used for feeding, melting, devolatilizing and pumping. Depending upon the intended manufacturing process either flood or starve fed extruders can be used. These involve use of continuous, high pressure pumps to generate thousands of pounds of pressure on viscous material during melting and mixing process **(Figure 9.3)**. The most of the extruder screws are driven from the hopper end. However, when screws are reduced to less than 18 mm, they become weak and solids transportation is far less reliable. To overcome these shortcomings, a vertical screw, driven from the discharge end, may be used.

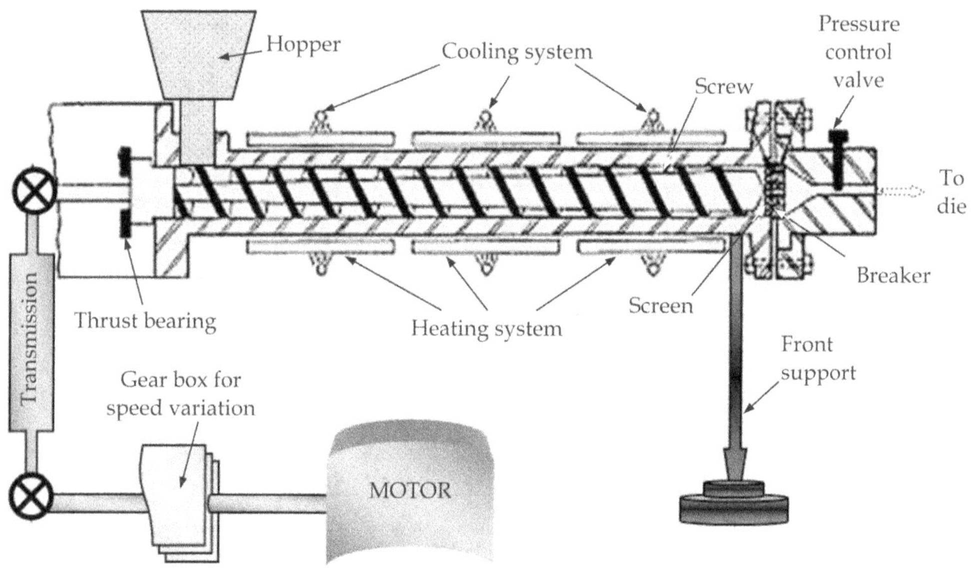

Fig. 9.3 Schematic representation of single screw extruder

Three basic function of a single screw extruder include solids conveying, melting and pumping. As a result of friction between the material and the feed section's bore the solid particles are forwarded in the early portion of the screw. After conveying of solids the flight depth begins to taper down and the energy from the heaters and shearing of heated barrel causes formation to melt. Ideally, the melt pool will increase as the solid bed reduces in size until all is molten at the end of the compression zone. Finally, the extrudate is form by pumping the molten materials against the die resistance.

(b)   *Twin screw extruder*

The Twin-screw extruder is yet another method; this offers several advantages over single screw extruder, including easier material feeding, dispersing capacities, high kneading, shorter transit time and fewer tendencies to over-heat.

In the late 1930's the first twin-screw extruder was developed in Italy, the concept occupied a combination of the machine actions of several available devices into a single unit. As the name suggests, twin-screw extruder involve two screws usually arranged side by side **(Figure 9.4)**. These screws permit number of different configurations and provide different conditions on all zones of the extruder, from the transfer of material from hopper to screw and all the way to the metered pumping zone. In this extruder the screws can rotate either in the same (co-rotating) or opposite (counter-rotating) direction. When very high shear regions are desired the counter-rotating extruder are utilized. Counter-rotating extruder suffers from drawbacks of potential air entrapment, generation of high pressure, low screw speeds and output. Co-rotating extruders are the most important type of extruders from industrial point of view. They can be operated at high screw speeds with high outputs, simultaneously maintenance of mixing and conveying characteristics.

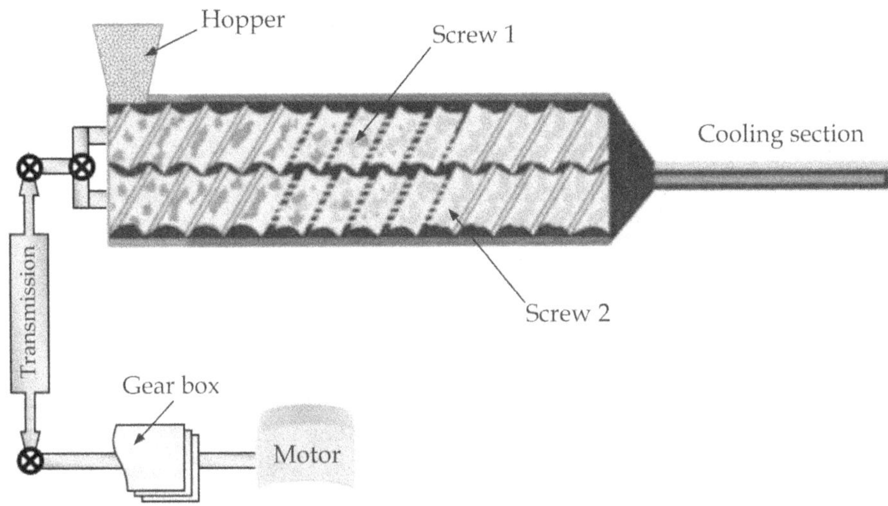

Fig. 9.4 Schematic representation of twin screw extruder

Further these two primary extruders can be classified as non-intermeshing and fully intermeshing. Fully intermeshing screw design is very popular as twin-screw extruders. This design minimizes the non-motion and prevents localized overheating of materials within the extruder and hence self-wiping by it. The material does not rotate along with the screw and hence extruder operates by first in/first out principle. On the other hand non-intermeshing extruders are used when large amount of volatiles need to be removed and process highly viscous materials. These extruders permit large volume devolatization via a vent opening as screws are positioned apart from one another.

Film casting method remains the manufacturing process of choice at laboratory scale. However hot melt extrusion method has been effectively utilized for producing bioadhesive films. Still so many possibilities are there in the designing of bioadhesive films like current application as platforms for nanoparticles delivery. Development of safe and patient friendly dosage forms with improved technologies are challenging to pharmaceutical scientists.

9.4 CHARACTERIZATION OF BIOADHESIVE PATCHES/FILMS

9.4.1 Film Weight and Thickness

The evaluation of film weight is carried out by collecting three films of every formulation batch and weigh individually on digital balance. The average weights are calculated. Similarly, three films of each formulation batch are taken and the film thickness is measured using Micrometer Screw Gauge at three different places and the mean value can be calculated.

9.4.2 Surface pH of Films

Three films of each formulation batch are allowed to swell for two hour on the surface of an agar plate. Surface pH is measured by using a pH paper placed on the surface of the swollen patch. Mean is calculated from observed values.

9.4.3 Percent Swelling

To determine percent swelling the samples are swelled on agar plate surface kept in an incubator and temperature is maintained at 37 °C. Increase in the weight of the films is determined at preset time intervals (1-5 h). The percent swelling (% S) is calculated using the following equation:

$$\text{Percent swelling (\%S)} = \left(\frac{X_t - X_0}{X_0} \right) \times 100$$

where,

X_t is the weight of the swollen film after time t and

X_0 is the initial film weight at time 0.

9.4.4 Folding Endurance

For determination of folding endurance three films of each formulation batch were cut into the size of 2 × 2 cm using sharp blade. Film strip is folded repeatedly at the same place till it breaks and the number of times the film can be folded at the same place without breaks gives the value of folding endurance.

9.4.5 *In-vitro* Residence Time

The USP disintegration apparatus is used to determine the *in-vitro* residence time. Phosphate buffer (pH 6.6) is used as disintegration medium and maintained at 37 ± 2 °C.

The segments of biological membranes (porcine skin/buccal mucosa) is taken, each of 3 cm length, and are glued to the surface of a glass slab, which is then vertically attached to the apparatus. Three bioadhesive films of each formulation batch are hydrated on one surface using phosphate buffer and the hydrated surface is brought in contact with the biological membrane. In the apparatus glass slab is vertically fixed and allowed to move up and down. The film is fully immersed in the buffer solution at the lowest point and was out at the highest point. The time required for complete erosion or detachment of the film from the biological surface is recorded.

9.4.6 Drug Content Uniformity

For determining the drug content uniformity three film units of each formulation batch were taken in separate 100 ml volumetric flasks; in this 100 ml of phosphate buffer pH 6.6 is added and continuously stirred for 24 h. After that the solutions are filtered, diluted suitably and are set to be analyzed for the drug content.

9.4.7 Vapor Transmission Test

Vapor transmission method is employed for the determination of vapor transmission from the patch. Glass-bottle (length = 5 cm, narrow mouth with internal diameter = 0.8 cm) filled with 2 g anhydrous calcium chloride and an adhesive spread across its rim. The patch was fixed over the adhesive and the assembly was placed in a constant humidity chamber, prepared using saturated solution of ammonium chloride and maintained at 37 °C. The difference in weight after 24 h, 3rd day and 1 week was calculated. The vapor transmission rate (VTR) was obtained as follow:

$$\text{Vapor transmission rate (VTR)} = \frac{\text{Amount of moisture transmitted}}{\text{Area} \times \text{Time}}$$

9.4.8 *In-vitro* Release Study

The dissolution apparatus is used for the *in-vitro* drug release study. Film is fixed to the central shaft using a cyanoacrylate adhesive. The dissolution medium consisted of 100 ml phosphate buffer pH 6.6. The release study is performed at 37 °C with a rotation speed of 50 rpm. At specific time intervals samples are withdrawn, filtered and then analyzed for the drug content.

9.4.9 *Ex-vivo* Permeation Studies

Generally, porcine skin/buccal mucosa is used as a barrier membrane. The skin/buccal pouch of freshly sacrificed animal is procured. The skin/buccal mucosa is excised and trimmed evenly from the sides. It is then washed in phosphate buffer pH 6.6 and used immediately. The *ex-vivo* permeation study of bioadhesive films through an excised layer of porcine skin/buccal mucosa is carried out using the Franz diffusion cell. Excised porcine buccal mucosa is kept in contact with 2.0 cm diameter film and the topside is covered as a backing membrane with aluminum foil. Receptor compartment is filled with phosphate buffer pH 7.4 and Teflon bead is placed in it. Stirring is done with a magnetic stirrer and temperature of 37 °C is maintained throughout the study. The samples are withdrawn periodically, filtered and then analyzed for drug content.

9.4.10 Measurement of Mechanical Properties

Films/patches mechanical properties like tensile strength and elongation at break is measured using a tensile tester. Film strip (dimensions 60 × 10 mm) devoid of any visual defects/cuts is positioned between two clamps separated by 3 cm distance. Clamps are designed to protect the patch without crushing it during the test. The lower clamp held immobile and the strips are pulled apart by the upper clamp moving at a rate of 2 mm/sec until strip breaks. The force and elongation of the film at the break point is recorded. The tensile strength (T) and elongation at break values are calculated using the formula:

$$\text{Tensile strength (T)} = \frac{m \times g}{b \times t} \text{ kg / mm}^2$$

where,

m is the mass in g,

g is the acceleration due to gravity

b is the breadth of the specimen in cm

t is the thickness of specimen in cm.

Tensile strength is the force at break (kg) per initial cross-sectional area of the specimen (mm^2).

9.4.11 Stability Studies

The stability studies are conducted for all the formulation batches at 40 °C and 75% RH to investigate the effect of temperature on the drug content in different formulation batches. The films are removed from the oven at the end of 0, 7, 14, 21 and 28 days and analyzed for drug content.

9.5 BIOADHESIVE PATCHES FOR TRANSDERMAL DELIVERY

A medicated adhesive patch is a transdermal patch that delivers a specific dose of medication through the skin and finally to the bloodstream when placed on the skin.

These patches are specifically designed to provide continuous controlled drug delivery. Patches avoid side effects like painful drug delivery, first pass metabolism associated with other drug delivery systems. Many drugs have been formulated in the form of transdermal patches that can be injected directly into the blood stream. The major benefits of this system are painless delivery and controlled drug release throughout the period. Currently transdermal drug delivery system has become a major field of interest due to their advantages. Various patches have been marketed for deliverance of therapeutic agents.

In December 1979 very first USFDA approved commercially available patch delivered scopolamine for motion sickness. Transdermal drug delivery system (TDDS) delivers drug to systemic circulation through the skin via diffusion process. As there is high concentration on the patch and low concentration in the blood, the drug diffuses into the blood for an extended period of time, and maintains the constant drug concentration in the blood flow. TDDS offers numerous advantages over conventional methods. It can be used as an alternative to oral route by avoiding gastrointestinal absorption with its associated pitfalls of enzymatic and pH deactivation. This approach also reduces pharmacological damaging due to shortened metabolism pathway as compared to gastrointestinal pathway. Transdermal patch also allows constant dosing with controlled release in spite of peaks and valleys that occurs with oral medication. Further advantages include multi-day therapy with a single application and possibility of dose termination via removal of patch.

Along with numerous advantages TDDS posses certain limitations like unsuitability for drugs that need high blood levels and skin irritation or sensitization. Sometimes adhesive not adhere to skin and may be uncomfortable to wear. High cost of the product also limits its wide acceptance.

9.5.1 Types of Transdermal Patches

9.5.1.1 Membrane permeation controlled systems

This system comprises of drug reservoir encapsulation in a shallow compartment fabricated from a drug impermeable metallic plastic laminate (backing film) and a rate controlling polymeric membrane **(Figure 9.5)** e.g. Ethylene vinyl acetate with defined drug permeability. Drug release is permitted only through the rate controlling polymeric membrane. Drug reservoir compartment may be dispersion of drug in a solid polymer matrix or suspension in a viscous liquid medium. Adhesive polymer is applied as a thin layer to the external surface of the rate controlling polymeric membrane to get an intimate contact of the system and skin surface. Examples of some marketed preparation: Transderm-Nitro®, Transderm-Scop®, Catapress-TTS®.

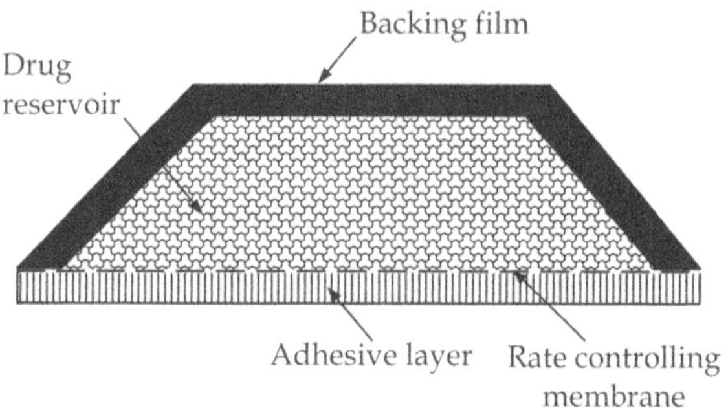

Fig. 9.5 Membrane permeation controlled system

9.5.1.2 Matrix diffusion-controlled systems

In this type of system drug reservoir is prepared by homogeneous dispersion of drug either in hydrophilic or lipophilic polymeric matrix followed by molding into a medicated disc with a defined surface area and controlled thickness. Drug reservoir containing polymer disc is then pasted on base plate in a compartment fabricated from a drug impermeable plastic backing film **(Figure 9.6)**. Further adhesive polymer is spread along the circumference to form a strip of adhesive rim around the medicated disc.

Example: Nitro-Dur® System.

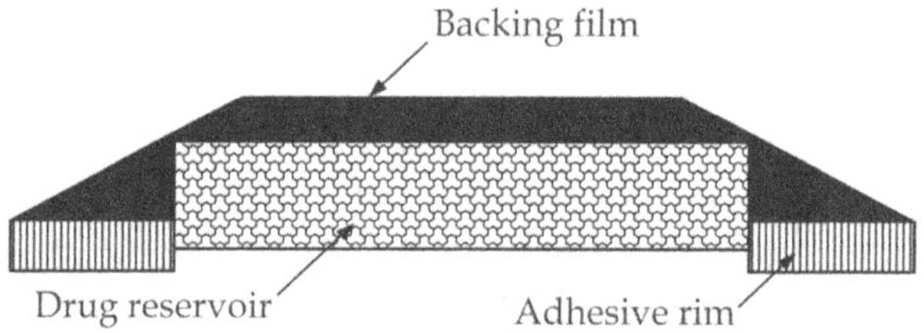

Fig. 9.6 Matrix diffusion-controlled system

9.5.1.3 Adhesive dispersion-type systems

This type of system is simplified version of membrane permeation-controlled system. In this approach drug reservoir is formulated by direct drug dispersion in an adhesive polymer e.g. Poly-isobutylene and then spreading the medicated adhesive, by solvent casting or hot melt onto a flat sheet of drug impermeable metallic plastic backing to fabricate a thin drug reservoir layer. On the top of the drug reservoir layer, thin layers of non-medicated, rate-controlling adhesive polymer of a specific permeability are applied to produce an adhesive diffusion-controlled delivery system **(Figure 9.7)**. Example: Deponit®, Frandol Tape.

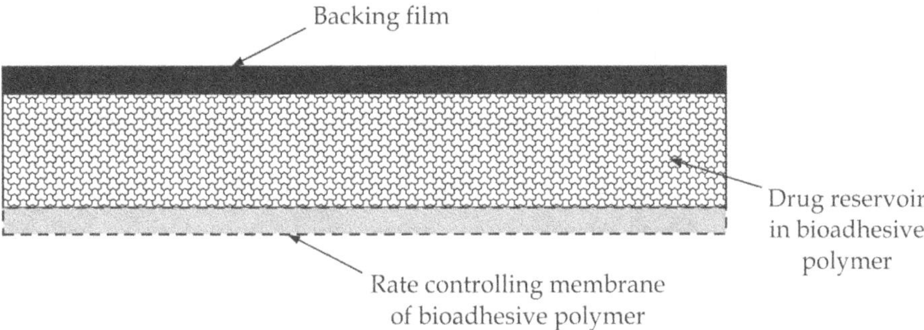

Fig. 9.7 Adhesive dispersion-type system

9.5.1.4 Micro-reservoir type or micro-sealed dissolution controlled systems

In this type of system drug reservoir is prepared by suspending the drug solids in an aqueous solution and then dispersing the drug suspension homogenously in a lipophilic polymer by high shear mechanical force to form a large number of micro-reservoirs. This thermodynamically unstable dispersion is stabilized quickly by immediate addition of cross linking polymers like glutaraldehyde which produces a medicated polymer disc with a constant surface area and a fixed thickness. A transdermal therapeutic system is produced by positioning the medicated disc at the center and surrounding it with an adhesive rim and then it is spread on to the occlusive base plate with adhesive foam pad **(Figure 9.8)**.

Example: Nitro-Disc® System.

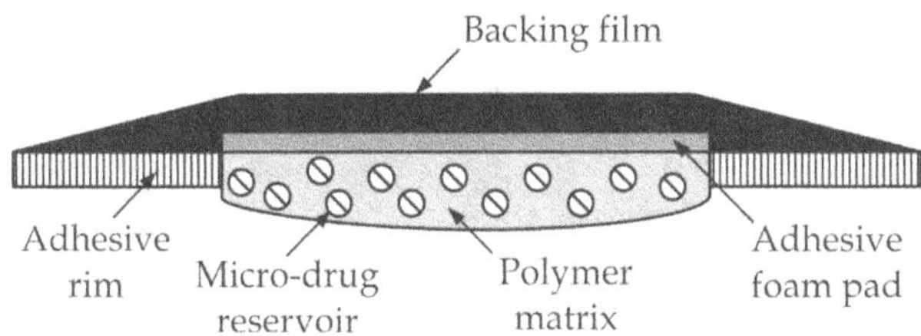

Fig. 9.8 Micro-reservoir type or micro-sealed dissolution controlled system

9.5.2 Mechanism of Permeation

The mechanism of permeation of drug across the skin to systemic circulation can involve the passage through the epidermis. It has been concluded that the three major possible channels by which a drug can reach systemic circulation via skin are SC, tran-follicular and glandular pathway. SC plays a vital role in the diffusion of drugs through skin. SC is around 12-15 µm layer composed of dead keratinized cells arranged in a brick fashion.

Drug basically follows two pathways i.e. paracellular or transcellular **(Figure 9.9)**. In *paracellular* pathway drug moves around the periphery of cells (does not traverse) and reaches systemic circulation; while in *transcellular* pathway the drug readily traverse across the cells and reaches blood stream and elicits a therapeutic response. Most substances diffuse across the SC via the intercellular lipoidal route. When drug to be permeated exists at SC, it enters the wet cell mass of the epidermis. As there is no direct blood supply to the epidermis, the drug is forced to diffuse across it and reach the vasculature beneath immediately. Permeation requires frequent crossings of cell membranes since epidermal cell membranes are tightly joined and there is small or negligible intercellular space for ions and polar non-electrolytes to squeeze through diffusion. Dermal region represents an ultimate obstacle for permeation to systemic entry. Drugs permeated through the dermis via interlocking channels of the ground substance and diffusion occurs through the gaps between collagen fibers.

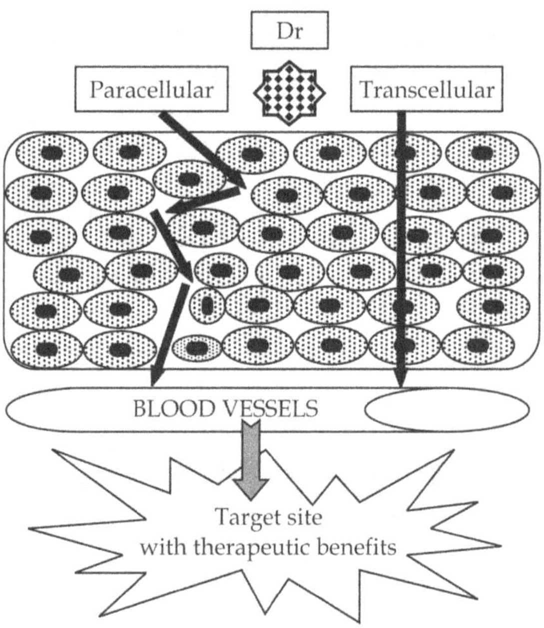

Fig. 9.9 Mechanism of drug permeation via skin

9.6 BIOADHESIVE PATCHES/FILMS FOR BUCCAL DELIVERY

Buccal route is an attractive route of administration for systemic drug delivery. Buccal bioadhesive films, releasing drugs in the oral cavity at a slow and predetermined rate, provide distinct advantages over traditional dosage forms for treatment of many diseases. Trans-mucosal routes of drug delivery (i.e. the mucosal linings of the nasal, rectal, vaginal, ocular and oral cavity) offer several advantages over oral administration for systemic drug delivery. These advantages include bypass of first pass effect, avoidance of pre systemic elimination within the GI tract and depending on the particular drug, a better enzymatic flora for drug absorption in the GI tract. Various bioadhesive dosage forms including tablets, films, patches, disks, strips, ointments and gels, have recently been developed. However, buccal patch offer greater flexibility and comfort in comparison to other dosage forms. In addition, a bioadhesive patch can circumvent the problem of the relatively short residence time of oral gels on mucosa, since the gels are easily washed away by saliva.

Buccal route of drug delivery system provides the direct access to the systemic circulation through the jugular vein that bypassing the first pass hepatic metabolism leading to high bioavailability. Other advantages of buccal route are excellent accessibility, low enzymatic activity, and suitability for drugs or excipients. This reversibly damage or irritate the mucosa, painless administration, easy withdrawal, facility to include permeation enhancer/ enzyme inhibitor or pH modifier in the formulation, these buccal route versatility in designing as multidirectional or unidirectional release system for local or systemic action.

9.6.1 Advantages of Buccal Patches

- The buccal mucosa has having a rich blood supply. The drugs are absorbed from the oral cavity through the mucosal surface and transported through the deep lingual or facial vein, internal jugular vein and brachio-cephalic vein into the systemic circulation.

- After buccal administration, the drug gets direct entry into the systemic circulation thereby bypassing the first-pass effect. Contact with the digestive fluids of gastrointestinal tract is avoided. This may lead to stability of many drugs like insulin or other proteins, peptides and steroids. In addition, the rate of drug absorption is not influenced by food or gastric emptying rate.

- The area of buccal membrane is sufficiently large to allow a delivery system to be placed at different occasions. Additionally; there are two areas of buccal membranes per mouth, which would allow buccal drug delivery systems to be placed, alternatively on the left and right buccal membranes.

- Buccal patch has been well known for its advantage as good accessibility to the membranes that line the oral cavity, which makes application painless and with comfort.

- The novel buccal dosage forms exhibits better patient compliance. The buccal drug delivery system easily administered into the buccal cavity. Patients can control the period of administration or terminate delivery in case of emergencies.

9.6.2 Mechanism of Buccal Absorption

Mechanism of buccal drug absorption occurs by passive diffusion of the non-ionized species, a process governed primarily by a concentration gradient, through the intercellular spaces of the epithelium. The primary transport mechanism in buccal cavity is the passive transport of non-ionic species across the lipid membrane. The buccal mucosa has been said to be a lipoidal barrier to the passage of drugs. The dynamics of buccal absorption of drugs could be adequately described by first order rate process. Several potential barriers to buccal drug absorption have been identified. In the year 1971 two scientists Dearden and Tomlison pointed out that salivary secretion alters the buccal absorption kinetics from drug solution by changing the concentration of drug in the mouth. The linear relationship between salivary secretion and time is given as follows:

$$-\frac{dm}{dt} = KC / V_i V_t$$

where,

    m is the mass of drug in mouth at time t

    K is proportionality constant

    C is the concentration of drug in mouth

    V_i is the volume of solution put into mouth and

    V_t is the salivary secretion rate

9.6.3 Factors Affecting Buccal Absorption

The oral cavity is a complex environment for drug delivery as there are many interdependent and independent factors which reduce the absorbable concentration at the site of absorption.

9.6.3.1 Membrane factors

This involves degree of keratinization, surface area available for absorption, mucus layer of salivary pellicle, intercellular lipids of epithelium, basement membrane and lamina propria. In addition, the absorptive membrane thickness, blood supply/lymph drainage, cell renewal and enzyme content will all contribute to reducing the rate and amount of drug entering the systemic circulation.

9.6.3.2 Environmental factors

(a) *Saliva:* The thin film of saliva coats throughout the lining of buccal mucosa and is called salivary pellicle or film. The thickness of salivary film is 0.07 to 0.10 mm. The thickness, composition and movement of this film affect the rate of buccal absorption.

(b) *Salivary glands***:** The minor salivary glands are located in epithelial or deep epithelial region of buccal mucosa. They constantly secrete mucus on surface of buccal mucosa. Although, mucus helps to retain mucoadhesive dosage forms, it is potential barrier to drug penetration.

(c) *Movement of buccal tissues***:** Buccal region of oral cavity shows less active movements. The mucoadhesive polymers are to be incorporated to keep dosage form at buccal region for long periods to withstand tissue movements during talking and if possible during eating food or swallowing.

9.7 BIOADHESIVE PATCHES FOR LOCAL DELIVERY AND WOUND DRESSINGS

Wound dressings and devices form an important segment of the medical and pharmaceutical wound care market worldwide. In the past, traditional dressings such as natural or synthetic bandages, cotton wool, lint and gauzes all with varying degrees of absorbency were used for the management of wounds. Their primary function was to keep the wound dry by allowing evaporation of wound exudates and preventing entry of harmful bacteria into the wound. It has now been shown however, that having a warm moist wound environment achieves more rapid and successful wound healing. The variety of wound types has resulted in a wide range of wound dressings with new products frequently introduced to target different aspects of the wound healing process. The last two decades have witnessed the introduction of many dressings, with new ones becoming available each year.

The ideal dressing should achieve rapid healing at reasonable cost with minimal inconvenience to the patient. The common wound management dressings are combined with emerging technologies for achieving improved wound healing. Development in the field of wound dressings and novel polymers has provide the advantage of deliverance of drugs to acute, chronic and other types of wound in addition to the protective and other necessary functions **(Table 9.4)**. These polymers include hydrocolloids, alginates, hydrogels, polyurethane, collagen, chitosan, pectin and hyaluronic acid. Pharmacological agents such as antibiotics, vitamins, minerals, growth factors and other wound healing accelerators that take active part in the healing process are incorporated in dressings. Direct delivery of these agents to the wound site is desirable, particularly when systemic delivery could cause organ damage due to toxicological concerns associated with the preferred agents. General formulation approaches are innovated towards the achievement of optimum physical properties and controlled delivery characteristics for an active wound healing dressing.

Table 9.4 Desirable functions of wound dressings after Eccleston

Desirable functions	Clinical significance
Debridement (wound cleansing)	Enhanced leukocytes migration into the wound bed and accumulation of enzymes.
Balance of moisture to maintain a moist wound environment	Prevention of desiccation and cell death, enhancement of epidermal migration, angiogenesis promotion, connective tissue synthesis and autolysis support by rehydration of tissue.
Absorption, removal of blood and excess exudates	Excess exudates in chronic wounds containing tissue degrading enzymes that obstruct the proliferation and activity of cells, break down extracellular matrix materials and growth factors, thus delaying wound healing. Excess exudates can also macerate surrounding skin.
Gaseous exchange	Management of exudates by control of water vapor permeability. Stimulation of angiogenesis by low tissue oxygen levels. Stimulation of epithelialization and fibroblasts by raised tissue oxygen.
Prevention of infection: Wound protection from bacterial invasion	In this necrotic tissue, foreign bodies and particles prolong the inflammatory phase and serve as a medium for bacterial growth. Collagen synthesis delayed by infection inhibits epidermal migration and induces additional tissue damage.
Thermal insulation provision	Improvement of blood flow to the wound bed and enhancement of epidermal migration by normal tissue temperature.
Low adherence	Greater adherence of dressings may be painful and difficult to eliminate and cause further tissue damage.
Cost effective (reduced frequency of dressings change)	Comparison of dressings is based on cost of treatment rather than unit or pack costs should be made (cost-benefit-ratio).

Modern dressings are based on the concept of optimum environment creation which permit epithelial cells to move unimpeded, for wounds treatment. Optimum conditions include a wet or moist environment around the wound, effective circulation of oxygen to aid regenerating cells/tissues and a low bacterial load. The management of effective wound depends on understanding a number of different factors such as the type of wound being treated, the healing process, patient conditions in terms of health and disease (e.g. diabetes), environment and social setting, and the physical chemical properties of the available dressings. It is important therefore, different dressings be evaluated and tested in terms of their physical properties and clinical performance for a given type of wound and the stage of wound healing, before being considered for routine use.

9.7.1 Classification of Dressings

Usually dressings are classified as primary, secondary and island dressings. Classification can be done based on the type of material used to prepare dressing (hydrocolloid, alginate, collagen), the form of dressing (ointment, gel, film, foam) and their role (absorbent, occlusive, adherent, antibacterial). Primary dressings are those that come in direct contact with the wound surface while those hold or cover the primary dressings are known as secondary dressings. Dressings with central absorbent region and surrounded by an adhesive part known as island dressings. Further dressings may be classified like traditional dressings, modern and advanced dressings, skin replacement products and wound healing devices.

9.7.2 Modern Wound Dressings

These are classified as per the type of material employed for the production like hydrocolloids, alginates, and hydrogels. As name indicates they are nothing but modified version of traditional wound healing materials. The vital characteristic of these dressings is to create and maintain moist environment around the wound for wound healing. Modern dressings are available generally in the form of thin films, gels and foam sheets.

9.7.2.1 Hydrocolloid dressings

Hydrocolloid explained as products for wound management that are derived from colloidal substances (gel forming agents). These are mixed with other substances like elastomers and adhesives that provide flexibility to dressing. Materials that applied as gel forming agents are carboxymethylcellulose (CMC), gelatin and pectin. These materials come in the form of thin films and sheets or as composite dressings in combination with other substances like alginates. These dressings are amongst the widely utilized dressings include Granuflex^{TM} and Aquacel^{TM} (Conva Tec, Hounslow, UK), Comfeel^{TM} (Coloplast, Peterborough, UK) and Tegasorb^{TM} (3M Healthcare, Loughborough, UK). Hydrocolloid dressings are applied on light to moderate exuding wounds like pressure sores, minor burns and traumatic injuries and also used clinically due to their adherence to moist as well as dry sites.

They are found to be advantageous for the management of leg ulcers by treatment of wounds which do not respond to compression therapy alone. Hydrocolloid dressings are impermeable to water vapor in its intact state but a change in physical state may occur after formation of a gel covering the wound up on absorption of wound exudates. As the gel forms they turn out to be progressively more permeable to water and air. They are also useful in pediatric wound care for management of acute as well as chronic wounds because they do not cause pain on removal.

When hydrocolloid dressings were compared with paraffin gauze in randomized trial upon application to skin draft donor sites they achieved quick healing with minimum pain. In another research when hydrocolloid dressing was compared with non-adherent dressing on patients with lacerations, abrasions and minor operation incisions and equal time provided for healing, they reported minimum pain; minimum analgesia required and could manage their routine activities like bathing or showering without disturbing the wound or dressing.

9.7.2.2 Alginate dressings

These dressings are prepared usually from the sodium and calcium salts of alginic acid, a polysaccharide with mannuronic and guluronic acid units. Dressings may be obtained in the form of flexible fibers or freeze dried porous sheets. Use of alginate as dressings is based on the formation of gels up on contact with wound exudates (high absorbency). Due to strong hydrophilic gel formation high absorption occurs that restricts wound secretions and minimizes bacterial contamination.

Mannuronate rich alginates such as Sorbsan^{TM} (Maersk, Suffolk, UK) upon hydration produce soft flexible gels while guluronic acid rich alginates like Kaltostat^{TM} (Conva Tec) upon absorption of wound exudates produce firmer gels. Some contain calcium alginate fiber such as Sorbsan^{TM} and Tegagen^{TM} (3M Healthcare). Comfeel Plus^{TM} is a hydrocolloid/alginate combination dressing. Up on application to wounds these dressings may cause exchange of ions that present in the alginate fiber with ions present in blood and exudates to produce protective gel film. This protective film helps to retain the lesion at an optimum moisture content and healing temperature. Alginate gelling property is attributed to the existence of calcium ions which help to produce cross-linked polymeric gel that degrades slowly. Calcium alginate dressings are considered ideal materials as scaffolds for tissue engineering due to the capability of calcium ions to cross-links with the alginic acid polymer.

Alginate dressings as fibers when trapped in a wound found to be quickly biodegradable and can be rinsed away with saline irrigation. These dressings are helpful for all stages of wound healing and can be used for moderate to heavily exuding wounds. Their subsequent removal does not destroy granulation tissue and change of dressing remains virtually painless. These are not applied usually for dry wounds and hard necrotic tissue covered wounds as require moist condition for effective functioning. It may dehydrate the wound and delays the wound healing so it is the major drawback observed with these dressings.

Schmidt and Turner investigated the role of calcium alginate in the wound healing process and suggested its utility in the mouse fibroblast production. Further Doyle et al. modeled this process *in-vitro* and showed improved fibroblasts proliferation by calcium alginate. Alginates dressings were also compared with hydrocolloids in one study and it was observed that these may remain present for a prolonged period on wound than hydrocolloids. Alginate dressings may activate human macrophages for production of tumor necrosis factor-$^{TM}\alpha$ (TNF α) required for initiation of inflammatory signals, as part of the wound healing process has been reported by Thomas et al.

9.7.2.3 Hydrogel dressings

Hydrogels may be defined as hydrophilic materials with swellable yet insoluble property and are generally made of PVPs or PMAs which belong to class of synthetic polymers. These are applied as gels, sheets or as elastic film. The gels are used as primary dressings while the films may be used as primary or secondary dressing. The hydrogels contain high percentage of water (up to 90%), therefore are useful for less exuding wounds where less absorption is needed. They also lack sufficient mechanical strength, require gauze backing, are difficult to handle and hence exhibit poor patient compliance. The films/sheets are made of crosslinked polymers, hence can absorb significant amount of liquid exudates, fit to the wounds flexibly and control water vapor transmission through it. These hydrogel dressings are non-irritant, non-reactive to tissue, metabolite permeable and are suitable for use at all the four stages of wound healing.

9.7.2.4 Semi-permeable adhesive film dressings

These types of dressings are in use since long time and their Semi-permeable adhesive film dressings have been used for a long time and their effects on moist wound healing were first investigated by Winter, Maibach and Hinman. Originally, being made of nylon derivatives along with polyethylene adhesive frame to provide occlusiveness but suffered from poor ability to absorb large quantity of exudates. This caused accumulation of excess exudates beneath the dressing causing skin maceration and bacterial growth and infection. The use of nylon dressing is now discontinued owing to frequent changing, saline irrigation required of the wound, difficulty to apply and wrinkling while removal from the packs. A thin polyurethane semi permeable film; Opsite^{TM} (Smith and Nephew, Hull, UK) covered with hypoallergenic acrylic derivatives is available. It is more porous and permeable to water vapor and gases but no liquid from exudates. This film is transparent, elastic, flexible and is contour confirming to areas as knees and elbows and do not require additional support and taping. However, they are relatively thin to be used for deep or cavity wounds and only suitable for rather shallow wounds.

9.8 CURRENT RESEARCH IN THE FIELD OF BIOADHESIVE PATCHES

9.8.1 Testosterone Transdermal Patch

Testosterone daily production in premenopausal women is approximately 300 μg. Approximately half of which is derived from the ovaries and half from the adrenal glands. Young women with spontaneous premature ovarian failure (sPOF) may have lower androgen levels as compared to normal ovulatory women. Testosterone transdermal patch (TTP) has been designed to deliver the normal ovarian production rate of testosterone.

9.8.2 Oxybutynin Transdermal Patch for Over Active Bladder (OAB)

Oxybutynin hydrochloride transdermal patch is approved in US as Oxytrol® and in Europe as Kentra®. Oxytrol is applied to the abdomen, hip or buttock as thin, flexible and clear patch twice weekly. It provides continuous and consistent delivery of oxybutynin over a 3-4 day interval. Oxytrol offers effective bladder control in OAB patient's with fewer side effects like dry mouth and constipation.

9.8.3 Transdermal Patch for Menstrual Problems

Patch is usually 4.5 cm^2 in size and having three layers: the inner release liner, a layer containing hormones, and an outer protective polyester layer. The patch consists of progestin (6 mg) and ethinyle estradiol (0.75 mg) which is applied on the skin. Through skin, hormones are absorbed during menstrual cycle to provide continuous flow of hormones. The patch is marketed as Ortho Evra™ by Ortho McNeil Pharmaceutical.

9.8.4 Transdermal Patches for Parkinson's Disease

Transdermal patch of Rotigotine is used for symptom control in Parkinson's disease. The patches can be effective in reducing the symptoms of early Parkinson's disease and in reducing "off" time in advanced Parkinson's disease. It is available in market as NeuproR.

9.8.5 Bioadhesive Buccal Films

Erodible bioadhesive buccal films containing glipizide for systemic delivery indicates enormous potential with an added advantage of circumventing the hepatic first pass metabolism. The result shows that therapeutic levels of glipizide can be delivered buccally. It may be concluded that the film containing 5 mg glipizide in 4.9 % w/v HPMC with 1.5 % w/v SCMC, shows good swelling, a convenient residence time and promising controlled drug release. Thus seems to be a potential candidate for the development of buccal film for effective therapeutic use.

9.8.6 Sustained Release Bioadhesive Buccal Patches

A new buccoadhesive patch for sustained released of Verapamil hydrochloride was developed with chitosan. Chitosan has not only film forming ability but good bioadhesion properties as well. The drug release rate increases on inclusion of PVP K-30 into the chitosan base matrix system. So, chitosan with PVP K-30 can meet the ideal requirement for buccal devices, which can be good way to bypass the extensive hepatic first pass metabolism and increase bioavailability.

Bibliography

- Abu-Dahab, R., Schafer, U.F., Lehr, C.M., 2001. Lectin-functionalized liposomes for pulmonary drug delivery: effect of nebulization on stability and bioadhesion. Eur. J. Pharm. Sci., 14, 37-46.

- Abu-Lail, N.I., Camesano, T.A., 2003. Role of ionic strength on the relationship of biopolymer conformation, DLVO contributions, and steric interactions to bioadhesion of Pseudomonas putida KT2442. Biomacromolecules., 4, 1000-1012.

- Acarturk, F., 2009. Mucoadhesive vaginal drug delivery systems. Recent Pat Drug Deliv. Formul., 3, 193-205.

- Achouri, D., Alhanout, K., Piccerelle, P., Andrieu, V., 2013. Recent advances in ocular drug delivery. Drug Dev. Ind. Pharm., 39, 1599-1617.

- Agueros, M., Areses, P., Campanero, M.A., Salman, H., Quincoces, G., Penuelas, I., Irache, J.M., 2009. Bioadhesive properties and biodistribution of cyclodextrin-poly(anhydride) nanoparticles. Eur. J. Pharm. Sci., 37, 231-240.

- Agueros, M., Ruiz-Gaton, L., Vauthier, C., Bouchemal, K., Espuelas, S., Ponchel, G., Irache, J.M., 2009. Combined hydroxypropyl-beta-cyclodextrin and poly(anhydride) nanoparticles improve the oral permeability of paclitaxel. Eur. J. Pharm. Sci., 38, 405-413.

- Ahmad, F.J., Alam, M.A., Khan, Z.I., Khar, R.K., Ali, M., 2008. Development and *in-vitro* evaluation of an acid buffering bioadhesive vaginal gel for mixed vaginal infections. Acta Pharm., 58, 407-419.

- Ahmed, A., Bonner, C., Desai, T.A., 2002. Bioadhesive microdevices with multiple reservoirs: a new platform for oral drug delivery. J. Control Release, 81, 291-306.

- Ahuja, M., Kumar, S., Kumar, A., 2013. Evaluation of mucoadhesive potential of gum cordia, an anionic polysaccharide. Int. J. Biol. Macromol., 55, 109-112.

- Ahuja, M., Kumar, S., Yadav, M., 2010. Evaluation of mimosa seed mucilage as bucoadhesive polymer. Yakugaku Zasshi, 130, 937-944.

- Ahuja, M., Singh, S., Kumar, A., 2013. Evaluation of carboxymethyl gellan gum as a mucoadhesive polymer. Int. J. Biol. Macromol., 53, 114-121.

- Ainslie, K.M., Lowe, R.D., Beaudette, T.T., Petty, L., Bachelder, E.M., Desai, T.A., 2009. Microfabricated devices for enhanced bioadhesive drug delivery: attachment to and small-molecule release through a cell monolayer under flow. Small, 5, 2857-2863.

- Akbari, J., Nokhodchi, A., Farid, D., Adrangui, M., Siahi-Shadbad, M.R., Saeedi, M., 2004. Development and evaluation of buccoadhesive propranolol hydrochloride tablet formulations: effect of fillers. Farmaco, 59, 155-161.

- Akiyoshi, K., 2007. Nanogel-based materials for drug delivery system. Eur. Cells and Mater., 14, 36.

- Alam, M.A., Ahmad, F.J., Khan, Z.I., Khar, R.K., Ali, M., 2007. Development and evaluation of acid-buffering bioadhesive vaginal tablet for mixed vaginal infections. AAPS. Pharm Sci Tech., 8, E109.

- Albertini, B., Passerini, N., Di, S.M., Vitali, B., Brigidi, P., Rodriguez, L., 2009. Polymer-lipid based mucoadhesive microspheres prepared by spray-congealing for the vaginal delivery of econazole nitrate. Eur. J. Pharm. Sci., 36, 591-601.

- Aldred, N., Ekblad, T., Andersson, O., Liedberg, B., Clare, A.S., 2011. Real-time quantification of microscale bioadhesion events *in-situ* using imaging surface plasmon resonance (iSPR). ACS Appl. Mater. Interfaces., 3, 2085-2091.

- Allion, A., Baron, J.P., Boulange-Petermann, L., 2006. Impact of surface energy and roughness on cell distribution and viability. Biofouling., 22, 269-278.

- Alonso, M.J., Sanchez, A., 2003. The potential of chitosan in ocular drug delivery. J. Pharm. Pharmacol., 55, 1451-1463.

- Alsarra, I.A., Alanazi, F.K., Mahrous, G.M., Abdel Rahman, A.A., Al Hezaimi, K.A., 2007. Clinical evaluation of novel buccoadhesive film containing ketorolac in dental and post-oral surgery pain management. Pharmazie, 62, 773-778.

- Ameye, D., Voorspoels, J., Foreman, P., Tsai, J., Richardson, P., Geresh, S., Remon, J.P., 2002. *Ex-vivo* bioadhesion and *in-vivo* testosterone bioavailability study of different bioadhesive formulations based on starch-g-poly(acrylic acid) copolymers and starch/poly(acrylic acid) mixtures. J. Control Release, 79, 173-182.

- Ammar, H.O., Ghorab, M., El-Nahhas, S.A., Kamel, R., 2009. Polymeric matrix system for prolonged delivery of tramadol hydrochloride, part II: biological evaluation. AAPS. Pharm Sci Tech., 10, 1065-1070.

- Anlar, S., Capan,Y., Hincal, A.A., 1993. Physico-chemical and bioadhesive properties of polyacrylic acid polymers. Pharmazie, 48, 285-287.

- Ansel's Pharmaceutical Dosage Forms and Drug Delivery Systems. 2010, 9th Revised edition, Lippincott Williams and Wilkins. USA.

- Arangoa, M.A., Campanero, M.A., Renedo, M.J., Ponchel, G., Irache, J.M., 2001. Gliadin nanoparticles as carriers for the oral administration of lipophilic drugs.

Relationships between bioadhesion and pharmacokinetics. Pharm. Res., 18, 1521-1527.

- Attama, A.A., Onuigbo, E.B., 2007. Properties of cotrimoxazole microparticles prepared with carbopol 941 and exogenous mucin. Scientific Res. and Essay, 2, 421-25.

- Attama, A.A., Adikwu, M.U., 1999. Bioadhesive delivery of hydrochlorothiazide using tacca starch/SCMC and tacca starch/Carbopols 940 and 941 admixtures. Boll. Chim. Farm., 138, 343-350.

- Attama, A.A., Adikwu, M.U., Okoli, N.D., 2000. Studies on bioadhesive granules I: granules formulated with Prosopis africana (prosopis) gum. Chem. Pharm. Bull. (Tokyo), 48, 734-737.

- Avachat, A.M., Gujar, K.N., Wagh, K.V., 2013. Development and evaluation of tamarind seed xyloglucan-based mucoadhesive buccal films of rizatriptan benzoate. Carbohydr. Polym., 91, 537-542.

- Bachhav, Y.G., Patravale, V.B., 2009a. Microemulsion based vaginal gel of fluconazole: formulation, *in-vitro* and *in-vivo* evaluation. Int. J. Pharm., 365, 175-179.

- Bachhav, Y.G., Patravale, V.B., 2009b. Microemulsion-based vaginal gel of clotrimazole: formulation, *in-vitro* evaluation, and stability studies. AAPS. PharmSciTech., 10, 476-481.

- Bahri, S., Jonsson, C.M., Jonsson, C.L., Azzolini, D., Sverjensky, D.A., Hazen, R.M., 2011. Adsorption and surface complexation study of L-DOPA on Rutile (alpha-TiO(2)) in NaCl solutions. Environ. Sci. Technol., 45, 3959-3966.

- Baier, R.E., 1982. Conditioning surfaces to suit the biomedical environment: recent progress. J. Biomech. Eng, 104, 257-271.

- Baier, R.E., 1987. Selected methods of investigation for blood-contact surfaces. Ann. N. Y. Acad. Sci., 516, 68-77.

- Baier, R.E., 1988. Advanced biomaterials development from "natural products". J. Biomater. Appl., 2, 615-626.

- Baier, R.E., 1999. Physical and biomechanical issues in graft design. Semin. Vasc. Surg., 12, 8-17.

- Baier, R.E., 2006. Surface behaviour of biomaterials: the theta surface for biocompatibility. J. Mater. Sci. Mater. Med., 17, 1057-1062.

- Baier, R.E., Meyer, A.E., 1988. Future directions in surface preparation of dental implants. J. Dent. Educ., 52, 788-791.

- Balaguer-Fernandez, C., Padula, C., Femenia-Font, A., Merino, V., Santi, P., Lopez-Castellano, A., 2010. Development and evaluation of occlusive systems employing polyvinyl alcohol for transdermal delivery of sumatriptan succinate. Drug Deliv., 17, 83-91.

- Balamurugan, S., Ista, L.K., Yan, J., Lopez, G.P., Fick, J., Himmelhaus, M., Grunze, M., 2005. Reversible protein adsorption and bioadhesion on monolayers terminated with mixtures of oligo(ethylene glycol) and methyl groups. J. Am. Chem. Soc., 127, 14548-14549.

- Baloglu, E., Ozyazici, M., Hizarcioglu, S.Y., Karavana, H.A., 2003. An *in-vitro* investigation for vaginal bioadhesive formulations: bioadhesive properties and swelling states of polymer mixtures. Farmaco, 58, 391-396.

- Banker GS. Rhodes CT. (Ed.). Modern pharmaceutics. 2002. 4th edition, Marcel Dekker, Inc., USA.

- Barauskas, J., Christerson, L., Wadsater, M., Lindstrom, F., Lindqvist, A.K., Tiberg, F., 2014. Bioadhesive Lipid Compositions: Self-Assembly Structures, Functionality and Medical Applications. Mol. Pharm..

- Bassi, P., Kaur, G., 2012. Innovations in bioadhesive vaginal drug delivery system. Expert. Opin. Ther. Pat, 22, 1019-1032.

- Batchelor, H., Dettmar, P., Hampson, F., Jolliffe, I., Craig, D., 2004. Microscopic techniques as potential tools to quantify the extent of bioadhesion of liquid systems. Eur. J. Pharm. Sci., 22, 341-346.

- Batchelor, H.K., Banning, D., Dettmar, P.W., Hampson, F.C., Jolliffe, I.G., Craig, D.Q., 2002. An *in-vitro* mucosal model for prediction of the bioadhesion of alginate solutions to the oesophagus. Int. J. Pharm., 238, 123-132.

- Batchelor, H.K., Tang, M., Dettmar, P.W., Hampson, F.C., Jolliffe, I.G., Craig, D.Q., 2004. Feasibility of a bioadhesive drug delivery system targeted to oesophageal tissue. Eur. J. Pharm. Biopharm., 57, 295-298.

- Berglin, M., Lonn, N., Gatenholm, P., 2003. Coating modulus and barnacle bioadhesion. Biofouling., 19 Suppl, 63-69.

- Bernkop-Schnurch, A., Gabor, F., Spiegl, P., 1997. Bacterial adhesins as a drug carrier: covalent attachment of K99 fimbriae to 6-methylprednisolone. Pharmazie, 52, 41-44.

- Bertholon, I., Ponchel, G., Labarre, D., Couvreur, P., Vauthier, C., 2006. Bioadhesive properties of poly(alkylcyanoacrylate) nanoparticles coated with polysaccharide. J. Nanosci. Nanotechnol., 6, 3102-3109.

- Bertram, U., Bodmeier, R., 2006. *In-situ* gelling, bioadhesive nasal inserts for extended drug delivery: *in-vitro* characterization of a new nasal dosage form. Eur. J. Pharm. Sci., 27, 62-71.

- Bertram, U., Bodmeier, R., 2012. Effect of polymer molecular weight and of polymer blends on the properties of rapidly gelling nasal inserts. Drug Dev. Ind. Pharm., 38, 659-669.

- Betageri, G.V., Deshmukh, D.V., Gupta, R.B., 2001. Oral sustained-release bioadhesive tablet formulation of didanosine. Drug Dev. Ind. Pharm., 27, 129-136.

- Bhabani, S.N., Prasant, K.R., Udaya, K.N., Benoy, B.B., 2010. Development and characterization of bioadhesive gel of microencapsulated metronidazole for vaginal use. Iran J. Pharm. Res., 9, 209-219.

- Bhadra, D., Gupta, G., Bhadra, S., Umamaheshwari, R.B., Jain, N., 2004. Multicomposite ultrathin capsules for sustained ocular delivery of ciprofloxacin hydrochloride. J. Pharm. Pharm. Sci., 7, 241-251.

- Bhakdi, S., Kuller, G., Muhly, M., Fromm, S., Seibert, G., Parrisius, J., 1987. Formation of transmural complement pores in serum-sensitive Escherichia coli. Infect. Immun., 55, 206-210.

- Bies, C., Lehr, C.M., Woodley, J.F., 2004. Lectin-mediated drug targeting: history and applications. Adv. Drug Deliv. Rev., 56, 425-435.

- Biradar, S.V., Dhumal, R.S., Shah, M.H., Paradkar, A.R., Yamamura, S., 2009. Preparation of multiparticulate vaginal tablet using glyceryl monooleate for sustained progesterone delivery. Pharm. Dev. Technol., 14, 38-49.

- Birudaraj, R., Mahalingam, R., Li, X., Jasti, B.R., 2005. Advances in buccal drug delivery. Crit Rev. Ther. Drug Carrier Syst., 22, 295-330.

- Blanco-Fuente, H., Esteban-Fernandez, B., Blanco-Mendez, J., Otero-Espinar, F.J., 2002. Use of beta-cyclodextrins to prevent modifications of the properties of carbopol hydrogels due to carbopol-drug interactions. Chem. Pharm. Bull. (Tokyo), 50, 40-46.

- Boateng, J.S., 2008. Wound healing dressings and drug delivery systems: A review. J. Pharm. Sci., 97, 2892-2923.

- Bosch van den, E., Gielens C., 2003. Gelatin degradation at elevated temperature. Int. J. Biol. Macromol., 32, 129-138.

- Bottenberg, P., Cleymaet, R., de, M.C., Remon, J.P., Coomans, D., Michotte, Y., Slop, D., 1991. Development and testing of bioadhesive, fluoride-containing slow-release tablets for oral use. J. Pharm. Pharmacol., 43, 457-464.

- Bouckaert, S., Lefebvre, R.A., Colardyn, F., Remon, J.P., 1993a. Influence of the application site on bioadhesion and slow-release characteristics of a bioadhesive buccal slow-release tablet of miconazole. Eur. J. Clin. Pharmacol., 44, 331-335.

- Bouckaert, S., Lefebvre, R.A., Remon, J.P., 1993b. *In-vitro/in-vivo* correlation of the bioadhesive properties of a buccal bioadhesive miconazole slow-release tablet. Pharm. Res., 10, 853-856.

- Bouckaert, S., Remon, J.P., 1993. *In-vitro* bioadhesion of a buccal, miconazole slow-release tablet. J. Pharm. Pharmacol., 45, 504-507.

- Boulane-Petermann, L., 1996. Processes of bioadhesion on stainless steel surfaces and cleanability: A review with special reference to the food industry. Biofouling., 10, 275-300.

- Bozzini, S., Petrini, P., Tanzi, M.C., Arciola, C.R., Tosatti, S., Visai, L., 2011. Poly(ethylene glycol) and hydroxy functionalized alkane phosphate self-assembled monolayers reduce bacterial adhesion and support osteoblast proliferation. Int. J. Artif. Organs, 34, 898-907.

- Brady, R.F., Singer, I.L., 2000. Mechanical factors favoring release from fouling release coatings. Biofouling., 15, 73-81.

- Bravo-Osuna, I., Millotti, G., Vauthier, C., Ponchel, G., 2007. *In-vitro* evaluation of calcium binding capacity of chitosan and thiolated chitosan poly(isobutyl cyanoacrylate) core-shell nanoparticles. Int. J. Pharm., 338, 284-290.

- Bredenberg, S., Nystrom, C., 2003. *In-vitro* evaluation of bioadhesion in particulate systems and possible improvement using interactive mixtures. J. Pharm. Pharmacol., 55, 169-177.

- Briandet, R., Herry, J., Bellon-Fontaine, M., 2001. Determination of the van der Waals, electron donor and electron acceptor surface tension components of static Gram-positive microbial biofilms. Colloids Surf. B Biointerfaces., 21, 299-310.

- Briandet, R., Meylheuc, T., Maher, C., Bellon-Fontaine, M.N., 1999. Listeria monocytogenes Scott A: cell surface charge, hydrophobicity, and electron donor and acceptor characteristics under different environmental growth conditions. Appl. Environ. Microbiol., 65, 5328-5333.

- Bruck, A., Abu-Dahab, R., Borchard, G., Schafer, U.F., Lehr, C.M., 2001. Lectin-functionalized liposomes for pulmonary drug delivery: interaction with human alveolar epithelial cells. J. Drug Target, 9, 241-251.

- Bruinsma, R., Behrisch, A., Sackmann, E., 2000. Adhesive switching of membranes: experiment and theory. Phys. Rev. E. Stat. Phys. Plasmas. Fluids Relat Interdiscip. Topics., 61, 4253-4267.

- Bruschi, M.L., de, F.O., 2005. Oral bioadhesive drug delivery systems. Drug Dev. Ind. Pharm., 31, 293-310.

- Buchan, B., Kay, G., Heneghan, A., Matthews, K.H., Cairns, D., 2010. Gel formulations for treatment of the ophthalmic complications in cystinosis. Int. J. Pharm., 392, 192-197.

- Burzio, L.O., Burzio, V.A., Silva, T., Burzio, L.A., Pardo, J., 1997. Environmental bioadhesion: themes and applications. Curr. Opin. Biotechnol., 8, 309-312.

- Cardile, V., Frasca, G., Rizza, L., Bonina, F., Puglia, C., Barge, A., Chiambretti, N., Cravotto, G., 2008. Improved adhesion to mucosal cells of water-soluble chitosan tetraalkylammonium salts. Int. J. Pharm., 362, 88-92.

- Carman, M.L., Estes, T.G., Feinberg, A.W., Schumacher, J.F., Wilkerson, W., Wilson, L.H., Callow, M.E., Callow, J.A., Brennan, A.B., 2006. Engineered antifouling microtopographies – correlating wettability with cell attachment. Biofouling., 22, 11-21.

- Carvalho, F.C., Calixto, G., Hatakeyama, I.N., Luz, G.M., Gremiao, M.P., Chorilli, M., 2013. Rheological, mechanical, and bioadhesive behavior of hydrogels to optimize skin delivery systems. Drug Dev. Ind. Pharm., 39, 1750-1757.

- Caswell, M., Kane, M., 2002. Comparison of the moisturization efficacy of two vaginal moisturizers: Pectin versus polycarbophil technologies. J. Cosmet. Sci., 53, 81-87.

- Cattani, V.B., Fiel, L.A., Jager, A., Jager, E., Colome, L.M., Uchoa, F., Stefani, V., Dalla, C.T., Guterres, S.S., Pohlmann, A.R., 2010. Lipid-core nanocapsules restrained the indomethacin ethyl ester hydrolysis in the gastrointestinal lumen and wall acting as mucoadhesive reservoirs. Eur. J. Pharm. Sci., 39, 116-124.

- Cavallari, C., Fini, A., Ospitali, F., 2013. Mucoadhesive multiparticulate patch for the intrabuccal controlled delivery of lidocaine. Eur. J. Pharm. Biopharm., 83, 405-414.

- Cevher, E., Sensoy, D., Zloh, M., Mulazimoglu, L., 2008. Preparation and characterisation of natamycin: gamma-cyclodextrin inclusion complex and its evaluation in vaginal mucoadhesive formulations. J. Pharm. Sci., 97, 4319-4335.

- Chakraborty, P., Dey, S., Parcha, V., Bhattacharya, S.S., Ghosh, A., 2013. Design expert supported mathematical optimization and predictability study of buccoadhesive pharmaceutical wafers of Loratadine. Biomed. Res. Int., 2013, 197398.

- Chary, R.B., Rao, Y.M., 2000. Formulation and evaluation of Methocel K15M bioadhesive matrix tablets. Drug Dev. Ind. Pharm., 26, 901-906.

- Chary, R.B., Vani, G., Rao, Y.M., 1999. *In-vitro* and *in-vivo* adhesion testing of mucoadhesive drug delivery systems. Drug Dev. Ind. Pharm., 25, 685-690.

- Chavanpatil, M.D., Jain, P., Chaudhari, S., Shear, R., Vavia, P.R., 2006. Novel sustained release, swellable and bioadhesive gastroretentive drug delivery system for ofloxacin. Int. J. Pharm., 316, 86-92.

- Chavda, H., Modhia, I., Mehta, A., Patel, R., Patel, C., 2013. Development of bioadhesive chitosan superporous hydrogel composite particles based intestinal drug delivery system. Biomed. Res. Int., 2013, 563651.

- Chawla, V., Saraf, S.A., 2012. Rheological studies on solid lipid nanoparticle based carbopol gels of aceclofenac. Colloids Surf. B Biointerfaces., 92, 293-298.

- Chelladurai, S., Mishra, M., Mishra, B., 2008. Design and evaluation of bioadhesive *in-situ* nasal gel of ketorolac tromethamine. Chem. Pharm. Bull. (Tokyo), 56, 1596-1599.

- Cheng, Y., Gao, Y., Rao, T., Li, Y., Xu, T., 2007. Dendrimer-based prodrugs: design, synthesis, screening and biological evaluation. Comb. Chem. High Throughput. Screen., 10, 336-349.

- Cheng, Z., Lai, H., Du, Y., Fu, K., Hou, R., Li, C., Zhang, N., Sun, K., 2014. pH-Induced Reversible Wetting Transition between the Underwater Superoleophilicity and Superoleophobicity. ACS Appl. Mater. Interfaces., 6, 636-641.

- Chickering, D., Jacob, J., Mathiowitz, E., 1996. Poly(fumaric-co-sebacic) microspheres as oral drug delivery systems. Biotechnol. Bioeng., 52, 96-101.

- Chickering, D.E., III, Harris, W.P., Mathiowitz, E., 1995. A microtensiometer for the analysis of bioadhesive microspheres. Biomed. Instrum. Technol., 29, 501-512.

- Chirra, H.D., Desai, T.A., 2012. Multi-reservoir bioadhesive microdevices for independent rate-controlled delivery of multiple drugs. Small, 8, 3839-3846.

- Ch'ng, H.S., Park, H., Kelly, P., Robinson, J.R., 1985. Bioadhesive polymers as platforms for oral controlled drug delivery II: synthesis and evaluation of some swelling, water-insoluble bioadhesive polymers. J. Pharm. Sci., 74, 399-405.

- Cho, C.W., Choi, J.S., Shin, S.C., 2011. Enhanced local anesthetic action of mepivacaine from the bioadhesive gels. Pak. J. Pharm. Sci., 24, 87-93.

- Cilurzo, F., Minghetti, P., Selmin, F., Casiraghi, A., Montanari, L., 2003. Polymethacrylate salts as new low-swellable mucoadhesive materials. J. Control Release, 88, 43-53.

- Claro-Pereira, D., Sampaio-Maia, B., Ferreira, C., Rodrigues, A., Melo, L.F., Vasconcelos, M.R., 2011. *In-situ* evaluation of a new silorane-based composite resin's bioadhesion properties. Dent. Mater., 27, 1238-1245.

- Cochrane, C., Rippon, M.G., Rogers, A., Walmsley, R., Knottenbelt, D., Bowler, P., 1999. Application of an *in-vitro* model to evaluate bioadhesion of fibroblasts and epithelial cells to two different dressings. Biomaterials, 20, 1237-1244.

- Collaud, S., Warloe, T., Jordan, O., Gurny, R., Lange, N., 2007. Clinical evaluation of bioadhesive hydrogels for topical delivery of hexylaminolevulinate to Barrett's esophagus. J. Control Release, 123, 203-210.

- Colonna, C., Genta, I., Perugini, P., Pavanetto, F., Modena, T., Valli, M., Muzzarelli, C., Conti, B., 2006. 5-methyl-pyrrolidinone chitosan films as carriers for buccal administration of proteins. AAPS. PharmSciTech., 7, 70.

- Cooperstein, M.A., Canavan, H.E., 2010. Biological cell detachment from poly(N-isopropyl acrylamide) and its applications. Langmuir, 26, 7695-7707.

- Csaba, N., Garcia-Fuentes, M., Alonso, M.J., 2006. The performance of nanocarriers for transmucosal drug delivery. Expert. Opin. Drug Deliv., 3, 463-478.

- Cvetkovic, N., Nesic, M., Moracic, V., Rosic, M., 1997. Design of a method for *in-vitro* studies of polymer adhesion. Pharmazie, 52, 536-537.

- Darwish, A.M., El-Sayed, A.M., El-Harras, S.A., Khaled, K.A., Ismail, M.A., 2008. Clinical efficacy of novel unidirectional buccoadhesive vs. vaginoadhesive bromocriptine mesylate discs for treating pathologic hyperprolactinemia. Fertil. Steril., 90, 1864-1868.

- Darwish, M.K., Elmeshad, A.N., 2009. Buccal mucoadhesive tablets of flurbiprofen: Characterization and optimization. Drug Discov. Ther., 3, 181-189.

- de la Fuente, M., Seijo, B., Alonso, M.J., 2008. Bioadhesive hyaluronan-chitosan nanoparticles can transport genes across the ocular mucosa and transfect ocular tissue. Gene Ther., 15, 668-676.

- Dehghan, M.H., Girase, M., 2012. Freeze-dried Xanthan/Guar Gum Nasal Inserts for the Delivery of Metoclopramide Hydrochloride. Iran J. Pharm. Res., 11, 513-521.

- Dhiman, M.K., Yedurkar, P.D., Sawant, K.K., 2008. Buccal bioadhesive delivery system of 5-fluorouracil: optimization and characterization. Drug Dev. Ind. Pharm., 34, 761-770.

- Di Simone, M.P., Baldi, F., Vasina, V., Scorrano, F., Bacci, M.L., Ferrieri, A., Poggioli, G., 2012. Barrier effect of Esoxx (R) on esophageal mucosal damage: experimental study on *ex-vivo* swine model. Clin. Exp. Gastroenterol., 5, 103-107.

- Ding, J.S., Jiang, X.H., Yuan, M., 2001. [Improving bioavailability of naftopidil by using bioadhesion in dogs]. Yao Xue. Xue. Bao., 36, 377-380.

- Dittgen, M., Oestereich,S., Dittrich, F., 1989. The effect of mucous excipient concentration on bioadhesion *ex-vivo*. Pharmazie, 44, 460-462.

- Dittgen, M., Oestereich, S., Eckhardt, D., 1991. The effect of bioadhesiveness of viscous solutions with naphazoline hydrochloride on the elimination of the drug from the eye of swine. Pharmazie, 46, 716-718.

- Dong, Y., Feng, S.S., 2005. Poly(d,l-lactide-co-glycolide)/montmorillonite nanoparticles for oral delivery of anticancer drugs. Biomaterials, 26, 6068-6076.

- Doundoulakis, J.H., 1987. Surface analysis of titanium after sterilization: role in implant-tissue interface and bioadhesion. J. Prosthet. Dent., 58, 471-478.

- Drotlef, D.M., Blumler, P., Del, C.A., 2013. Magnetically Actuated Patterns for Bioinspired Reversible Adhesion (Dry and Wet). Adv. Mater.

- Duchene, D., Ponchel, G., 1992. Principle and investigation of the bioadhesion mechanism of solid dosage forms. Biomaterials, 13, 709-714.

- Dufrene, Y.F., Boonaert, C.J., Rouxhet, P.G., 1999. Surface analysis by X-ray photoelectron spectroscopy in study of bioadhesion and biofilms. Methods Enzymol., 310, 375-389.

- Dunn, H.K., King, R., Andrade, J.D., Jr., De Vries, K.L., 1973. Polyester textile bioadhesion to muscle and bone. J. Biomed. Mater. Res., 7, 109-135.

- Eftaiha, A.F., Qinna, N., Rashid, I.S., Al Remawi, M.M., Al Shami, M.R., Arafat,T.A., Badwan, A.A., 2010. Bioadhesive controlled metronidazole release matrix based on chitosan and xanthan gum. Mar. Drugs, 8, 1716-1730.

- El-Kamel, A.H., Ashri, L.Y., Alsarra, I.A., 2007. Micromatricial metronidazole benzoate film as a local mucoadhesive delivery system for treatment of periodontal diseases. AAPS. Pharm Sci Tech., 8, E75.

- Elkheshen, S., Yassin, A.E., Alkhaled, F., 2003. Per-oral extended-release bioadhesive tablet formulation of verapamil HCl. Boll. Chim. Farm., 142, 226-231.

- Emami, J., Shetabboushehri, M.A., Varshosaz, J., Eisaei, A., 2013. Preparation and characterization of a sustained release buccoadhesive system for delivery of terbutaline sulfate. Res. Pharm. Sci., 8, 219-231.

- Ertl, B., Heigl, F., Wirth, M., Gabor, F., 2000. Lectin-mediated bioadhesion: preparation, stability and caco-2 binding of wheat germ agglutinin-functionalized Poly(D,L-lactic-co-glycolic acid)-microspheres. J. Drug Target, 8, 173-184.

- Escobar-Chavez, J.J., Merino,V., Diez-Sales, O., Nacher-Alonso, A., Ganem-Quintanar, A., Herraez, M., Merino-Sanjuan, M., 2011. Transdermal nortriptyline hydrocloride patch formulated within a chitosan matrix intended to be used for smoking cessation. Pharm. Dev. Technol., 16, 162-169.

- Evans, L.V., 1989. Mucilaginous substances from macroalgae: an overview. Symp. Soc. Exp. Biol., 43, 455-461.

- Fabri, F.V., Cupertino, R.R., Hidalgo, M.M., de Oliveira, R.M., Bruschi, M.L., 2011. Preparation and characterization of bioadhesive systems containing propolis or sildenafil for dental pulp protection. Drug Dev. Ind. Pharm., 37, 1446-1454.

- Falconi, M., Focaroli, S., Teti, G., Salvatore, V., Durante, S., Nicolini, B., Orienti, I., 2013. Novel PLA microspheres with hydrophilic and bioadhesive surfaces for the controlled delivery of fenretinide. J. Microencapsul.

- Fang, N., Chan, V., 2003. Interaction of liposome with immobilized chitosan during main phase transition. Biomacromolecules., 4, 581-588.

- Fei, D.T., Lowe, J., Bodary, S., Bunting, S., McLean, J.W., Napier, M., Chen, A.B., 1993. RGD-containing peptides inhibit adhesion of 293 cells transfected with GpIIb/IIIa to fibrinogen: comparison to inhibition of platelet aggregation. Blood Coagul. Fibrinolysis, 4, 255-262.

- Fisher, O.Z., 2008, Novel pH-responsive microgels and nanogels as intelligent polymer therapeutics. Dissertation submitted for the degree of Doctor of philosophy to The University of Texas, Austin.

- Flammang, P., Santos, R., Haesaerts, D., 2005. Echinoderm adhesive secretions: from experimental characterization to biotechnological applications. Prog. Mol. Subcell. Biol., 39, 201-220.

- Florence, A.T., Hussain, N., 2001. Transcytosis of nanoparticle and dendrimer delivery systems: evolving vistas. Adv. Drug Deliv. Rev., 50 Suppl 1, S69-S89.

- Francius, G., Henry, R., Duval, J.F., Bruneau, E., Merlin, J., Fahs, A., Leblond-Bourget, N., 2013. Thermo-regulated adhesion of the Streptococcus thermophilus Deltargg0182 strain. Langmuir, 29, 4847-4856.

- Gabor, F., Stangl, M., Wirth, M., 1998. Lectin-mediated bioadhesion: binding characteristics of plant lectins on the enterocyte-like cell lines Caco-2, HT-29 and HCT-8. J. Control Release, 55, 131-142.

- Gabriella, F., 2012. Human serum albumin: From bench to bedside. Mol. Aspects of Med., 33, 209-290.

- Galaleldeen, A., Taylor, A.B., Chen, D., Schuermann, J.P., Holloway,S.P., Hou, S., Gong,S., Zhong,G., Hart,P.J., 2013. Structure of the Chlamydia trachomatis immunodominant antigen Pgp3. J. Biol. Chem., 288, 22068-22079.

- Gangurde, H.H., Chordiya, M.A., Tamizharasi, S., Senthilkumaran, K., Sivakumar, T., 2011. Formulation and evaluation of sustained release bioadhesive tablets of ofloxacin using 3(2) factorial design. Int. J. Pharm. Investig., 1, 148-156.

- Garcia, J., Ghaly, E.S., 2001. Evaluation of bioadhesive glipizide spheres and compacts from spheres prepared by extruder/marumerizer technique. Pharm. Dev. Technol., 6, 407-417.

- Garg, S., Jambu, L., Vermani, K., 2007. Development of novel sustained release bioadhesive vaginal tablets of povidone iodine. Drug Dev. Ind. Pharm., 33, 1340-1349.

- Garg, S., Tambwekar, K.R., Vermani, K., Kandarapu, R., Garg, A., Waller, D.P., Zaneveld, L.J., 2003. Development pharmaceutics of microbicide formulations. Part II: formulation, evaluation, and challenges. AIDS Patient. Care STDS., 17, 377-399.

- Genc, L., Oguzlar, C., Guler, E., 2000. Studies on vaginal bioadhesive tablets of acyclovir. Pharmazie, 55, 297-299.

- Genta, I., Perugini, P., Pavanetto, F., Modena, T., Conti, B., Muzzarelli, R.A., 1999. Microparticulate Drug Delivery Systems. EXS, 87, 305-313.

- Geraghty, P.B., Attwood, D., Collett, J.H., Sharma, H., Dandiker, Y., 1997. An investigation of the parameters influencing the bioadhesive properties of Myverol 18-99/water gels. Biomaterials, 18, 63-67.

- Ghavamzadeh, R., Haddadi-Asl, V., Mirzadeh, H., 2004. Bioadhesion and biocompatibility evaluations of gelatin and polyacrylic acid as a crosslinked hydrogel *in-vitro*. J. Biomater. Sci. Polym. Ed, 15, 1019-1031.

- Ghugare, S.V., Chiessi, E., Telling, M.T., Deriu, A., Gerelli, Y., Wuttke, J., Paradossi, G., 2010. Structure and dynamics of a thermoresponsive microgel around its volume phase transition temperature. J. Phys. Chem. B, 114, 10285-10293.

- Giaouris, E., Chapot-Chartier, M.P., Briandet, R., 2009. Surface physicochemical analysis of natural Lactococcus lactis strains reveals the existence of hydrophobic and low charged strains with altered adhesive properties. Int. J. Food Microbiol., 131, 2-9.

- Gilhotra, R.M., Gilhotra, N., Mishra, D.N., 2009. Piroxicam bioadhesive ocular inserts: physicochemical characterization and evaluation in prostaglandin-induced inflammation. Curr. Eye Res., 34, 1065-1073.

- Gilhotra, R.M., Mishra, D.N., 2008. Alginate-chitosan film for ocular drug delivery: effect of surface cross-linking on film properties and characterization. Pharmazie, 63, 576-579.

- Gilhotra, R.M., Nagpal, K., Mishra, D.N., 2011. Azithromycin novel drug delivery system for ocular application. Int. J. Pharm. Investig., 1, 22-28.

- Glantz, P.O., 1998a. Biomaterial considerations for the optimized therapy for the edentulous predicament. J. Prosthet. Dent., 79, 90-92.

- Glantz, P.O., 1998b. The choice of alloplastic materials for oral implants: does it really matter? Int. J. Prosthodont., 11, 402-407.

- Glantz, P.O., Arnebrant, T., Nylander, T., Baier, R.E., 1999. Bioadhesion – a phenomenon with multiple dimensions. Acta Odontol. Scand., 57, 238-241.

- Goecks, T., Werner, L., Mamalis, N., Fuller, S.R., Jensen, M., Kavoussi, S.C., Hill, M., Olson, R.J., 2012. Toxicity comparison of intraocular azithromycin with and without a bioadhesive delivery system in rabbit eyes. J. Cataract Refract. Surg., 38, 137-145.

- Gomez-Guillen, M.C., 2011. Functional and bioactive properties of collagen and gelatin from alternative sources: A review. Food Hydrocolloids, 25, 1813-1827.

- Gon, S., Kumar, K.N., Nusslein, K., Santore, M.M., 2012. How Bacteria Adhere to Brushy PEG Surfaces: Clinging to Flaws and Compressing the Brush. Macromolecules, 45, 8373-8381.

- Gon, S., Santore, M.M., 2011. Sensitivity of protein adsorption to architectural variations in a protein-resistant polymer brush containing engineered nanoscale adhesive sites. Langmuir, 27, 15083-15091.

- Goncalez, M.L., Correa, M.A., Chorilli, M., 2013. Skin delivery of kojic Acid-loaded nanotechnology-based drug delivery systems for the treatment of skin aging. Biomed. Res. Int., 2013, 271276.

- Gonda, I., Gipps, E., 1990. Model of disposition of drugs administered into the human nasal cavity. Pharm. Res., 7, 69-75.

- Gonjari, I.D., Hosmani, A.H., Karmarkar, A.B., Godage, A.S., Kadam, S.B., Dhabale, P.N., 2009. Formulation and evaluation of *in-situ* gelling thermoreversible mucoadhesive gel of fluconazole. Drug Discov. Ther., 3, 6-9.

- Gonjari, I.D., Karmarkar, A.B., Khade, T.S., Hosmani, A.H., Navale, R.B., 2010. Use of factorial design in formulation and evaluation of ophthalmic gels of gatifloxacin: Comparison of different mucoadhesive polymers. Drug Discov. Ther., 4, 423-434.

- Govender, S., Pillay, V., Chetty, D.J., Essack, S.Y., Dangor, C.M., Govender, T., 2005. Optimisation and characterisation of bioadhesive controlled release tetracycline microspheres. Int. J. Pharm., 306, 24-40.

- Graham, N.B., Cameron, A., 1998. Nanogels and microgels: The new polymeric materials playground. Pure and Applied Chem., 70, 1271-1275.

- Grand, I., Bellon-Fontaine, M.N., Herry, J.M., Hilaire, D., Moriconi, F.X., Naitali, M., 2011. Possible overestimation of surface disinfection efficiency by assessment methods based on liquid sampling procedures as demonstrated by *in-situ* quantification of spore viability. Appl. Environ. Microbiol., 77, 6208-6214.

- Gu, J.M., Robinson, J.R., Leung, S.H., 1988. Binding of acrylic polymers to mucin/epithelial surfaces: structure-property relationships. Crit Rev. Ther. Drug Carrier Syst., 5, 21-67.

- Guegan, C., Garderes, J., Le, P.G., Gaillard, F., Fay, F., Linossier, I., Herry, J.M., Fontaine, M.N., Rehel, K.V., 2014. Alteration of bacterial adhesion induced by the substrate stiffness. Colloids Surf. B Biointerfaces., 114, 193-200.

- Guillier, L., Nazer, A.I., Dubois-Brissonnet, F., 2007. Growth response of Salmonella typhimurium in the presence of natural and synthetic antimicrobials: estimation of MICs from three different models. J. Food Prot., 70, 2243-2250.

- Guillier, L., Stahl, V., Hezard, B., Notz, E., Briandet, R., 2008. Modelling the competitive growth between Listeria monocytogenes and biofilm microflora of smear cheese wooden shelves. Int. J. Food Microbiol., 128, 51-57.

- Guo, J.H., 1994. Investigating the surface properties and bioadhesion of buccal patches. J. Pharm. Pharmacol., 46, 647-650.

- Guo, J.H., Cooklock, K.M., 1998. Theoretical approaches and practical investigations in carbopol buccal patches for drug delivery. Drug Dev. Ind. Pharm., 24, 175-178.

- Gupta, N.V., Natasha, S., Getyala, A., Bhat, R.S., 2013. Bioadhesive vaginal tablets containing spray dried microspheres loaded with clotrimazole for treatment of vaginal Candidiasis. Acta Pharm., 63, 359-372.

- Haas, J., Lehr, C.M., 2002. Developments in the area of bioadhesive drug delivery systems. Expert. Opin. Biol. Ther., 2, 287-298.

- Habimana, O., Le, G.C., Juillard, V., Bellon-Fontaine, M.N., Buist, G., Kulakauskas, S., Briandet, R., 2007. Positive role of cell wall anchored proteinase PrtP in adhesion of lactococci. BMC. Microbiol., 7, 36.

- Haltner, E., Borchard, G., Lehr, C.M., 1998. Absorption enhancement by lectin-mediated endo- and transcytosis. Methods Mol. Med., 9, 567-581.

- Hannig, C., Gaeding, A., Basche, S., Richter, G., Helbig, R., Hannig, M., 2013. Effect of conventional mouthrinses on initial bioadhesion to enamel and dentin *in-situ*. Caries Res., 47, 150-161.

- Hannig, C., Hannig, M., 2009. The oral cavity – a key system to understand substratum-dependent bioadhesion on solid surfaces in man. Clin. Oral Investig., 13, 123-139.

- Harish, N.M., Prabhu, P., Charyulu, R.N., Gulzar, M.A., Subrahmanyam, E.V., 2009. Formulation and Evaluation of *in-situ* Gels Containing Clotrimazole for Oral Candidiasis. Indian J. Pharm. Sci., 71, 421-427.

- Hassan, E.E., Gallo, J.M., 1990. A simple rheological method for the *in-vitro* assessment of mucin-polymer bioadhesive bond strength. Pharm. Res., 7, 491-495.

- Helledi, L.S., Schubert, L., 2001. Release kinetics of acyclovir from a suspension of acyclovir incorporated in a cubic phase delivery system. Drug Dev. Ind. Pharm., 27, 1073-1081.

- Hoath, S.B., 1997. The stickiness of newborn skin: bioadhesion and the epidermal barrier. J. Pediatr., 131, 338-340.

- Hooda, A., Nanda, A., Jain, M., Kumar, V., Rathee, P., 2012. Optimization and evaluation of gastroretentive ranitidine HCl microspheres by using design expert software. Int. J. Biol. Macromol., 51, 691-700.

- Hou, S.Y., Cowles, V.E., Berner, B., 2003. Gastric retentive dosage forms: a review. Crit Rev. Ther. Drug Carrier Syst., 20, 459-497.

- Hu, C., Liu, S., Li, B., Yang, H., Fan, C., Cui, W., 2013. Micro-/nanometer rough structure of a superhydrophobic biodegradable coating by electrospraying for initial anti-bioadhesion. Adv. Healthc. Mater., 2, 1314-1321.

- Huang, Y., Leobandung, W., Foss, A., Peppas, N.A., 2000. Molecular aspects of muco- and bioadhesion: tethered structures and site-specific surfaces. J. Control Release, 65, 63-71.

- Ikinci, G., Capan,Y., Senel, S., Alaaddinoglu, E., Dalkara, T., Hincal, A.A., 2000. *In-vitro/in-vivo* studies on a buccal bioadhesive tablet formulation of carbamazepine. Pharmazie, 55, 762-765.

- Ikinci, G., Senel, S., Akincibay, H., Kas, S., Ercis, S., Wilson, C.G., Hincal, A.A., 2002. Effect of chitosan on a periodontal pathogen Porphyromonas gingivalis. Int. J. Pharm., 235, 121-127.

- Ikinci, G., Senel, S., Tokgozoglu, L., Wilson, C.G., Sumnu, M., 2006. Development and *in-vitro/in-vivo* evaluations of bioadhesive buccal tablets for nicotine replacement therapy. Pharmazie, 61, 203-207.

- Ikinci, G., Senel, S., Wilson, C.G., Sumnu, M., 2004. Development of a buccal bioadhesive nicotine tablet formulation for smoking cessation. Int. J. Pharm., 277, 173-178.

- Illum, L., 2006. Nasal clearance in health and disease. J. Aerosol Med., 19, 92-99.

- Irache, J.M., Durrer, C., Duchene, D., Ponchel, G., 1994. Preparation and characterization of lectin-latex conjugates for specific bioadhesion. Biomaterials, 15, 899-904.

- Irache, J.M., Durrer, C., Duchene, D., Ponchel, G., 1996. Bioadhesion of lectin-latex conjugates to rat intestinal mucosa. Pharm. Res., 13, 1716-1719.

- Jadhav, B.K., Khandelwal, K.R., Ketkar, A.R., Pisal, S.S., 2004. Formulation and evaluation of mucoadhesive tablets containing eugenol for the treatment of periodontal diseases. Drug Dev. Ind. Pharm., 30, 195-203.

- Jain, K.K. (Ed.), 2008. Drug Delivery Systems. Humana Press, USA.

- Jain, S.K., Jain, A., Gupta, Y., Kharya, A., 2008. Design and development of a mucoadhesive buccal film bearing progesterone. Pharmazie, 63, 129-135.

- Jaipal, A., Pandey, M.M., Abhishek, A., Vinay, S., Charde, S.Y., 2013. Interaction of calcium sulfate with xanthan gum: Effect on *in-vitro* bioadhesion and drug release behavior from xanthan gum based buccal discs of buspirone. Colloids Surf. B Biointerfaces., 111C, 644-650.

- Jayakumar, R., Prabaharan, M., Sudheesh, P.T., Nair, S.V., Furuike, T., Tamura, H., 2011. Novel Chitin and Chitosan Materials in Wound Dressing, Biomedical Engineering, Trends in Materials Science. Mr. Anthony Laskovski (Ed.), ISBN: 978-953-307-513-6, InTech, Available from: http://www.intechopen.com/books/biomedical-engineering-trends-in-materials-science/novel-chitin-andchitosan-materials-in-wound-dressing.

- Jelvehgari, M., Montazam, H., 2011. Evaluation of mechanical and rheological properties of metronidazole gel as local delivery system. Arch. Pharm. Res., 34, 931-940.

- Jones, D.S., Brown, A.F., Woolfson, A.D., 2001. Rheological characterization of bioadhesive, antimicrobial, semisolids designed for the treatment of periodontal diseases: transient and dynamic viscoelastic and continuous shear analysis. J. Pharm. Sci., 90, 1978-1990.

- Jones, D.S., Lawlor, M.S., Woolfson, A.D., 2004. Formulation and characterisation of tetracycline-containing bioadhesive polymer networks designed for the treatment of periodontal disease. Curr. Drug Deliv., 1, 17-25.

- Jones, D.S., Woolfson, A.D., Brown, A.F., 1998. Viscoelastic properties of bioadhesive, chlorhexidine-containing semi-solids for topical application to the oropharynx. Pharm. Res., 15, 1131-1136.

- Jones, D.S., Woolfson, A.D., Djokic, J., Coulter, W.A., 1996. Development and mechanical characterization of bioadhesive semi-solid, polymeric systems containing tetracycline for the treatment of periodontal diseases. Pharm. Res., 13, 1734-1738.

- Jug, M., Becirevic-Lacan, M., 2004. Influence of hydroxypropyl-beta-cyclodextrin complexation on piroxicam release from buccoadhesive tablets. Eur. J. Pharm. Sci., 21, 251-260.

- Jug, M., Becirevic-Lacan, M., Bengez, S., 2009. Novel cyclodextrin-based film formulation intended for buccal delivery of atenolol. Drug Dev. Ind. Pharm., 35, 796-807.

- Kakoulides, E.P., Smart, J.D., Tsibouklis, J., 1998. Azocrosslinked poly(acrylic acid) for colonic delivery and adhesion specificity: *in-vitro* degradation and preliminary *ex-vivo* bioadhesion studies. J. Control Release, 54, 95-109.

- Kalasin, S., Santore, M.M., 2009. Non-specific adhesion on biomaterial surfaces driven by small amounts of protein adsorption. Colloids Surf. B Biointerfaces., 73, 229-236.

- Kamel, R., Mahmoud, A., El-Feky, G., 2012. Double-phase hydrogel for buccal delivery of tramadol. Drug Dev. Ind. Pharm., 38, 468-483.

- Kamgang-Youbi, G., Herry, J.M., Brisset, J.L., Bellon-Fontaine, M.N., Doubla, A., Naitali, M., 2008. Impact on disinfection efficiency of cell load and of planktonic/adherent/detached state: case of Hafnia alvei inactivation by plasma activated water. Appl. Microbiol. Biotechnol., 81, 449-457.

- Kamgang-Youbi, G., Herry, J.M., Meylheuc, T., Brisset, J.L., Bellon-Fontaine, M.N., Doubla, A., Naitali, M., 2009. Microbial inactivation using plasma-activated water obtained by gliding electric discharges. Lett. Appl. Microbiol., 48, 13-18.

- Kang, C., Shin, S.C., 2012. Development of prilocaine gels for enhanced local anesthetic action. Arch. Pharm. Res., 35, 1197-1204.

- Kapil, R., Dhawan, S., Beg, S., Singh, B., 2013. Buccoadhesive films for once-a-day administration of rivastigmine: systematic formulation development and pharmacokinetic evaluation. Drug Dev. Ind. Pharm., 39, 466-480.

- Karavana, S.Y., Guneri, P., Ertan, G., 2009. Benzydamine hydrochloride buccal bioadhesive gels designed for oral ulcers: preparation, rheological, textural, mucoadhesive and release properties. Pharm. Dev. Technol., 14, 623-631.

- Kaur, A., Kaur, G., 2012. Mucoadhesive buccal patches based on interpolymer complexes of chitosan-pectin for delivery of carvedilol. Saudi. Pharm. J., 20, 21-27.

- Keegan, G.M., Smart, J.D., Ingram, M.J., Barnes, L.M., Burnett, G.R., Rees, G.D., 2012. Chitosan microparticles for the controlled delivery of fluoride. J. Dent., 40, 229-240.

- Keely, S., Rullay, A., Wilson, C., Carmichael, A., Carrington, S., Corfield, A., Haddleton, D.M., Brayden, D.J., 2005. *In-vitro* and *ex-vivo* intestinal tissue models to measure mucoadhesion of poly (methacrylate) and N-trimethylated chitosan polymers. Pharm. Res., 22, 38-49.

- Kelly, H.M., Deasy, P.B., Busquet, M., Torrance, A.A., 2004. Bioadhesive, rheological, lubricant and other aspects of an oral gel formulation intended for the treatment of xerostomia. Int. J. Pharm., 278, 391-406.

- Kennedy, A.J., Vasudevan, R., Pappas, D.D., Weiss, C.A., Hendrix, S.H., Baney, R.H., 2011. Efficacy of non-toxic surfaces to reduce bioadhesion in terrestrial gastropods. Pest. Manag. Sci., 67, 318-327.

- Kensche, A., Basche, S., Bowen, W.H., Hannig, M., Hannig, C., 2013. Fluorescence microscopic visualization of non cellular components during initial bioadhesion *in-situ*. Arch. Oral Biol., 58, 1271-1281.

- Kensche, A., Reich, M., Kummerer, K., Hannig, M., Hannig, C., 2013. Lipids in preventive dentistry. Clin. Oral Investig., 17, 669-685.

- Kesavan, K., Nath, G., Pandit, J., 2010a. Preparation and *in-vitro* antibacterial evaluation of gatifloxacin mucoadhesive gellan system. Daru., 18, 237-246.

- Kesavan, K., Nath, G., Pandit, J.K., 2010b. Sodium alginate based mucoadhesive system for gatifloxacin and its *in-vitro* antibacterial activity. Sci. Pharm., 78, 941-957.

- Keshavarz, M., Kaffashi, B., 2014. The ability of retention, drug release and rheological properties of nanogel bioadhesives based on cellulose derivatives. Pharm. Dev. Technol., 19, 952-959.

- Khullar, R., Kumar, D., Seth, N., Saini, S., 2012. Formulation and evaluation of mefenamic acid emulgel for topical delivery. Saudi. Pharm. J., 20, 63-67.

- Kim, G., Kim, H., Kim, I.J., Kim, J.R., Lee, J.I., Ree, M., 2009. Bacterial adhesion, cell adhesion and biocompatibility of Nafion films. J. Biomater. Sci. Polym. Ed, 20, 1687-1707.

- Koffi, A.A., Agnely, F., Besnard, M., Kablan, B.J., Grossiord, J.L., Ponchel, G., 2008. *In-vitro* and *in-vivo* characteristics of a thermogelling and bioadhesive delivery system intended for rectal administration of quinine in children. Eur. J. Pharm. Biopharm., 69, 167-175.

- Kotagale, N.R., Patel, C.J., Parkhe, A.P., Khandelwal, H.M., Taksande, J.B., Umekar, M.J., 2010. Carbopol 934-Sodium Alginate-Gelatin Mucoadhesive Ondansetron Tablets for Buccal Delivery: Effect of pH Modifiers. Indian J. Pharm. Sci., 72, 471-479.

- Krishnan, S., Ayothi, R., Hexemer, A., Finlay, J.A., Sohn, K.E., Perry, R., Ober, C.K., Kramer, E.J., Callow, M.E., Callow, J.A., Fischer, D.A., 2006. Anti-biofouling properties of comblike block copolymers with amphiphilic side chains. Langmuir, 22, 5075-5086.

- Kumar, K., Dhawan, N., Sharma, H., Vaidya, S., Vaidya, B., 2013. Bioadhesive polymers: Novel tool for drug delivery. Artif. Cells Nanomed. Biotechnol..

- Lachman, L., Liebermann, H.A., Kanig, J.L., 2010. The Theory and Practice of Industrial Pharmacy. CBS Publisher & Distributors P Ltd.

- Lamprecht, A., Schafer, U., Lehr, C.M., 2001. Size-dependent bioadhesion of micro- and nanoparticulate carriers to the inflamed colonic mucosa. Pharm. Res., 18, 788-793.

- Laulicht, B., Mancini, A., Geman, N., Cho, D., Estrellas, K., Furtado, S., Hopson, R., Tripathi, A., Mathiowitz, E., 2012. Bioinspired bioadhesive polymers: dopa-modified poly(acrylic acid) derivatives. Macromol. Biosci., 12, 1555-1565.

- Lavelle, E.C., 2001. Targeted delivery of drugs to the gastrointestinal tract. Crit Rev. Ther. Drug Carrier Syst., 18, 341-386.

- Lboutounne, H., Faivre, V., Falson, F., Pirot, F., 2004. Characterization of transport of chlorhexidine-loaded nanocapsules through hairless and wistar rat skin. Skin Pharmacol. Physiol, 17, 176-182.

- Le Ray, A.M., Iooss, P., Gouyette, A., Vonarx, V., Patrice, T., Merle, C., 1999. Development of a "continuous-flow adhesion cell" for the assessment of hydrogel adhesion. Drug Dev. Ind. Pharm., 25, 897-904.

- Le, C.S., Nguyen, K., Chen, Z., 2009. Sum Frequency Generation Studies on Bioadhesion: Elucidating the Molecular Structure of Proteins at Interfaces. J. Adhes., 85, 484-511.

- Lee, R.W., 2010. 'Micellar nanoparticles: Applications for topical and passive transdermal drug delivery' in Handbook of Non-Invasive Drug Delivery Systems. Elsevier Inc., 37-58.

- Lee, S.J., Kim, S.W., Chung, H., Park, Y.T., Choi, Y.W., Cho, Y.H., Yoon, M.S., 2005. Bioadhesive drug delivery system using glyceryl monooleate for the intravesical administration of paclitaxel. Chemotherapy, 51, 311-318.

- Legeay, G., Poncin-Epaillard, F., Arciola, C.R., 2006. New surfaces with hydrophilic/hydrophobic characteristics in relation to (no)bioadhesion. Int. J. Artif. Organs, 29, 453-461.

- Lehr, C.M., 1994. Bioadhesion technologies for the delivery of peptide and protein drugs to the gastrointestinal tract. Crit Rev. Ther. Drug Carrier Syst., 11, 119-160.

- Lehr, C.M., 1996. From sticky stuff to sweet receptors – achievements, limits and novel approaches to bioadhesion. Eur. J. Drug Metab Pharmacokinet., 21, 139-148.

- Lehr, C.M., 2000. Lectin-mediated drug delivery: the second generation of bioadhesives. J. Control Release, 65, 19-29.

- Lehr, C.M., Bouwstra, J.A., Kok, W., De Boer, A.G., Tukker, J.J., Verhoef, J.C., Breimer, D.D., Junginger, H.E., 1992a. Effects of the mucoadhesive polymer polycarbophil on the intestinal absorption of a peptide drug in the rat. J. Pharm. Pharmacol., 44, 402-407.

- Lehr, C.M., Bouwstra, J.A., Kok, W., Noach, A.B., De Boer, A.G., Junginger, H.E., 1992b. Bioadhesion by means of specific binding of tomato lectin. Pharm. Res., 9, 547-553.

- Lerebour, G., Cupferman, S., Bellon-Fontaine, M.N., 2004. Adhesion of Staphylococcus aureus and Staphylococcus epidermidis to the Episkin reconstructed epidermis model and to an inert 304 stainless steel substrate. J. Appl. Microbiol., 97, 7-16.

- Lerebour, G., Cupferman, S., Cohen, C., Bellon-Fontaine, M.N., 2000. Comparison of surface free energy between reconstructed human epidermis and *in-situ* human skin. Skin Res. Technol., 6, 245-249.

- Li, C., Bhatt, P.P., Johnston, T.P., 1998. Evaluation of a mucoadhesive buccal patch for delivery of peptides: *in-vitro* screening of bioadhesion. Drug Dev. Ind. Pharm., 24, 919-926.

- Li, K., Zhao, X., Xu, S., Pang, D., Yang, C., Chen, D., 2011. Application of Ulex europaeus agglutinin I-modified liposomes for oral vaccine: *Ex-vivo* bioadhesion and *in-vivo* immunity. Chem. Pharm. Bull. (Tokyo), 59, 618-623.

- Li, M.G., Lu, W.L., Wang, J.C., Zhang, X., Wang, X.Q., Zheng, A.P., Zhang, Q., 2007. Distribution, transition, adhesion and release of insulin loaded nanoparticles in the gut of rats. Int. J. Pharm., 329, 182-191.

- Li, N., Zhuang, C., Wang, M., Sun, X., Nie, S., Pan, W., 2009. Liposome coated with low molecular weight chitosan and its potential use in ocular drug delivery. Int. J. Pharm., 379, 131-138.

- Lian, H., Zhang, T., Sun, J., Liu, X., Ren, G., Kou, L., Zhang, Y., Han, X., Ding, W., Ai, X., Wu, C., Li, L., Wang, Y., Sun, Y., Wang, S., He, Z., 2013. Enhanced Oral Delivery of Paclitaxel Using Acetylcysteine Functionalized Chitosan-Vitamin E Succinate Nanomicelles Based on a Mucus Bioadhesion and Penetration Mechanism. Mol. Pharm..

- Liebau, M., Hildebrand, A., Neubert, R.H., 2001. Bioadhesion of supramolecular structures at supported planar bilayers as studied by the quartz crystal microbalance. Eur. Biophys. J., 30, 42-52.

- Lim, J.Y., Liu, X., Vogler, E.A., Donahue, H.J., 2004. Systematic variation in osteoblast adhesion and phenotype with substratum surface characteristics. J. Biomed. Mater. Res. A, 68, 504-512.

- Liu, B.S., 2009. Novel wound dressing of non-woven fabric coated with genipin-crosslinked chitosan and Bletilla Striata herbal extract. J. Med. Biol. Engg., 29, 60-67.

- Liu, P., Krishnan, T.R., 1999. Alginate-pectin-poly-L-lysine particulate as a potential controlled release formulation. J. Pharm. Pharmacol., 51, 141-149.

- Liu, Y., Wang, P., Sun, C., Feng, N., Zhou, W., Yang, Y., Tan, R., Chen, Z., Wu, S., Zhao, J., 2010. Wheat germ agglutinin-grafted lipid nanoparticles: preparation and *in-vitro* evaluation of the association with Caco-2 monolayers. Int. J. Pharm., 397, 155-163.

- Liu, Y., Wang, P., Sun, C., Zhao, J., Du, Y., Shi, F., Feng, N., 2011. Bioadhesion and enhanced bioavailability by wheat germ agglutinin-grafted lipid nanoparticles for oral delivery of poorly water-soluble drug bufalin. Int. J. Pharm., 419, 260-265.

- Llabot, J.M., Salman, H., Millotti, G., Bernkop-Schnurch, A., Allemandi, D., Manuel, I.J., 2011. Bioadhesive properties of poly(anhydride) nanoparticles coated with different molecular weights chitosan. J. Microencapsul., 28, 455-463.

- Lohbach, C., Neumann, D., Lehr, C.M., Lamprecht, A., 2006. Human vascular endothelial cells in primary cell culture for the evaluation of nanoparticle bioadhesion. J. Nanosci. Nanotechnol., 6, 3303-3309.

- Longer, M.A., Ch'ng, H.S., Robinson, J.R., 1985. Bioadhesive polymers as platforms for oral controlled drug delivery III: oral delivery of chlorothiazide using a bioadhesive polymer. J. Pharm. Sci., 74, 406-411.

- Lopez-Cervantes, M., Escobar-Chavez, J.J., Casas-Alancaster, N., Quintanar-Guerrero, D., Ganem-Quintanar, A., 2009. Development and characterization of a transdermal patch and an emulgel containing kanamycin intended to be used in the treatment of mycetoma caused by Actinomadura madurae. Drug Dev. Ind. Pharm., 35, 1511-1521.

- Lu, G., Ling, K., Zhao, P., Xu, Z., Deng, C., Zheng, H., Huang, J., Chen, J., 2010. A novel *in-situ*-formed hydrogel wound dressing by the photocross-linking of a chitosan derivative. Wound. Repair Regen., 18, 70-79.

- Lu, Y., Sarshar, M.A., Du, K., Chou, T., Choi, C.H., Sukhishvili, S.A., 2013. Large-Amplitude, Reversible, pH-Triggered Wetting Transitions Enabled by Layer-by-Layer Films. ACS Appl. Mater. Interfaces., 5, 12617-12623.

- Lukaszewska-Smyk, A., Kaluzny, J., 2010. [Lens platform]. Klin. Oczna, 112, 257-262.

- Luo, Q., Zhao, J., Zhang, X., Pan, W., 2011. Nanostructured lipid carrier (NLC) coated with Chitosan Oligosaccharides and its potential use in ocular drug delivery system. Int. J. Pharm., 403, 185-191.

- Luzardo, A.A., Blanco, G.E., Guerrero, C.F., Gomez, C.H., Blanco, M.J., 2012. *In-vitro* evaluation of the suppressive effect of chitosan/poly(vinyl alcohol) microspheres on attachment of C. parvum to enterocytic cells. Eur. J. Pharm. Sci., 47, 215-227.

- Madgulkar, A., Kadam, S., Pokharkar, V., 2009. Development of Buccal Adhesive Tablet with Prolonged Antifungal activity: Optimization and *ex-vivo* Deposition Studies. Indian J. Pharm. Sci., 71, 290-294.

- Madsen, K.D., Sander, C., Baldursdottir, S., Pedersen, A.M., Jacobsen, J., 2013. Development of an *ex-vivo* retention model simulating bioadhesion in the oral cavity using human saliva and physiologically relevant irrigation media. Int. J. Pharm., 448, 373-381.

- Maggi, L., Catellani, P.L., Fisicaro, E., Santi, P., Zani, F., Massimo, G., Colombo, P., 2000. Effect of drying methods on retention of moist sucralfate gel properties. AAPS. PharmSciTech., 1, E26.

- Mahajan, H.S., Tyagi, V.K., Patil, R.R., Dusunge, S.B., 2013. Thiolated xyloglucan: Synthesis, characterization and evaluation as mucoadhesive *in-situ* gelling agent. Carbohydr. Polym., 91, 618-625.

- Mahalingam, R., Jasti, B., Birudaraj, R., Stefanidis, D., Killion, R., Alfredson, T., Anne, P., Li, X., 2009. Evaluation of polyethylene oxide compacts as gastroretentive delivery systems. AAPS. PharmSciTech., 10, 98-103.

- Makhlof, A., Tozuka, Y., Takeuchi, H., 2011. Design and evaluation of novel pH-sensitive chitosan nanoparticles for oral insulin delivery. Eur. J. Pharm. Sci., 42, 445-451.

- Malik, S., Kumar, A., Ahuja, M., 2012. Synthesis of gum kondagogu-g-poly(N-vinyl-2-pyrrolidone) and its evaluation as a mucoadhesive polymer. Int. J. Biol. Macromol., 51, 756-762.

- Mansour, M., Mansour, S., Mortada, N.D., Abd Elhady, S.S., 2008. Ocular poloxamer-based ciprofloxacin hydrochloride *in-situ* forming gels. Drug Dev. Ind. Pharm., 34, 744-752.

- Marcato, P.D., Duran, N., 2008. New aspects of nanopharmaceutical delivery systems. J. Nanosci. Nanotech., 8, 1-14.

- Martin, L., Wilson, C.G., Koosha, F., Tetley, L., Gray, A.I., Senel, S., Uchegbu, I.F., 2002. The release of model macromolecules may be controlled by the hydrophobicity of palmitoyl glycol chitosan hydrogels. J. Control Release, 80, 87-100.

- Martini, A., Bonadeo, D., Bottoni, G., Caramella, C., Esposito, P., Gazzaniga, A., Merlo, M., Muggetti, L., Orlandi, R., Rossi, S., 1995. Bioadhesives: rationale, state of the art and therapeutic potential. Boll. Chim. Farm., 134, 595-603.

- Matsuda, S., Iwata, H., Se, N., Ikada, Y., 1999. Bioadhesion of gelatin films crosslinked with glutaraldehyde. J. Biomed. Mater. Res., 45, 20-27.

- Meenaghan, M.A., Natiella, J.R., Moresi, J.L., Flynn, H.E., Wirth, J.E., Baier, R.E., 1979. Tissue response to surface-treated tantalum implants: preliminary observations in primates. J. Biomed. Mater. Res., 13, 631-643.

- Mercier-Bonin, M., Ouazzani, K., Schmitz, P., Lorthois, S., 2004. Study of bioadhesion on a flat plate with a yeast/glass model system. J. Colloid Interface Sci., 271, 342-350.

- Meylheuc, T., Giovannacci, I., Briandet, R., Bellon-Fontaine, M.N., 2002. Comparison of the cell surface properties and growth characteristics of Listeria monocytogenes and Listeria innocua. J. Food Prot., 65, 786-793.

- Meylheuc, T., Methivier, C., Renault, M., Herry, J.M., Pradier, C.M., Bellon-Fontaine, M.N., 2006. Adsorption on stainless steel surfaces of biosurfactants produced by gram-negative and gram-positive bacteria: consequence on the bioadhesive behavior of Listeria monocytogenes. Colloids Surf. B Biointerfaces., 52, 128-137.

- Meylheuc, T., Renault, M., Bellon-Fontaine, M.N., 2006. Adsorption of a biosurfactant on surfaces to enhance the disinfection of surfaces contaminated with Listeria monocytogenes. Int. J. Food Microbiol., 109, 71-78.

- Meylheuc, T., van Oss, C.J., Bellon-Fontaine, M.N., 2001. Adsorption of biosurfactant on solid surfaces and consequences regarding the bioadhesion of Listeria monocytogenes LO28. J. Appl. Microbiol., 91, 822-832.

- Mididoddi, P.K., Prodduturi, S., Repka, M.A., 2006. Influence of tartaric acid on the bioadhesion and mechanical properties of hot-melt extruded hydroxypropyl cellulose films for the human nail. Drug Dev. Ind. Pharm., 32, 1059-1066.

- Mididoddi, P.K., Repka, M.A., 2007. Characterization of hot-melt extruded drug delivery systems for onychomycosis. Eur. J. Pharm. Biopharm., 66, 95-105.

- Mirza, M.A., Ahmad, S., Mallick, M.N., Manzoor, N., Talegaonkar, S., Iqbal, Z., 2013. Development of a novel synergistic thermosensitive gel for vaginal candidiasis: an *in-vitro*, *in-vivo* evaluation. Colloids Surf. B Biointerfaces., 103, 275-282.

- Mishra, S.K., Garud, N., Singh, R., 2011. Development and evaluation of mucoadhesive buccal patches of flurbiprofen. Acta Pol. Pharm., 68, 955-964.

- Mitra, A.K., (Ed.), 2003. Ophthalmic drug delivery systems. 2nd edition, Marcel Dekker, Inc. USA.

- Moes, A.J., 1993. Gastroretentive dosage forms. Crit Rev. Ther. Drug Carrier Syst., 10, 143-195.

- Mogal, V., Papper, V., Chaurasia, A., Feng, G., Marks, R., Steele, T., 2013. Novel On-Demand Bioadhesion to Soft Tissue in Wet Environments. Macromol. Biosci..

- Mohamed, S.P., Muzzammil, S., Pramod, K.T., 2011. Preparation of fluconazole buccal tablet and influence of formulation expedients on its properties. Yao Xue. Xue. Bao., 46, 460-465.

- Mohanraj, V.J., Chen, Y., 2006. Nanoparticles – A review. Tropical J. Pharma. Res., 5, 561-573.

- Molino, P.J., Hodson, O.M., Quinn, J.F., Wetherbee, R., 2008. The quartz crystal microbalance: a new tool for the investigation of the bioadhesion of diatoms to surfaces of differing surface energies. Langmuir, 24, 6730-6737.

- Mortazavi, SA., Aboofazeli, R., 2000. Preparation and *in-vitro* assessment of various mucosa-adhesive films for buccal delivery. DARU., 8, 9-18.

- Mulhbacher, J., Ispas-Szabo, P., Ouellet, M., Alex, S., Mateescu, M.A., 2006. Mucoadhesive properties of cross-linked high amylose starch derivatives. Int. J. Biol. Macromol., 40, 9-14.

- Muller, C., Luders, A., Hoth-Hannig, W., Hannig, M., Ziegler, C., 2010. Initial bioadhesion on dental materials as a function of contact time, pH, surface wettability, and isoelectric point. Langmuir, 26, 4136-4141.

- Murata, M., Yonamine, T., Tanaka, S., Tahara, K., Tozuka, Y., Takeuchi, H., 2013. Surface modification of liposomes using polymer-wheat germ agglutinin conjugates to improve the absorption of peptide drugs by pulmonary administration. J. Pharm. Sci., 102, 1281-1289.

- Murphy, D.J., Sankalia, M.G., Loughlin, R.G., Donnelly, R.F., Jenkins, M.G., Carron PA, M.C., 2012. Physical characterisation and component release of poly(vinyl alcohol)-tetrahydroxyborate hydrogels and their applicability as potential topical drug delivery systems. Int. J. Pharm., 423, 326-334.

- Mussard, W., Kebir, N., Kriegel, I., Esteve, M., Semetey, V., 2011. Facile and efficient control of bioadhesion on poly(dimethylsiloxane) by using a biomimetic approach. Angew. Chem. Int. Ed Engl., 50, 10871-10874.

- Nafee, N.A., Ismail, F.A., Boraie, N.A., Mortada, L.M., 2003. Mucoadhesive buccal patches of miconazole nitrate: *in-vitro/in-vivo* performance and effect of ageing. Int. J. Pharm., 264, 1-14.

- Nafee, N.A., Ismail, F.A., Boraie, N.A., Mortada, L.M., 2004a. Mucoadhesive delivery systems. I. Evaluation of mucoadhesive polymers for buccal tablet formulation. Drug Dev. Ind. Pharm., 30, 985-993.

- Nafee, N.A., Ismail, F.A., Boraie, N.A., Mortada, L.M., 2004b. Mucoadhesive delivery systems. II. Formulation and *in-vitro/in-vivo* evaluation of buccal mucoadhesive tablets containing water-soluble drugs. Drug Dev. Ind. Pharm., 30, 995-1004.

- Nakanishi, T., Kaiho, F., Hayashi, M., 1998. Improvement of drug release rate from carbopol 934P formulation. Chem. Pharm. Bull. (Tokyo), 46, 171-173.

- Nakhat, P.D., Kondawar, A.A., Rathi, L.G., Yeole, P.G., 2008. Development and *in-vitro* evaluation of buccoadhesive tablets of metoprolol tartrate. Indian J. Pharm. Sci., 70, 121-124.

- Narendra, C., Srinath, M.S., Prakash, R.B., 2005. Development of three layered buccal compact containing metoprolol tartrate by statistical optimization technique. Int. J. Pharm., 304, 102-114.

- Ndesendo, V.M., Pillay, V., Choonara, Y.E., du Toit, L.C., Kumar, P., Buchmann, E., Meyer, L.C., Khan, R.A., 2012. Optimization of a polymer composite employing molecular mechanic simulations and artificial neural networks for a novel intravaginal bioadhesive drug delivery device. Pharm. Dev. Technol., 17, 407-420.

- Ndesendo, V.M., Pillay, V., Choonara, Y.E., Khan, R.A., Meyer, L., Buchmann, E., Rosin, U., 2009. *In-vitro* and *ex-vivo* bioadhesivity analysis of polymeric intravaginal caplets using physicomechanics and computational structural modeling. Int. J. Pharm., 370, 151-159.

- Needleman, I.G., Martin, G.P., Smales, F.C., 1998. Characterisation of bioadhesives for periodontal and oral mucosal drug delivery. J. Clin. Periodontol., 25, 74-82.

- Needleman, I.G., Smales, F.C., 1994. Cultural technique for *in-vitro* modelling of prolonged bioadhesion. Biomaterials, 15, 950-952.

- Needleman, I.G., Smales, F.C., 1995. *In-vitro* assessment of bioadhesion for periodontal and buccal drug delivery. Biomaterials, 16, 617-624.

- Needleman, I.G., Smales, F.C., Martin, G.P., 1997. An investigation of bioadhesion for periodontal and oral mucosal drug delivery. J. Clin. Periodontol., 24, 394-400.

- Negi, J.S., Trivedi, A., Khanduri, P., Negi, V., Kasliwal, N., 2011. Effect of bioadhesion on initial *in-vitro* buoyancy of effervescent floating matrix tablets of ciprofloxacin HCL. J. Adv. Pharm. Technol. Res., 2, 121-127.

- Neutsch, L., Plattner, V.E., Polster-Wildhofen, S., Zidar, A., Chott, A., Borchard, G., Zechner, O., Gabor, F., Wirth, M., 2011. Lectin mediated biorecognition as a novel strategy for targeted delivery to bladder cancer. J. Urol., 186, 1481-1488.

- Ngo, T.C., Kalinova, R., Cossement, D., Hennebert, E., Mincheva, R., Snyders, R., Flammang, P., Dubois, P., Lazzaroni, R., Leclere, P., 2014. Modification of the adhesive properties of silicone-based coatings by block copolymers. Langmuir, 30, 358-368.

- Nielsen, L.S., Schubert, L., Hansen, J., 1998. Bioadhesive drug delivery systems. I. Characterisation of mucoadhesive properties of systems based on glyceryl mono-oleate and glyceryl monolinoleate. Eur. J. Pharm. Sci., 6, 231-239.

- Nikumbh, K.V., Sevankar, S.G., Patil, M.P., 2013. Formulation development, *in-vitro* and *in-vivo* evaluation of microemulsion-based gel loaded with ketoprofen. Drug Deliv..

- Norowski, P.A., Jr., Bumgardner, J.D., 2009. Biomaterial and antibiotic strategies for peri-implantitis: a review. J. Biomed. Mater. Res. B Appl. Biomater., 88, 530-543.

- Nunez, J.L., Ballesteros, M.P., Lastres, J.L., Castro, R.M., 2000. Interaction of poly methyl vinyl ether/maleic anhydride-dimiristoyl phosphatidylcholine: a model bioadhesion study. Biomaterials, 21, 2131-2135.

- Onoue, S., Ochi, M., Yamada, S., 2011. Development of (-)-epigallocatechin-3-gallate (EGCG)-loaded enteric microparticles with intestinal mucoadhesive property. Int. J. Pharm., 410, 111-113.

- Owens, T.S., Dansereau, R.J., Sakr, A., 2005. Development and evaluation of extended release bioadhesive sodium fluoride tablets. Int. J. Pharm., 288, 109-122.

- Ozturk, E., Eroglu, M., Ozdemir, N., Denkbas, E.B., 2004. Bioadhesive drug carriers for postoperative chemotherapy in bladder cancer. Adv. Exp. Med. Biol., 553, 231-242.

- Pal, S., Nagy, S., Bozo, T., Kocsis, B., Devay, A., 2013. Technological and biopharmaceutical optimization of nystatin release from a multiparticulate based bioadhesive drug delivery system. Eur. J. Pharm. Sci., 49, 258-264.

- Palacio, M.L., Bhushan, B., 2012. Bioadhesion: a review of concepts and applications. Philos. Trans. A Math. Phys. Eng Sci., 370, 2321-2347.

- Palacio, M.L., Schricker, S.R., Bhushan, B., 2011. Bioadhesion of various proteins on random, diblock and triblock copolymer surfaces and the effect of pH conditions. J. R. Soc. Interface, 8, 630-640.

- Palem, C.R., Gannu, R., Doodipala, N., Yamsani, V.V., Yamsani, M.R., 2011a. Transmucosal delivery of domperidone from bilayered buccal patches: *in-vitro, ex-vivo* and *in-vivo* characterization. Arch. Pharm. Res., 34, 1701-1710.

- Palem, C.R., Gannu, R., Yamsani, S.K., Yamsani, V.V., Yamsani, M.R., 2011b. Development of bioadhesive buccal tablets for felodipine and pioglitazone in combined dosage form: *in-vitro, ex-vivo,* and *in-vivo* characterization. Drug Deliv., 18, 344-352.

- Palem, C.R., Kumar, B.S., Gannu, R., Yamsani, V.V., Repka, M.A., Yamsani, M.R., 2012. Role of cyclodextrin complexation in felodipine-sustained release matrix tablets intended for oral transmucosal delivery: *in-vitro* and *ex-vivo* characterization. Pharm. Dev. Technol., 17, 321-332.

- Palem, C.R., Kumar, B.S., Maddineni, S., Gannu, R., Repka, M.A., Yamsani, M.R., 2013. Oral transmucosal delivery of domperidone from immediate release films produced via hot-melt extrusion technology. Pharm. Dev. Technol., 18, 186-195.

- Panigrahi, L., Pattnaik, S., Ghosal, S.K., 2004. Design and characterization of mucoadhesive buccal patches of salbutamol sulphate. Acta Pol. Pharm., 61, 351-360.

- Park, B.J., Abu-Lail, N.I., 2011. The role of the pH conditions of growth on the bioadhesion of individual and lawns of pathogenic Listeria monocytogenes cells. J. Colloid Interface Sci., 358, 611-620.

- Park, J.H., Robinson, J.R., 2008. Effect of a hydrophobic phospholipid lining of the gastric mucosa in bioadhesion. Pharm. Res., 25, 16-24.

- Parodi, B., Russo, E., Gatti, P., Cafaggi, S., Bignardi, G., 1999. Development and *in-vitro* evaluation of buccoadhesive tablets using a new model substrate for bioadhesion measures: the eggshell membrane. Drug Dev. Ind. Pharm., 25, 289-295.

- Pedrazzi, V., Del Ciampo, J.O., Panzeri, H., Lara, E.H., Issa, J.P., Do, N.C., 2009. Shear-bond strength between a new format of intra-buccal acrylic bioadhesive drug delivery system and adhesive systems. Minerva Stomatol., 58, 145-150.

- Pedrazzi, V., Lara, E.H., Dal Ciampo, J.O., Panzeri, H., 2001. Tensile bond strength of a polymeric intra-buccal bioadhesive: the mucin role. Boll. Chim. Farm., 140, 471-474.

- Peh, K.K., Wong, C.F., 1999. Polymeric films as vehicle for buccal delivery: swelling, mechanical, and bioadhesive properties. J. Pharm. Pharm. Sci., 2, 53-61.

- Peppas, N.A., 2000. Edith mathiowitz, donald E. Chickering III, and claus-michael lehr. eds., bioadhesive drug delivery systems. Fundamentals, novel applications and development, M. Dekker, new york, NY, xv+670 pages, $195.00. J. Control Release, 68, 135.

- Peppas, N.A., Sahlin, J.J., 1996. Hydrogels as mucoadhesive and bioadhesive materials: a review. Biomaterials, 17, 1553-1561.

- Pepper, L.R., Parthasarathy, R., Robbins, G.P., Dang, N.N., Hammer, D.A., Boder, E.T., 2013. Isolation of alphaL I domain mutants mediating firm cell adhesion using a novel flow-based sorting method. Protein Eng Des Sel, 26, 515-521.

- Perioli, L., Ambrogi, V., Venezia, L., Giovagnoli, S., Pagano, C., Rossi, C., 2009. Formulation studies of benzydamine mucoadhesive formulations for vaginal administration. Drug Dev. Ind. Pharm., 35, 769-779.

- Perioli, L., Pagano, C., Mazzitelli, S., Rossi, C., Nastruzzi, C., 2008. Rheological and functional characterization of new antiinflammatory delivery systems designed for buccal administration. Int. J. Pharm., 356, 19-28.

- Petrone, L., 2013. Molecular surface chemistry in marine bioadhesion. Adv. Colloid Interface Sci., 195-196, 1-18.

- Pham, T.T., Loiseau, P.M., Barratt, G., 2013. Strategies for the design of orally bioavailable antileishmanial treatments. Int. J. Pharm., 454, 539-552.

- Pillai, S., Arpanaei, A., Meyer, R.L., Birkedal, V., Gram, L., Besenbacher, F., Kingshott, P., 2009. Preventing protein adsorption from a range of surfaces using an aqueous fish protein extract. Biomacromolecules., 10, 2759-2766.

- Pliszczak, D., Bordes, C., Bourgeois, S., Marote, P., Zahouani, H., Tupin, S., Mattei, C.P., Lanteri, P., 2012. Mucoadhesion evaluation of polysaccharide gels for vaginal application by using rheological and indentation measurements. Colloids Surf. B Biointerfaces., 92, 168-174.

- Ponchel, G., Irache, J., 1998. Specific and non-specific bioadhesive particulate systems for oral delivery to the gastrointestinal tract. Adv. Drug Deliv. Rev., 34, 191-219.

- Poncin-Epaillard, F., Herry, J.M., Marmey, P., Legeay, G., Debarnot, D., Bellon-Fontaine, M.N., 2013. Elaboration of highly hydrophobic polymeric surface – a potential strategy to reduce the adhesion of pathogenic bacteria? Mater. Sci. Eng C. Mater. Biol. Appl., 33, 1152-1161.

- Poncin-Epaillard, F., Legeay, G., 2003. Surface engineering of biomaterials with plasma techniques. J. Biomater. Sci. Polym. Ed, 14, 1005-1028.

- Poncin-Epaillard, F., Shavdina, O., Debarnot, D., 2013. Elaboration and surface modification of structured poly(L-lactic acid) thin film on various substrates. Mater. Sci. Eng C. Mater. Biol. Appl., 33, 2526-2533.

- Porfire, A.S., Zabaleta, V., Gamazo, C., Leucuta, S.E., Irache, J.M., 2010. Influence of dextran on the bioadhesive properties of poly(anhydride) nanoparticles. Int. J. Pharm., 390, 37-44.

- Prinderre, P., Sauzet, C., Fuxen, C., 2011. Advances in gastro retentive drug-delivery systems. Expert. Opin. Drug Deliv., 8, 1189-1203.

- Rajinikanth, P.S., Sankar, C., Mishra, B., 2003. Sodium alginate microspheres of metoprolol tartrate for intranasal systemic delivery: development and evaluation. Drug Deliv., 10, 21-28.

- Ranade, V.V., Hollinger, M.A., 2004. Drug delivery systems. 2nd edition, CRC Press, USA.

- Rasool, B.K., Aziz, U.S., Sarheed, O., Rasool, A.A., 2011. Design and evaluation of a bioadhesive film for transdermal delivery of propranolol hydrochloride. Acta Pharm., 61, 271-282.

- Rastogi, R., Sultana, Y., Aqil, M., Ali, A., Kumar, S., Chuttani, K., Mishra, A.K., 2007. Alginate microspheres of isoniazid for oral sustained drug delivery. Int. J. Pharm., 334, 71-77.

- Rathbone, M.J., (Ed.), 2003. Modified-release drug delivery technology. Marcel Dekker, Inc. USA.

- Ratzinger, G., Wang, X., Wirth, M., Gabor, F., 2010. Targeted PLGA microparticles as a novel concept for treatment of lactose intolerance. J. Control Release, 147, 187-192.

- Refai, H., Tag, R., 2011. Development and characterization of sponge-like acyclovir ocular minitablets. Drug Deliv., 18, 38-45.

- Reich, M., Kummerer, K., Al-Ahmad, A., Hannig, C., 2013. Fatty acid profile of the initial oral biofilm (pellicle): an in-situ study. Lipids, 48, 929-937.

- Reineke, J., Cho, D.Y., Dingle, Y.L., Cheifetz, P., Laulicht, B., Lavin, D., Furtado, S., Mathiowitz, E., 2013. Can bioadhesive nanoparticles allow for more effective particle uptake from the small intestine? J. Control Release, 170, 477-484.

- Reis, C.P., 2006. Nanoencapsulation I. Methods for preparation of drug-loaded polymeric nanoparticles. Nanomedicine: Nanotechnology, Biology and Medicine., 2, 8-21.

- Repka, M.A., McGinity, J.W., 2000. Physical-mechanical, moisture absorption and bioadhesive properties of hydroxypropylcellulose hot-melt extruded films. Biomaterials, 21, 1509-1517.

- Repka, M.A., McGinity, J.W., 2001. Bioadhesive properties of hydroxypropylcellulose topical films produced by hot-melt extrusion. J. Control Release, 70, 341-351.

- Repka, M.A., Mididoddi, P.K., Stodghill, S.P., 2004. Influence of human nail etching for the assessment of topical onychomycosis therapies. Int. J. Pharm., 282, 95-106.

- Richardson, J.C., Bowtell, R.W., Mader, K., Melia, C.D., 2005. Pharmaceutical applications of magnetic resonance imaging (MRI). Adv. Drug Deliv. Rev., 57, 1191-1209.

- Richardson, J.C., Dettmar, P.W., Hampson, F.C., Melia, C.D., 2004. Oesophageal bioadhesion of sodium alginate suspensions: particle swelling and mucosal retention. Eur. J. Pharm. Sci., 23, 49-56.

- Richardson, J.C., Dettmar, P.W., Hampson, F.C., Melia, C.D., 2005. Oesophageal bioadhesion of sodium alginate suspensions 2. Suspension behaviour on oesophageal mucosa. Eur. J. Pharm. Sci., 24, 107-114.

- Ridolfi, D.M., Marcato, P.D., Justo, G.Z., Cordi, L., Machado, D., Duran, N., 2012. Chitosan-solid lipid nanoparticles as carriers for topical delivery of tretinoin. Colloids Surf. B Biointerfaces., 93, 36-40.

- Rodriguez-Tenreiro, C., Diez-Bueno, L., Concheiro, A., Torres-Labandeira, J.J., Alvarez-Lorenzo, C., 2007. Cyclodextrin/carbopol micro-scale interpenetrating networks (ms-IPNs) for drug delivery. J. Control Release, 123, 56-66.

- Rolin, G., Placet, V., Jacquet, E., Tauzin, H., Robin, S., Pazart, L., Viennet, C., Saas, P., Muret, P., Binda, D., Humbert, P., 2012. Development and characterization of a human dermal equivalent with physiological mechanical properties. Skin Res. Technol., 18, 251-258.

- Romoren, K., Thu, B.J., Evensen, O., 2002. Immersion delivery of plasmid DNA. II. A study of the potentials of a chitosan based delivery system in rainbow trout (Oncorhynchus mykiss) fry. J. Control Release, 85, 215-225.

- Rosca, I.D., Vergnaud, J.M., 2008. Evaluation of the characteristics of oral dosage forms with release controlled by erosion. Comput. Biol. Med., 38, 668-675.

- Rossi, A.M., Saidel, W.M., Marotta, R., Saglam, N., Shain, D.H., 2013. Operculum ultrastructure in leech cocoons. J. Morphol., 274, 940-946.

- Sajeesh, S., Bouchemal, K., Sharma, C.P., Vauthier, C., 2010. Surface-functionalized polymethacrylic acid based hydrogel microparticles for oral drug delivery. Eur. J. Pharm. Biopharm., 74, 209-218.

- Sakeer, K., Al-Zein, H., Hassan, I., Desai, S., Nokhodchi, A., 2010a. Enhancement of dissolution of nystatin from buccoadhesive tablets containing various surfactants and a solid dispersion formulation. Arch. Pharm. Res., 33, 1771-1779.

- Sakeer, K., Al-Zein, H., Hassan, I., Martin, G.P., Nokhodchi, A., 2010b. Use of xanthan and its binary blends with synthetic polymers to design controlled release formulations of buccoadhesive nystatin tablets. Pharm. Dev. Technol., 15, 360-368.

- Salman, H.H., Gamazo, C., Campanero, M.A., Irache, J.M., 2006. Bioadhesive mannosylated nanoparticles for oral drug delivery. J. Nanosci. Nanotechnol., 6, 3203-3209.

- Salman, H.H., Gamazo, C., de Smidt, P.C., Russell-Jones, G., Irache, J.M., 2008. Evaluation of bioadhesive capacity and immunoadjuvant properties of vitamin B(12)-Gantrez nanoparticles. Pharm. Res., 25, 2859-2868.

- Sander, C., Madsen, K.D., Hyrup, B., Nielsen, H.M., Rantanen, J., Jacobsen, J., 2013. Characterization of spray dried bioadhesive metformin microparticles for oromucosal administration. Eur. J. Pharm. Biopharm., 85, 682-688.

- Sander, C., Nielsen, H.M., Jacobsen, J., 2013. Buccal delivery of metformin: TR146 cell culture model evaluating the use of bioadhesive chitosan discs for drug permeability enhancement. Int. J. Pharm., 458, 254-261.

- Sankar, C., Mishra, B., 2003. Development and *in-vitro* evaluations of gelatin A microspheres of ketorolac tromethamine for intranasal administration. Acta Pharm., 53, 101-110.

- Sankar, C., Rani, M., Srivastava, A.K., Mishra, B., 2001. Chitosan based pentazocine microspheres for intranasal systemic delivery: development and biopharmaceutical evaluation. Pharmazie, 56, 223-226.

- Santos, C.A., Freedman, B.D., Ghosn, S., Jacob, J.S., Scarpulla, M., Mathiowitz, E., 2003. Evaluation of anhydride oligomers within polymer microsphere blends and their impact on bioadhesion and drug delivery *in-vitro*. Biomaterials, 24, 3571-3583.

- Santos, C.A., Jacob, J.S., Hertzog, B.A., Freedman, B.D., Press, D.L., Harnpicharnchai, P., Mathiowitz, E., 1999. Correlation of two bioadhesion assays: the everted sac technique and the CAHN microbalance. J. Control Release, 61, 113-122.

- Sareen, R., Kumar, S., Gupta, G.D., 2011. Meloxicam carbopol-based gels: characterization and evaluation. Curr. Drug Deliv., 8, 407-415.

- Schmidgall, J., Hensel, A., 2002. Bioadhesive properties of polygalacturonides against colonic epithelial membranes. Int. J. Biol. Macromol., 30, 217-225.

- Schmidgall, J., Schnetz, E., Hensel, A., 2000. Evidence for bioadhesive effects of polysaccharides and polysaccharide-containing herbs in an *ex-vivo* bioadhesion assay on buccal membranes. Planta Med., 66, 48-53.

- Sekhar, K.C., Naidu, K.V., Vishnu, Y.V., Gannu, R., Kishan, V., Rao, Y.M., 2008. Transbuccal delivery of chlorpheniramine maleate from mucoadhesive buccal patches. Drug Deliv., 15, 185-191.

- Sen, M., Avci, E.N., 2005. Radiation synthesis of poly(N-vinyl-2-pyrrolidone)-kappa-carrageenan hydrogels and their use in wound dressing applications. I. Preliminary laboratory tests. J. Biomed. Mater. Res. A, 74, 187-196.

- Sezer, A.D., Cevher, E., Hatipoglu, F., Ogurtan, Z., Bas, A.L., Akbuga, J., 2008a. Preparation of fucoidan-chitosan hydrogel and its application as burn healing accelerator on rabbits. Biol. Pharm. Bull., 31, 2326-2333.

- Sezer, A.D., Cevher, E., Hatipoglu, F., Ogurtan, Z., Bas, A.L., Akbuga, J., 2008b. The use of fucosphere in the treatment of dermal burns in rabbits. Eur. J. Pharm. Biopharm., 69, 189-198.

- Sezer, A.D., Hatipoglu, F., Cevher, E., Ogurtan, Z., Bas, A.L., Akbuga, J., 2007. Chitosan film containing fucoidan as a wound dressing for dermal burn healing: preparation and *in-vitro/in-vivo* evaluation. AAPS. Pharm Sci Tech., 8, Article.

- Sezgin, Z., Yuksel, N., Baykara, T., 2007. Investigation of pluronic and PEG-PE micelles as carriers of meso-tetraphenyl porphine for oral administration. Int. J. Pharm., 332, 161-167.

- Shah, M.H., Paradkar, A., 2007. Effect of HLB of additives on the properties and drug release from the glyceryl monooleate matrices. Eur. J. Pharm. Biopharm., 67, 166-174.

- Shanker, G., Kumar, C.K., Gonugunta, C.S., Kumar, B.V., Veerareddy, P.R., 2009. Formulation and evaluation of bioadhesive buccal drug delivery of tizanidine hydrochloride tablets. AAPS. Pharm Sci Tech., 10, 530-539.

- Shargel, L., Yu, A., Wu-Pong, S., 2012. Applied Biopharmaceutics & Pharmacokinetics. 6th Edition, McGraw-Hill Medical. USA.

- Sharma, G., Jain, S., Tiwary, A.K., Kaur, G., 2006. Once daily bioadhesive vaginal clotrimazole tablets: design and evaluation. Acta Pharm., 56, 337-345.

- Shastri, D.H., Prajapati, S.T., Patel, L.D., 2010a. Design and Development of Thermoreversible Ophthalmic *In-situ* Hydrogel of Moxifloxacin HCl. Curr. Drug Deliv..

- Shastri, D.H., Prajapati, S.T., Patel, L.D., 2010b. Studies on Poloxamer Based Mucoadhesive Insitu Ophthalmic Hydrogel of Moxifloxacin HCL. Curr. Drug Deliv..

- Shastri, D.H., Prajapati, S.T., Patel, L.D., 2010c. Thermoreversible mucoadhesive ophthalmic *in-situ* hydrogel: Design and optimization using a combination of polymers. Acta Pharm., 60, 349-360.

- Sheikh, N., Mirzadeh, H., Katbab, A.A., Salehian, P., Daliri, M., Amanpour, S., 2001. Isocyanate-terminated urethane prepolymer as bioadhesive material: evaluation of bioadhesion and biocompatibility, *in-vitro* and *in-vivo* assays. J. Biomater. Sci. Polym. Ed, 12, 707-719.

- Shekaran, A., Garcia, A.J., 2011. Nanoscale engineering of extracellular matrix-mimetic bioadhesive surfaces and implants for tissue engineering. Biochim. Biophys. Acta, 1810, 350-360.

- Shi, J., Wang, X., Jiang, Z., Liang, Y., Zhu, Y., Zhang, C., 2012. Constructing spatially separated multienzyme system through bioadhesion-assisted bio-inspired mineralization for efficient carbon dioxide conversion. Bioresour. Technol., 118, 359-366.

- Shi, Z., Li, Y., Chen, X., Han, H., Yang, G., 2013. Double network bacterial cellulose hydrogel to build a biology-device interface. Nanoscale., 6, 970-977.

- Shimoda, J., Onishi, H., Machida, Y., 2001. Bioadhesive characteristics of chitosan microspheres to the mucosa of rat small intestine. Drug Dev. Ind. Pharm., 27, 567-576.

- Shin, S.C., Cho, C.W., 2006. Enhanced transdermal delivery of pranoprofen from the bioadhesive gels. Arch. Pharm. Res., 29, 928-933.

- Shirsand, S., Suresh, S., Keshavshetti, G., Swamy, P., Reddy, P.V., 2012. Formulation and optimization of mucoadhesive bilayer buccal tablets of atenolol using simplex design method. Int. J. Pharm. Investig., 2, 34-41.

- Sin, M.C., Sun, Y.M., Chang, Y., 2014. Zwitterionic-based stainless steel with well-defined polysulfobetaine brushes for general bioadhesive control. ACS Appl. Mater. Interfaces., 6, 861-873.

- Singh, B., Ahuja, N., 2002. Development of controlled-release buccoadhesive hydrophilic matrices of diltiazem hydrochloride: optimization of bioadhesion, dissolution, and diffusion parameters. Drug Dev. Ind. Pharm., 28, 431-442.

- Singh, B., Chakkal, S.K., Ahuja, N., 2006. Formulation and optimization of controlled release mucoadhesive tablets of atenolol using response surface methodology. AAPS. Pharm Sci Tech., 7, E3.

- Singh, B., Pahuja, S., Kapil, R., Ahuja, N., 2009. Formulation development of oral controlled release tablets of hydralazine: optimization of drug release and bioadhesive characteristics. Acta Pharm., 59, 1-13.

- Singh, M., O'Hagan, D., 1998. The preparation and characterization of polymeric antigen delivery systems for oral administration. Adv. Drug Deliv. Rev., 34, 285-304.

- Singh, M., Tiwary, A.K., Kaur, G., 2010. Investigations on interpolymer complexes of cationic guar gum and xanthan gum for formulation of bioadhesive films. Res. Pharm. Sci., 5, 79-87.

- Singh, S., Jain, S., Muthu, M.S., Tilak, R., 2008a. Preparation and evaluation of buccal bioadhesive tablets containing clotrimazole. Curr. Drug Deliv., 5, 133-141.

- Singh, S., Jain, S., Muthu, M.S., Tiwari, S., Tilak, R., 2008b. Preparation and evaluation of buccal bioadhesive films containing clotrimazole. AAPS. Pharm Sci Tech., 9, 660-667.

- Singh, S., Parhi, R., Garg, A., 2011. Formulation of topical bioadhesive gel of aceclofenac using 3-level factorial design. Iran J. Pharm. Res., 10, 435-445.

- Singh, S., Soni, R., Rawat, M.K., Jain, A., Deshpande, S.B., Singh, S.K., Muthu, M.S., 2010. *In-vitro* and *in-vivo* evaluation of buccal bioadhesive films containing salbutamol sulphate. Chem. Pharm. Bull. (Tokyo), 58, 307-311.

- Sinko, P.J., 2010. Martin's Physical Pharmacy and Pharmaceutical Sciences. 6th Edition, Lippincott Williams and Wilkins, USA.

- Skulason, S., Asgeirsdottir, M.S., Magnusson, J.P., Kristmundsdottir, T., 2009. Evaluation of polymeric films for buccal drug delivery. Pharmazie, 64, 197-201.

- Smith, B.J., Rawal, A., Funkhouser, G.P., Roberts, L.R., Gupta, V., Israelachvili, J.N., Chmelka, B.F., 2011. Origins of saccharide-dependent hydration at aluminate, silicate, and aluminosilicate surfaces. Proc. Natl. Acad. Sci. U. S. A, 108, 8949-8954.

- Soane, R.J., Hinchcliffe, M., Davis, S.S., Illum, L., 2001. Clearance characteristics of chitosan based formulations in the sheep nasal cavity. Int. J. Pharm., 217, 183-191.

- Sohn, E.H., Ahn, J., Bhang, S.H., Kang, J., Yoon, J., Kim, B.S., Lee, J.C., 2012. Bacterial adhesion-resistant poly(2-hydroxyethyl methacrylate) derivative for mammalian cell cultures. Macromol. Biosci., 12, 211-217.

- Song, J., Kong, H., Jang, J., 2009. Enhanced antibacterial performance of cationic polymer modified silica nanoparticles. Chem. Commun. (Camb.), 5418-5420.

- Song, L., Zhao, J., Jin, J., Ma, J., Liu, J., Luan, S., Yin, J., 2014. Fabricating antigen recognition and anti-bioadhesion polymeric surface via a photografting polymerization strategy. Mater. Sci. Eng C. Mater. Biol. Appl., 36, 57-64.

- Souza, L.K., Bruno, C.H., Lopes, L., Pulcinelli, S.H., Santilli, C.V., Chiavacci, L.A., 2013. Ureasil-polyether hybrid film-forming materials. Colloids Surf. B Biointerfaces., 101, 156-161.

- Stabenfeldt, S.E., LaPlaca, M.C., 2011. Variations in rigidity and ligand density influence neuronal response in methylcellulose-laminin hydrogels. Acta Biomater., 7, 4102-4108.

- Sudhakar, Y., Kuotsu, K., Bandyopadhyay, A.K., 2006. Buccal bioadhesive drug delivery – a promising option for orally less efficient drugs. J. Control Release, 114, 15-40.

- Sulak, O., Cioci, G., Delia, M., Lahmann, M., Varrot, A., Imberty, A., Wimmerova, M., 2010. A TNF-like trimeric lectin domain from Burkholderia cenocepacia with specificity for fucosylated human histo-blood group antigens. Structure., 18, 59-72.

- Sultana, S., Talegaonkar, S., Singh, D., Ahmad, R., Manukonda, V., Bhatnagar, A., Ahmad, F.J., 2013. An approach for lacidipine loaded gastroretentive formulation prepared by different methods for gastroparesis in diabetic patients. Saudi. Pharm. J., 21, 293-304.

- Sun, W., Mao, S., Wang, Y., Junyaprasert, V.B., Zhang, T., Na, L., Wang, J., 2010. Bioadhesion and oral absorption of enoxaparin nanocomplexes. Int. J. Pharm., 386, 275-281.

- Sung, H.W., Huang, D.M., Chang, W.H., Huang, R.N., Hsu, J.C., 1999. Evaluation of gelatin hydrogel crosslinked with various crosslinking agents as bioadhesives: *in-vitro* study. J. Biomed. Mater. Res., 46, 520-530.

- Takayama, K., Hirata, M., Machida, Y., Masada, T., Sannan, T., Nagai, T., 1990. Effect of interpolymer complex formation on bioadhesive property and drug release phenomenon of compressed tablet consisting of chitosan and sodium hyaluronate. Chem. Pharm. Bull. (Tokyo), 38, 1993-1997.

- Tan, Y.T., Peh, K.K., Al-Hanbali, O., 2000. Effect of Carbopol and polyvinylpyrrolidone on the mechanical, rheological, and release properties of bioadhesive polyethylene glycol gels. AAPS. Pharm Sci Tech., 1, E24.

- Tansel, B., Tansel, D.Z., 2013. Adhesion strength and spreading characteristics of EPS on membrane surfaces during lateral and central growth. Colloids Surf. B Biointerfaces., 111C, 594-599.

- Tao, S.L., Desai, T.A., 2005. Gastrointestinal patch systems for oral drug delivery. Drug Discov. Today, 10, 909-915.

- Taware, C.P., Mazumdar, S., Pendharkar, M., Adani, M.H., Devarajan, P.V., 1997. A bioadhesive delivery system as an alternative to infiltration anesthesia. Oral Surg. Oral Med. Oral Pathol. Oral Radiol. Endod., 84, 609-615.

- Thanos, C.G., Liu, Z., Reineke, J., Edwards, E., Mathiowitz, E., 2003. Improving relative bioavailability of dicumarol by reducing particle size and adding the adhesive poly(fumaric-co-sebacic) anhydride. Pharm. Res., 20, 1093-1100.

- Thermes, F., Grove, J., Rozier, A., Plazonnet, B., Constancis, A., Bunel, C., Vairon, J.P., 1992. Mucoadhesion of copolymers and mixtures containing polyacrylic acid. Pharm. Res., 9, 1563-1567.

- Thumma, S., Majumdar, S., Elsohly, M.A., Gul, W., Repka, M.A., 2008a. Chemical stability and bioadhesive properties of an ester prodrug of Delta 9-tetrahydrocannabinol in poly(ethylene oxide) matrices: effect of formulation additives. Int. J. Pharm., 362, 126-132.

- Thumma, S., Majumdar, S., Elsohly, M.A., Gul, W., Repka, M.A., 2008b. Preformulation studies of a prodrug of Delta9-tetrahydrocannabinol. AAPS. Pharm Sci Tech., 9, 982-990.

- Thumma, S., Repka, M.A., 2009. Compatibility studies of promethazine hydrochloride with tablet excipients by means of thermal and non-thermal methods. Pharmazie, 64, 183-189.

- Tiwari, D., Goldman, D., Sause, R., Madan, P.L., 1999. Evaluation of polyoxyethylene homopolymers for buccal bioadhesive drug delivery device formulations. AAPS. Pharm Sci., 1, E13.

- Toegel, S., Harrer, N., Plattner, V.E., Unger, F.M., Viernstein, H., Goldring, M.B., Gabor, F., Wirth, M., 2007. Lectin binding studies on C-28/I2 and T/C-28a2 chondrocytes provide a basis for new tissue engineering and drug delivery perspectives in cartilage research. J. Control Release, 117, 121-129.

- Tokarova, V., Pittermannova, A., Kral, V., Rezacova, P., Stepanek, F., 2013. Feasibility and constraints of particle targeting using the antigen-antibody interaction. Nanoscale., 5, 11490-11498.

- Torchilin, V.P., (Ed.), 2006. Nanoparticulates as drug carriers. Imperial College Press, London.

- Truby, K., Wood, C., Stein, J., Cella, J., Carpenter, J., Kavanagh, C., Swain, G., Wiebe, D., Lapota, D., Meyer, A., Holm, E., Wendt, D., Smith, C., Montemarano, J., 2000. Evaluation of the performance enhancement of silicone biofouling-release coatings by oil incorporation. Biofouling., 15, 141-150.

- Turker, S., Onur, E., Ozer, Y., 2004. Nasal route and drug delivery systems. Pharm. World Sci., 26, 137-142.

- Vaghani, S.S., Patel, S.G., Jivani, R.R., Jivani, N.P., Patel, M.M., Borda, R., 2012. Design and optimization of a stomach-specific drug delivery system of repaglinide: application of simplex lattice design. Pharm. Dev. Technol., 17, 55-65.

- van Dijk, L.J., Weerkamp, A.H., Busscher, H.J., 1986. Bioadhesion and the development of dental plaque. Microbial and physical-chemical aspects. Ned. Tijdschr. Tandheelkd., 93 Spec No, 412-416.

- van Hoogmoed, C.G., Busscher, H.J., de, V.P., 2003. Fourier transform infrared spectroscopy studies of alginate-PLL capsules with varying compositions. J. Biomed. Mater. Res. A, 67, 172-178.

- Varshosaz, J., Dehghan, Z., 2002. Development and characterization of buccoadhesive nifedipine tablets. Eur. J. Pharm. Biopharm., 54, 135-141.

- Varshosaz, J., Jaffarian, D.A., Golafshan, S., 2006. Colon-specific delivery of mesalazine chitosan microspheres. J. Microencapsul., 23, 329-339.

- Varshosaz, J., Sadrai, H., Heidari, A., 2006. Nasal delivery of insulin using bioadhesive chitosan gels. Drug Deliv., 13, 31-38.

- Vasir, J.K., Tambwekar, K., Garg, S., 2003. Bioadhesive microspheres as a controlled drug delivery system. Int. J. Pharm., 255, 13-32.

- Vennat, B., Lardy, F., Arvouet-Grand, A., Pourrat, A., 1998. Comparative texturometric analysis of hydrogels based on cellulose derivatives, carraghenates, and alginates: evaluation of adhesiveness. Drug Dev. Ind. Pharm., 24, 27-35.

- Venugopalan, P., Sapre, A., Venkatesan, N., Vyas, S.P., 2001. Pelleted bioadhesive polymeric nanoparticles for buccal delivery of insulin: preparation and characterization. Pharmazie, 56, 217-219.

- Vermani, K., Garg, S., Zaneveld, L.J., 2002. Assemblies for *in-vitro* measurement of bioadhesive strength and retention characteristics in simulated vaginal environment. Drug Dev. Ind. Pharm., 28, 1133-1146.

- Vishnu, Y.V., Chandrasekhar, K., Ramesh, G., Rao, Y.M., 2007. Development of mucoadhesive patches for buccal administration of carvedilol. Curr. Drug Deliv., 4, 27-39.

- Viyoch, J., Patcharaworakulchai, P., Songmek, R., Pimsan, V., Wittaya-Areekul, S., 2003. Formulation and development of a patch containing tamarind fruit extract by using the blended chitosan-starch as a rate-controlling matrix. Int. J. Cosmet. Sci., 25, 113-125.

- Vlachou, M., Choulis, N.H., Efentakis, M., Andreopoulos, A.G., 1996. The effect of modification of acrylic resins on controlled release and bioadhesion. J. Biomater. Appl., 10, 217-229.

- Vogler, E.A., 1999. Water and the acute biological response to surfaces. J. Biomater. Sci. Polym. Ed, 10, 1015-1045.

- Voorspoels, J., Remon, J.P., Eechaute, W., De, S.W., 1996. Buccal absorption of testosterone and its esters using a bioadhesive tablet in dogs. Pharm. Res., 13, 1228-1232.

- Vyas, S.P., Gupta, P.N., 2007. Implication of nanoparticles/microparticles in mucosal vaccine delivery. Expert. Rev. Vaccines., 6, 401-418.

- Vyas, S.P., Jain, C.P., 1992. Bioadhesive polymer-grafted starch microspheres bearing isosorbide dinitrate for buccal administration. J. Microencapsul., 9, 457-464.

- Waite, J.H., 1999. Reverse engineering of bioadhesion in marine mussels. Ann. N. Y. Acad. Sci., 875, 301-309.

- Walter, F., Scholl, I., Untersmayr, E., Ellinger, A., Boltz-Nitulescu, G., Scheiner, O., Gabor, F., Jensen-Jarolim, E., 2004. Functionalisation of allergen-loaded microspheres with wheat germ agglutinin for targeting enterocytes. Biochem. Biophys. Res. Commun., 315, 281-287.

- Wang, L., Tang, X., 2008. A novel ketoconazole bioadhesive effervescent tablet for vaginal delivery: design, *in-vitro* and '*in-vivo*' evaluation. Int. J. Pharm., 350, 181-187.

- Wang, X., Gu, Y., Ren, T., Tian, B., Zhang, Y., Meng, L., Tang, X., 2013. Increased absorption of mangiferin in the gastrointestinal tract and its mechanism of action by absorption enhancers in rats. Drug Dev. Ind. Pharm., 39, 1408-1413.

- Wang, X.Q., Zhang, Q., 2012. pH-sensitive polymeric nanoparticles to improve oral bioavailability of peptide/protein drugs and poorly water-soluble drugs. Eur. J. Pharm. Biopharm., 82, 219-229.

- Wang, X.Y., Pichl, C., Gabor, F., Wirth, M., 2013. A novel cell-based microfluidic multichannel setup-impact of hydrodynamics and surface characteristics on the bioadhesion of polystyrene microspheres. Colloids Surf. B Biointerfaces., 102, 849-856.

- Waring, M., 2009. Skin adhesion properties of three dressings used for acute wounds. Wounds U.K., 5, 22-31.

- Wattanakorn, N., Asavapichayont, P., Nunthanid, J., Limmatvapirat, S., Sungthongjeen, S., Chantasart, D., Sriamornsak, P., 2010. Pectin-based bioadhesive delivery of carbenoxolone sodium for aphthous ulcers in oral cavity. AAPS. Pharm Sci Tech., 11, 743-751.

- Wearley, L.L., 1991. Recent progress in protein and peptide delivery by noninvasive routes. Crit Rev. Ther. Drug Carrier Syst., 8, 331-394.

- Wei, W., Ma, G.H., Wang, L.Y., Wu, J., Su, Z.G., 2010. Hollow quaternized chitosan microspheres increase the therapeutic effect of orally administered insulin. Acta Biomater., 6, 205-209.

- Wei, W., Wang, L.Y., Yuan, L., Yang, X.D., Su, Z.G., Ma, G.H., 2008. Bioprocess of uniform-sized crosslinked chitosan microspheres in rats following oral administration. Eur. J. Pharm. Biopharm., 69, 878-886.

- Weis, C., Odermatt, E.K., Kressler, J., Funke, Z., Wehner, T., Freytag, D., 2004. Poly(vinyl alcohol) membranes for adhesion prevention. J. Biomed. Mater. Res. B Appl. Biomater., 70, 191-202.

- Weissenboeck, A., Bogner, E., Wirth, M., Gabor, F., 2004. Binding and uptake of wheat germ agglutinin-grafted PLGA-nanospheres by caco-2 monolayers. Pharm. Res., 21, 1917-1923.

- Werle, M., Makhlof, A., Takeuchi, H., 2010. Carbopol-lectin conjugate coated liposomes for oral peptide delivery. Chem. Pharm. Bull. (Tokyo), 58, 432-434.

- Witschi, C., Mrsny, R.J., 1999. *In-vitro* evaluation of microparticles and polymer gels for use as nasal platforms for protein delivery. Pharm. Res., 16, 382-390.

- Wong, C.F., Yuen, K.H., Peh, K.K., 1999. An *in-vitro* method for buccal adhesion studies: importance of instrument variables. Int. J. Pharm., 180, 47-57.

- Woodley, J., 2001. Bioadhesion: new possibilities for drug administration? Clin. Pharmacokinet., 40, 77-84.

- Woodley, J.F., 2000. Lectins for gastrointestinal targeting – 15 years on. J. Drug Target, 7, 325-333.

- Yamsani, V.V., Gannu, R., Kolli, C., Rao, M.E., Yamsani, M.R., 2007. Development and *in-vitro* evaluation of buccoadhesive carvedilol tablets. Acta Pharm., 57, 185-197.

- Yassin, A.E., Alkhaled, F., al-Suwayeh, S., Elkheshen, S., 2003. Intra-gastric performance and bioavailability study of a new per-oral bioadhesive Verapamil HCl matrix tablet in dogs. Boll. Chim. Farm., 142, 285-289.

- Yedurkar, P., Dhiman, M.K., Petkar, K., Sawant, K., 2013. Biopolymeric mucoadhesive bilayer patch of pravastatin sodium for buccal delivery and treatment of patients with atherosclerosis. Drug Dev. Ind. Pharm., 39, 670-680.

- Yehia, S.A., El-Gazayerly, O.N., Basalious, E.B., 2009. Fluconazole mucoadhesive buccal films: *in-vitro/in-vivo* performance. Curr. Drug Deliv., 6, 17-27.

- Yin, Y., Chen, D., Qiao, M., Lu, Z., Hu, H., 2006. Preparation and evaluation of lectin-conjugated PLGA nanoparticles for oral delivery of thymopentin. J. Control Release, 116, 337-345.

- Yin, Y., Chen, D., Qiao, M., Wei, X., Hu, H., 2007a. Lectin-conjugated PLGA nanoparticles loaded with thymopentin: *ex-vivo* bioadhesion and *in-vivo* biodistribution. J. Control Release, 123, 27-38.

- Yin, Y.S., Chen, D.W., Qiao, M.X., Hu, H.Y., Qin, J., 2007b. Preparation of lectin-conjugated PLGA nanoparticles and evaluation of their *in-vitro* bioadhesive activity. Yao Xue. Xue. Bao., 42, 550-556.

- Zaman, H.U., Islam, J.M., Khan, M.A., Khan, R.A., 2011. Physico-mechanical properties of wound dressing material and its biomedical application. J. Mech. Behav. Biomed. Mater., 4, 1369-1375.

- Zaman, M.A., Martin, G.P., Rees, G.D., 2008. Mucoadhesion, hydration and rheological properties of non-aqueous delivery systems (NADS) for the oral cavity. J. Dent., 36, 351-359.

- Zaman, M.A., Martin, G.P., Rees, G.D., 2010. Bioadhesion and retention of non-aqueous delivery systems in a dental hard tissue model. J. Dent., 38, 757-764.

- Zhang, L., Shi, J., Jiang, Z., Jiang, Y., Meng, R., Zhu, Y., Liang, Y., Zheng, Y., 2011. Facile preparation of robust microcapsules by manipulating metal-coordination interaction between biomineral layer and bioadhesive layer. ACS Appl. Mater. Interfaces., 3, 597-605.

- Zhang, X., Sun, M., Zheng, A., Cao, D., Bi, Y., Sun, J., 2012. Preparation and characterization of insulin-loaded bioadhesive PLGA nanoparticles for oral administration. Eur. J. Pharm. Sci., 45, 632-638.

- Zhang, Z., Chao, T., Liu, L., Cheng, G., Ratner, B.D., Jiang, S., 2009. Zwitterionic hydrogels: an *in-vivo* implantation study. J. Biomater. Sci. Polym. Ed, 20, 1845-1859.

- Zhang, Z.R., Fu, J., Huang, Y., Duan, Y.S., 2001. Investigation of the bioadhesion of carbopol and hydroxypropyl methylcellulose to rat gastrointestinal mucosa *in-vivo* and *in-vitro*. Yao Xue. Xue. Bao., 36, 543-546.

- Zhao, J., Song, L., Yin, J., Ming, W., 2013. Anti-bioadhesion on hierarchically structured, superhydrophobic surfaces. Chem. Commun. (Camb.), 49, 9191-9193.

- Zhou, Y.Z., Cao, Y., Liu, W., Chu, C.H., Li, Q.L., 2012. Polydopamine-induced tooth remineralization. ACS Appl. Mater. Interfaces., 4, 6901-6910.

- Zhu, X., Qi, X., Wu, Z., Zhang, Z., Xing, J., Li, X., 2014. Preparation of multiple-unit floating-bioadhesive cooperative minitablets for improving the oral bioavailability of famotidine in rats. Drug Deliv.

- Zielinska-Jurek, A., Reszczynska, J., Grabowska, E., Zaleska, A., 2012. Nanoparticles preparation using microemulsion systems, Microemulsions – An Introduction to Properties and Applications, Dr. Reza Najjar (Ed.), ISBN: 978-953-51-0247-2, InTech, Available from: http://www.intechopen.com/books/microemulsions-an-introduction-to-properties-andapplications/nanoparticles-preparation-using-microemulsion-systems.

- Zumpano, B.J., Jacobs, L.R., Hall, J.B., Margolis, G., Sachs E Jr, 1982. Bioadhesive and histotoxic properties of ethyl-2-cyanoacrylate. Surg. Neurol., 18, 452-457.

INDEX

9 789352 301287